AF585060

Air Fryer Healthy

225+

RECIPES TO ABSOLUTELY NAIL IT

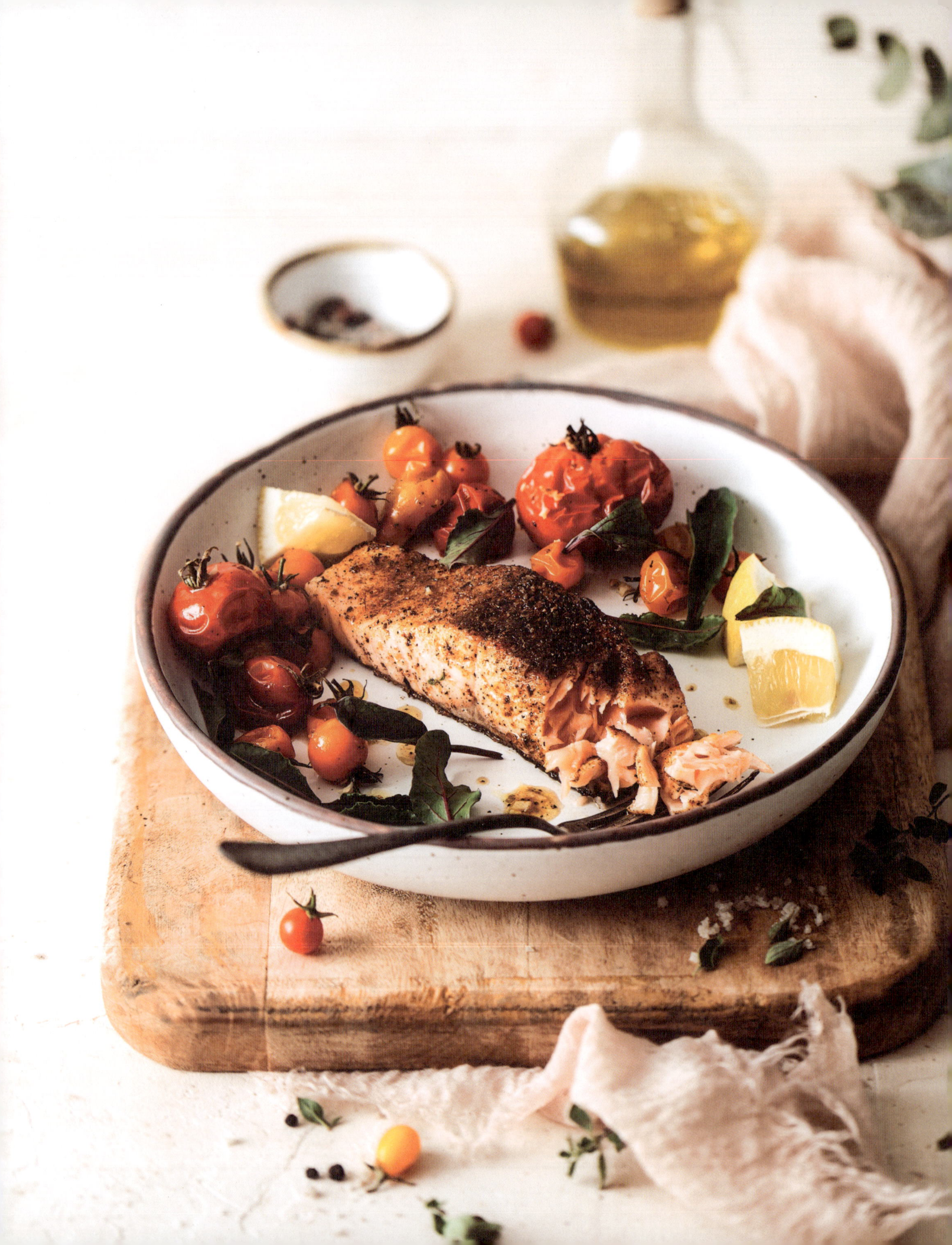

Contents

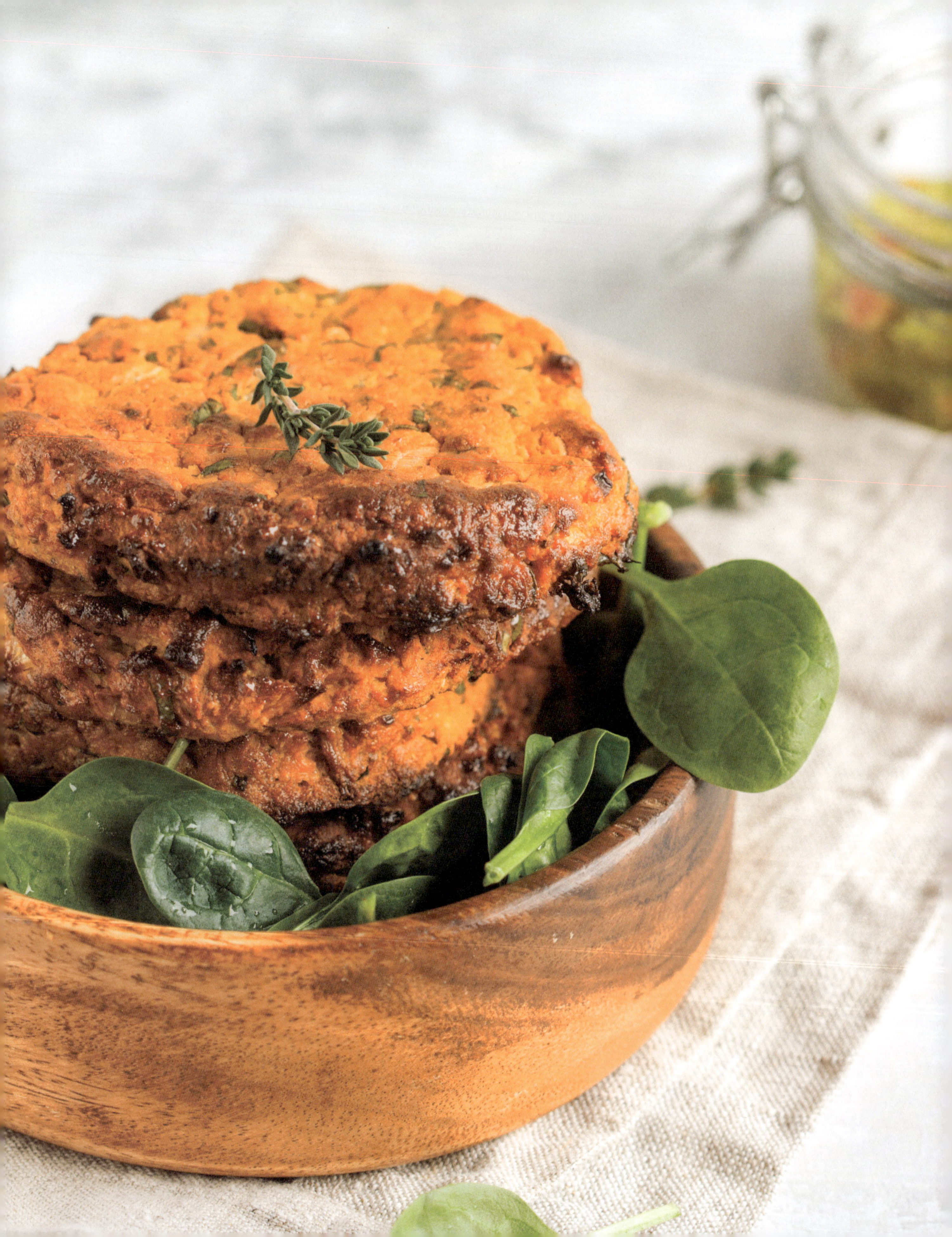

Welcome to the Healthy Air Fryer cookbook.

If a healthier diet is where you're headed, then the air fryer is your golden ticket to getting there. The principle is simple and easy to grasp: with an air fryer you need less fat to deliver the same crispy, crunchy and delicious results as traditional frying.

In that way, the air fryer is a healthier choice regardless of what you put in it. However what you put in in does make a big difference to the quality of your diet. (Chips and nuggets will only deliver so many nutrients – you know it!) That's why in this book we've gone the extra mile. The recipes you find here will help you to cook meals based on the general principles of healthy eating.

Think of your air fryer as a one-stop-shop for delivering nutritious food for yourself and others. Whether it's a power breakfast to help you get going (and keep going) through your busy day, an energy-packed snack, or a fresh and tasty lite meal, your air fryer can deal with it, and you'll find all the recipes you need here.

Eating less meat, reducing carbs, eliminating gluten (known to contribute to leaky gut) and eating more (and then more) veggies are pillars of a healthy eating lifestyle. That's why we've included sections in this book on paleo-style food (you'll find plenty of meat and fish recipes here), keto-style meals (for people keen to stick to a low-carb diet), gluten-free and vegetarian meals.

A not-to-so-well-kept secret is the air fryer's capacity for creating desserts and cakes. In this cookbook, you'll find a range of delicious low sugar treats to try in your air fryer. If you haven't experimented with desserts yet, you'll be amazed and delighted in the process.

Embrace your air fryer. It has the capacity to transform your cooking, making it easier and faster to get healthier food on the table. With the recipes in this book, we guarantee you'll absolutely nail it.

Why air fry?

HEALTHIER

Air fryers are well known for providing a healthier alternative to deep-frying food, but with similar (some say even better) results. That's why they are such a hit with families who want to keep on eating their favourite crispy chips and nuggets (whether homemade or pre-packaged) but with little or no fat. The health benefit of an air fryer is number one for many people, especially those looking to conserve calories or make the shift to a healthier diet, but there are other worthwhile benefits too.

SPEEDIER

For busy people, the air fryer delivers the benefit of speed. Ready-made food can be cooked in about half the time a conventional oven would take. Food can be cooked from frozen too, so you save on defrosting time (and you don't have to remember to get it out of the freezer in advance). It's so easy as well!

MORE VERSATILE

It's called a 'fryer', but this machine can grill, bake and roast foods as well so it's definitely not limited to chicken nuggets and chips. It is extremely versatile and should be viewed like a conventional oven in terms of its capability to cook different foods. You can bake a cake in it, roast a chicken, sear scallops, cook a quiche or make a perfect souffle. And that's just five ideas from over 225 recipes in this book.

LESS HASSLE

Last but certainly not least for busy people, is the ease of clean up. Traditional fryers and even ovens tend to use a lot of oil and make a splashy mess around the place. The air fryer, by contrast, uses little oil and all 'mess' is contained within the appliance. Most have been designed to be very easy to clean, with removable nonstick parts that are dishwasher friendly.

Healthy air fryer cooking tips

OIL SPARINGLY

For many people the deep-fried result without the deep-frying is the air fryer's number one asset. You do still need to use a little oil, however, otherwise your food will be very dry. A good rule of thumb is 1-2 teaspoons for most foods, or 1-2 tablespoons for breaded items that you want to get really crispy.

USE AN OIL SPRAY

Using a spray is a good way of ensuring a light, even coating of oil without the risk of being heavy handed.

CONSIDER FROZEN VEGGIES

Frozen veggies tend to contain a little more moisture thanks to the freezing process, which can be an advantage in air fryer cooking as they cook well on the inside before browning on the outside. Sometimes in an air fryer the opposite can occur with fresh veggies. The high heat levels can brown the outside of the vegetables while the inside is still crunchy. For perfectly cooked veggies, experiment with times and temperatures too.

EXPERIMENT WITH 'DRY COATINGS'

You can't use a traditional wet batter in an air fryer because it will seep through the holes in the basket, but that's all good because dry coatings offer a healthier alternative, with a wide array of options for flavour and texture. Experiment with nut flours, corn flour, semolina, Parmesan or whatever base you like and add in seasonings and herbs and you may discover that the 'healthy choice' is the tastiest too.

DON'T FORGET THE GOLDEN RULE ...

... which is that the air fryer is only as healthy as the food you put in it!

Choosing an air fryer

The two factors to consider when choosing the best air fryer for you are size (capacity) and wattage (power).

Size is measured by litre capacity. Air fryers come in three main sizes - small, medium and large. The small sizes range between 3L and 3.5L, the medium between 4L and 5L and large sizes range from 7L to 12L in capacity. These larger versions take up more bench space, but they often come with extra features such as a rotisserie or dehydrator.

If you have a large family to cook for, you will probably want to opt for a medium or large air fryer, or maybe even more than one. For couples or small families, a small air fryer may be enough. Do your homework and decide what's best for you.

Power is an important consideration during your research too. Power is measured by wattage. A higher wattage means greater power which means food will cook more quickly. If this is a priority, look for an air fryer with a high wattage.

Cooking times and temperatures

If you want to experiment with recipes beyond those in this book, you can find excellent tools online to assist with converting conventional oven temperatures to air fryer temperatures. Just google 'air fryer calculator'. A good rule of thumb to bear in mind though is the 20:20 rule: that you will generally reduce the temperature by approximately 20°C and reduce the cook time by 20%.

As with conventional cooking, the size of an ingredient, such as a potato, will influence the cooking time. Likewise, the extent to which you fill muffin trays or the size of your pies will influence cooking times. Check regularly until you are very familiar with your machine.

Air fryer cooking tips

PREHEAT

If a recipe specifies preheating, you can use the preheat setting on your air fryer or, if it doesn't have one, simply set to the desired temperature and let it run for 3 minutes.

PAT DRY

Use paper towel to pat foods dry before cooking to avoid splattering and excess smoke.

SPRITZ

Lightly spritz foods with cooking spray or toss in a small amount of oil to minimise the chance of sticking to the basket and to maximise results.

SPRITZ AGAIN DURING COOKING

You don't need to do this on fatty foods, such as steak, but for anything that's coated in breadcrumbs give an extra spritz with oil during cooking, especially on any dry, floury areas, for a crispier result.

DON'T OVERCROWD THE BASKET

Give food plenty of space so that the air can circulate. This will deliver the best and crispiest results. Cook in batches or use a double layer accessory to maximise available space.

SHAKE THE BASKET

For best results, shake the basket and/or rotate food every 5-10 minutes. This will allow the air to circulate better and will result in more uniform cooking.

Accessories

The great news is that you don't have to make a big investment in air fryer accessories up front. You can use any existing dish, ramekin, cake tin, bowl or other utensil in your air fryer so long as it is made from an ovenproof material such as glass, ceramic, metal or silicone and fits in your air fryer basket. Likewise you can use baking paper, patty pans (paper or silicone) and aluminium foil in your air fryer, just as long as this does not completely cover the bottom of the basket, which would disrupt air flow.

However, you might decide to invest in extras designed specifically for the air fryer that you feel would be helpful. Experiment with the recipes in this book and see what you most need. We have provided a list of the basics opposite. Or, if you are a complete beginner, you might prefer to invest in a starter pack, which will generally include a cake tin with a convenient handle, a double layer accessory (to expand your cooking surfaces), a pizza pan, a cooking rack with skewer holders, and a silicone mat to protect cooking surfaces. You can also buy accessory kits to suit your cooking interests, such as baking accessory kits or grilling accessory kits.

Note: One of the best things about appliances made specifically for the air fryer is their shape and size. They are designed to fit in the air fryer, whereas utensils designed for the oven tend to be bigger.

COMMON AIR FRYER ACCESSORIES

Baking pan

Cake tin

Pizza pan

Ramekins

Grill pan

Double layer accessory (or metal rack)

Bread rack

Silicone muffin or cupcake moulds

Silicone mat

The double layer accessory is especially useful because it doubles the space you have available to cook in. As the air fryer is small compared to the conventional oven, it will enable you to create food for the family without having to cook in batches.

Note: For the purposes of this book, we have assumed that you don't have any special air fryer accessories. Where a utensil is required, we have listed it in the ingredients. You will need to ensure that it fits in your air fryer and is ovenproof.

COOKING WITH PANS AND TINS

When placing a pan or tin in the air fryer basket, leave a little space around it so that the air can circulate. For the same reason, always put the pan into the air fryer basket and never directly into the air fryer. Use oven mitts when removing pans and tins from the air fryer.

COOKING SPRAY

Not exactly an accessory, cooking oil spray is nonetheless an essential ingredient for cooking in an air fryer. Invest in a sprayer bottle (or two) that you can refill. Depending on how and what you cook, you might like to have one filled with a nonstick cooking oil and the other with olive oil (for flavour as well as its nonstick properties).

PASTRY BRUSH

A pastry brush is handy for applying oil to food and glaze or egg wash to pies and pastries.

THERMOMETER

A great investment if you are serious about cooking in an air fryer is an instant-read kitchen thermometer. This will be particularly helpful for cooking meat, helping you achieve the best (and safest) results with the least fuss.

Sometimes meat and fish are simply cooked to preference, such as rare or well done (see below), but some meat, such as chicken, needs to reach a certain temperature to be safe. Chicken is cooked when the internal temperature reaches 74°C, but note that a thicker piece of meat might require a few more minutes' cooking.

Practice makes perfect, but a good rule of thumb for cooking red meat is:

For rare meat: 50°C.

For medium meat: 55°C.

For well-done meat: 60°C.

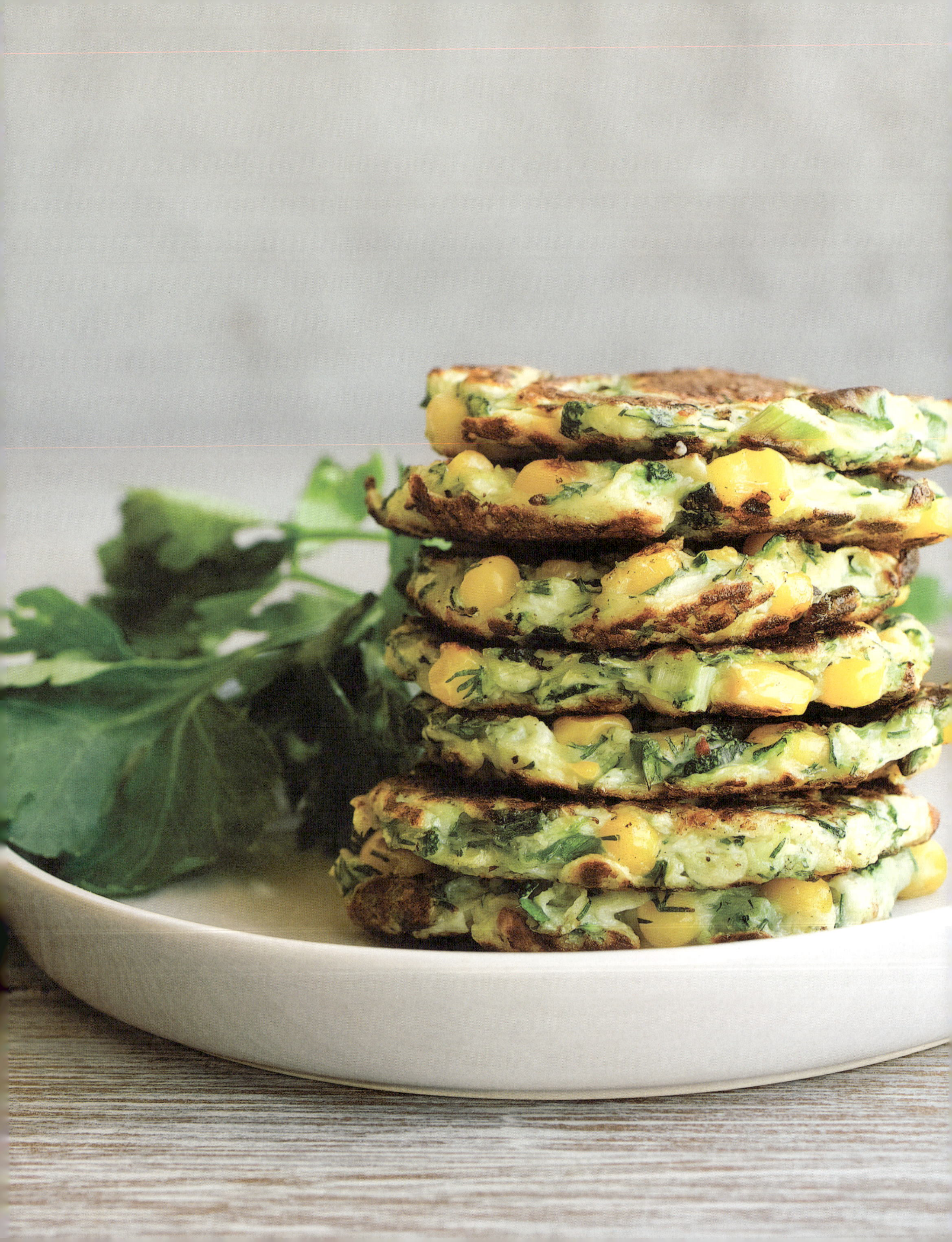

Breakfast

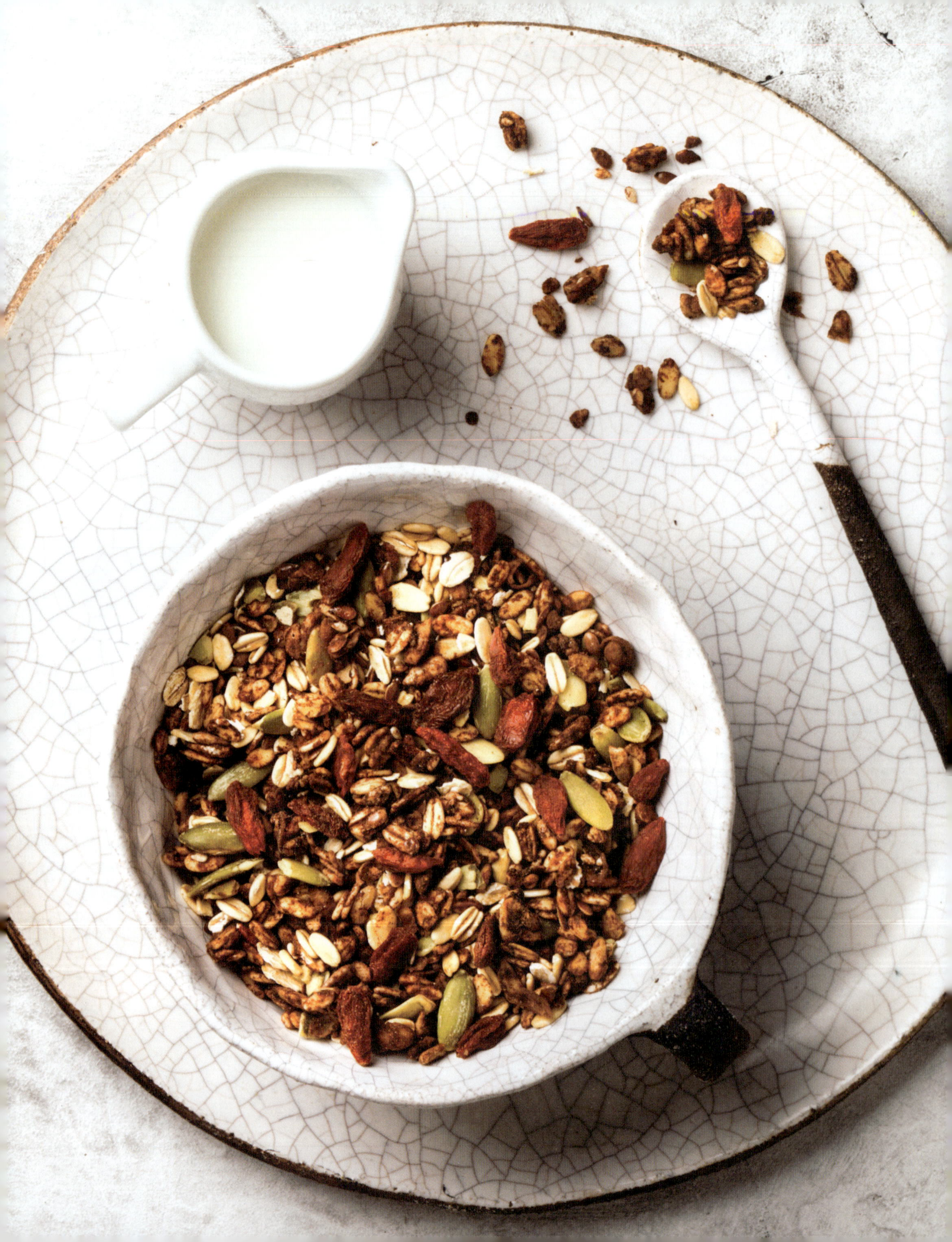

Cinnamon Granola

1½ cups (130g) rolled oats

½ cup (60g) walnuts, chopped

½ cup (60g) almonds, chopped

½ cup (60g) sunflower seeds

½ cup (60g) pepitas (pumpkin seeds)

¼ cup (80g) maple syrup or honey

1 tbsp coconut oil

2 tsps cinnamon

½ tsp salt

½ cup (50g) goji berries

Place all ingredients except the goji berries in a large bowl and mix to combine.

Place the granola mixture in the air fryer basket and cook for 35 minutes at 120°C, stirring every 10 minutes.

Remove from air fryer and spread out on a baking tray to cool for 30 minutes.

Pour into a large bowl, add goji berries and mix.

SERVES 12

Oat and Quinoa Muesli Bars

1 cup (90g) rolled oats

½ cup (80g) uncooked quinoa, rinsed

3 tbsps chia seeds

¼ tsp salt

1 tsp cinnamon

1 large banana, mashed

½ tsp vanilla extract

½ cup (60g) sunflower seeds

¼ cup (40g) raisins

¼ cup (65g) almond butter or tahini

2 tbsps honey or maple syrup

Cake tin, greased and lined

In a large bowl, combine oats, quinoa, chia seeds, salt and cinnamon. Add banana and vanilla and stir well. Fold in sunflower seeds and raisins.

Place almond butter or tahini and honey or maple syrup in a small saucepan over low heat for 2-3 minutes and stir until warm and well combined. Pour into granola bar mixture and mix well.

Preheat air fryer to 160°C.

Pour mixture into prepared tin and press down firmly. Place tin in the air fryer and cook for 20 minutes or until edges turn golden brown.

Allow to cool completely before cutting into bars.

MAKES 8

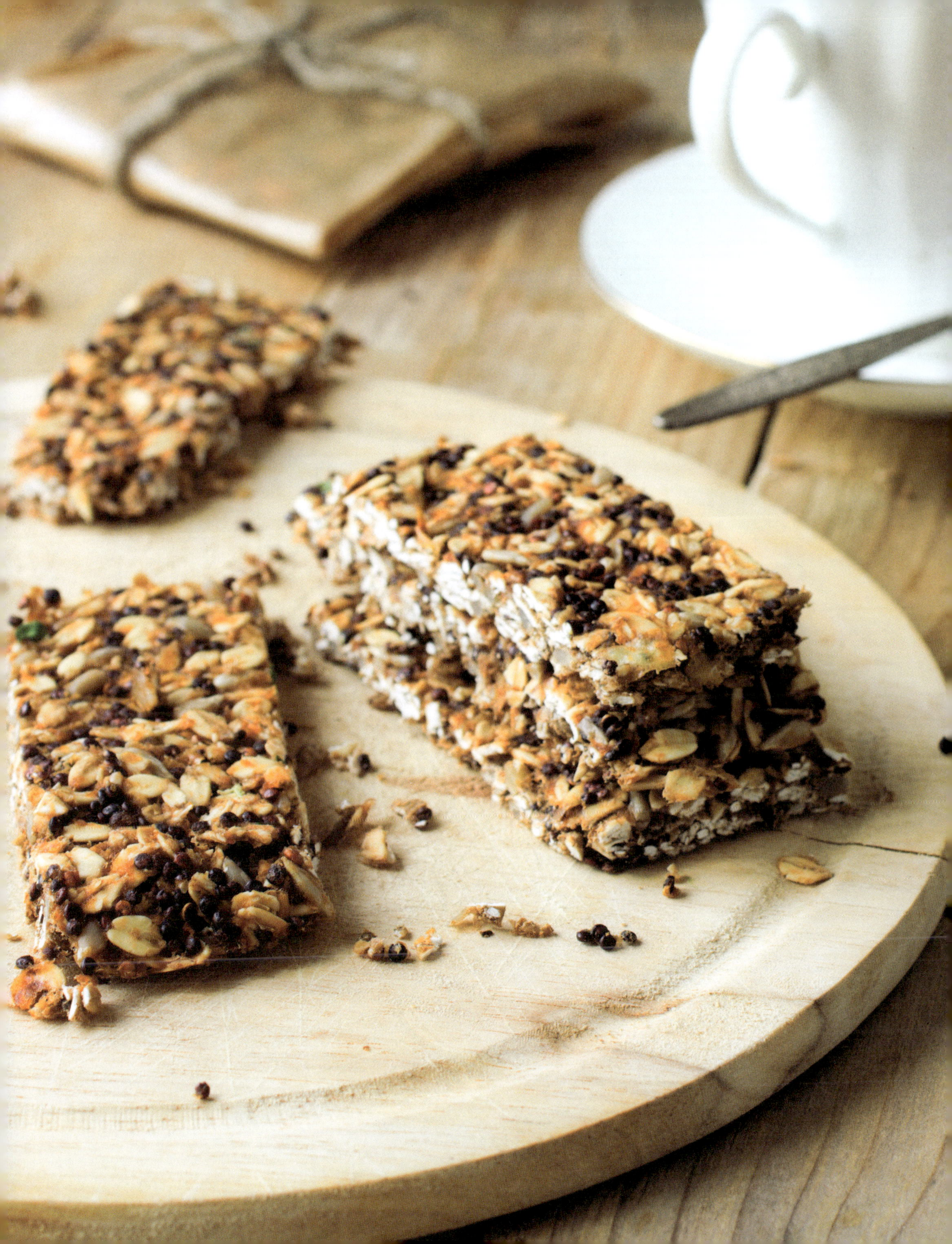

Baked Eggs

2 large eggs

⅛ tsp paprika

Salt and pepper to taste

Olive oil cooking spray

2 ramekins

Preheat air fryer to 180°C. Spray the ramekins with nonstick spray.

Crack each egg into a small ramekin. Sprinkle with paprika, salt and pepper to taste.

Bake the eggs for 5-8 minutes or until the eggs have cooked to desired consistency.

SERVES 2

Asparagus Frittata

Olive oil cooking spray

5 eggs

½ cup (125g) ricotta

½ cup (50g) Cheddar cheese, grated

¼ cup (25g) Parmesan cheese, grated

Zest of 1 lemon

6 asparagus spears

2 cherry tomatoes

Salt and pepper to taste

Baking pan

Preheat the air fryer to 160°C. Line the pan with greaseproof paper and spray with cooking spray.

Whisk together eggs, ricotta, Cheddar, Parmesan and lemon zest. Stir to combine.

Pour mixture into baking pan. Arrange asparagus and tomatoes in pan then place inside air fryer basket.

Cook for 12-16 minutes or until eggs are set.

SERVES 4

Mushroom Frittata

Olive oil cooking spray

4 eggs

3 tbsps double cream

½ cup (50g) Cheddar cheese, grated

200g mushrooms, sliced

1 small head of broccoli, divided into florets

½ cup (15g) watercress, to serve

Salt and pepper to taste

Baking pan

Preheat the air fryer to 180°C. Line the pan with greaseproof paper and spray with cooking spray.

In a bowl, whisk together eggs and cream.

Add the rest of the ingredients to the bowl and stir to combine.

Pour mixture into the baking pan and place inside air fryer basket.

Cook for 12-16 minutes or until eggs are set.

SERVES 4

Cheese and Pumpkin Mini Muffins

2 cups (450g) mashed cooked pumpkin

1 tsp baking powder

1 cup (125g) Cheddar cheese, grated

2 eggs, whisked

1 cup (125g) plain flour

Salt and pepper to taste

Mini-muffin tray or silicone moulds

Preheat air fryer to 160°C.

Place pumpkin, baking powder, cheese, eggs and flour in a large bowl. Season with salt and pepper and mix well.

Working in batches, pour mixture into the greased muffin tray.

Place in air fryer and cook for 18-20 minutes until puffed and golden.

Repeat with remaining mixture.

Serve warm or at room temperature.

MAKES 12

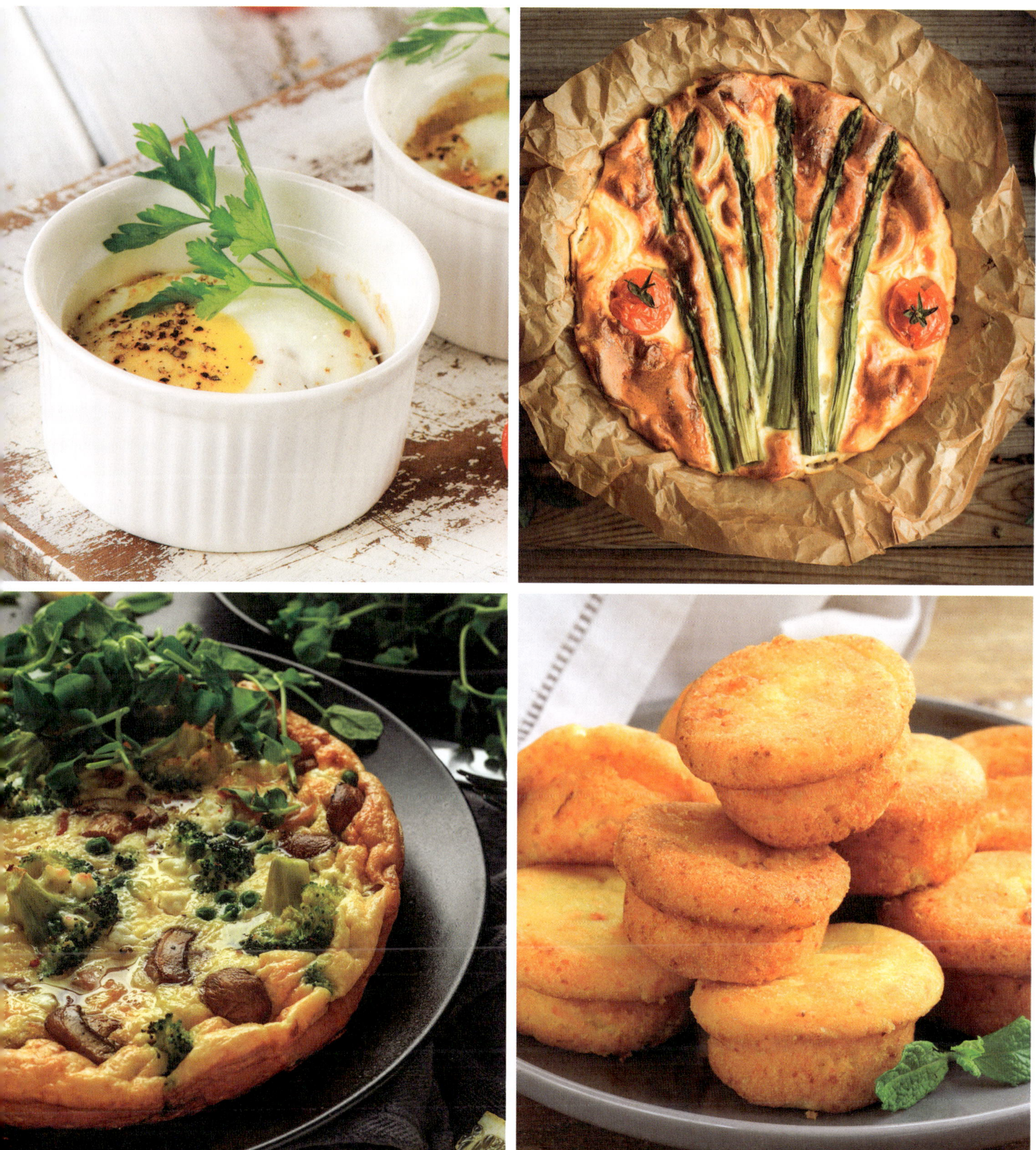

Korean Pajeon (Spring Onion) Pancakes

DIPPING SAUCE

⅓ cup (80ml) soy sauce

2 tbsps honey

2 tbsps rice wine vinegar

2 tbsps water

1 tbsp toasted sesame oil

2 cloves garlic, minced

½ tsp chilli flakes

PANCAKES

1 cup (125g) plain flour

2 tbsps cornflour

¼ tsp sugar

½ tsp salt

1 cup (250ml) cold sparkling water

1 egg, beaten

2 cloves garlic, minced

8 spring onions, halved lengthways and cut into 5cm pieces

1 carrot, julienned

Avocado or olive oil cooking spray

Combine sauce ingredients in a small pan over medium heat. Bring to a boil, then stir and reduce heat to medium-low. Simmer for 5-7 minutes, until slightly thickened.

In a large mixing bowl, whisk together flour, cornflour, sugar and salt. Make a well in the centre and pour in water, egg and garlic. Stir gently until just combined. Gently fold in spring onions and carrot.

Line base and sides of air fryer basket with greaseproof paper. Spray with cooking spray. Spoon a ladleful of batter onto the paper.

Cook for 6-8 minutes without flipping, at 160°C, until brown. Repeat with remaining batter, spraying each batch.

SERVES 2

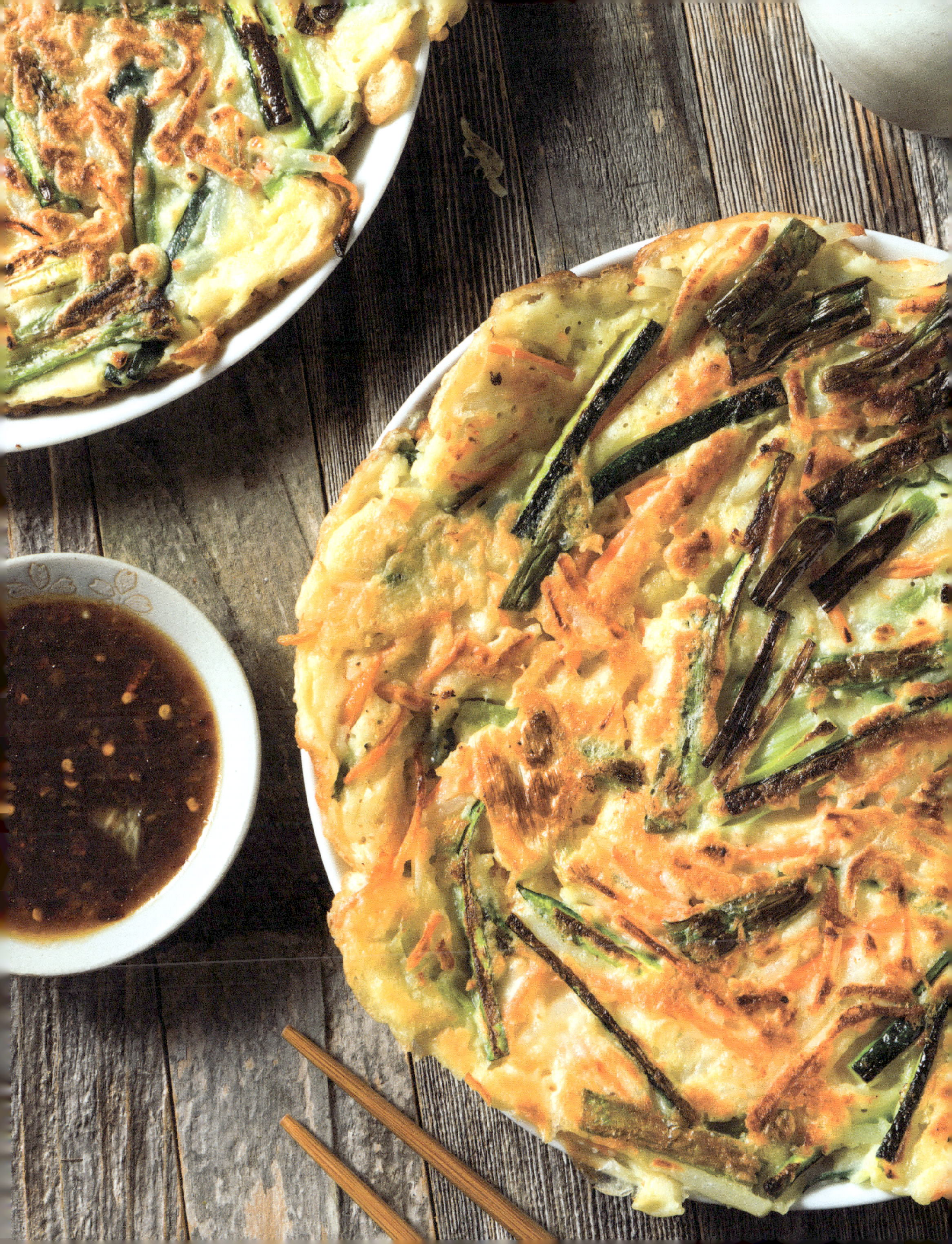

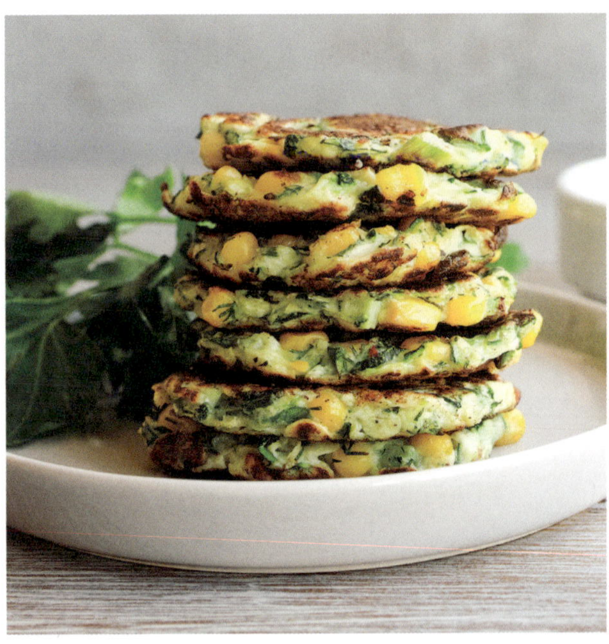

Corn Fritters

2 medium zucchinis, grated

Salt and pepper to taste

½ cup (130g) cooked mashed potato

1 cup (175g) corn kernels

2 tbsps chickpea flour

3 cloves garlic, minced

2 tbsps olive oil

In a large bowl mix grated zucchini with a ½ teaspoon salt and leave for 15 minutes. Then place on a clean tea towel and twist to squeeze out excess liquid.

Combine zucchini, potato, corn, chickpea flour, garlic, salt and pepper in a mixing bowl. Mix well.

Use your hands to shape the mixture into patties. Brush each fritter with olive oil.

Preheat air fryer to 180°C.

Arrange fritters in one layer in air fryer basket. Cook in batches or use a double layer accessory if necessary. Cook for 8 minutes then flip and cook for a further 3-4 minutes until brown.

SERVES 4

Tofu Scramble

300g silken tofu

¼ tsp garlic powder

1 tbsp nutritional yeast flakes

1 tsp dried oregano

¼ tsp dried chilli flakes

⅛ tsp turmeric

Salt and pepper to taste

200g mushrooms, sliced

2 spring onions, sliced

Baking pan

Preheat air fryer to 180°C.

Spray pan with cooking spray. Add tofu and mash with a fork, then stir through garlic powder, nutritional yeast, herbs and spices. Season with salt and pepper. Add the mushrooms and spring onions and stir to combine.

Place pan in air fryer basket and cook for 15 minutes.

SERVES 2

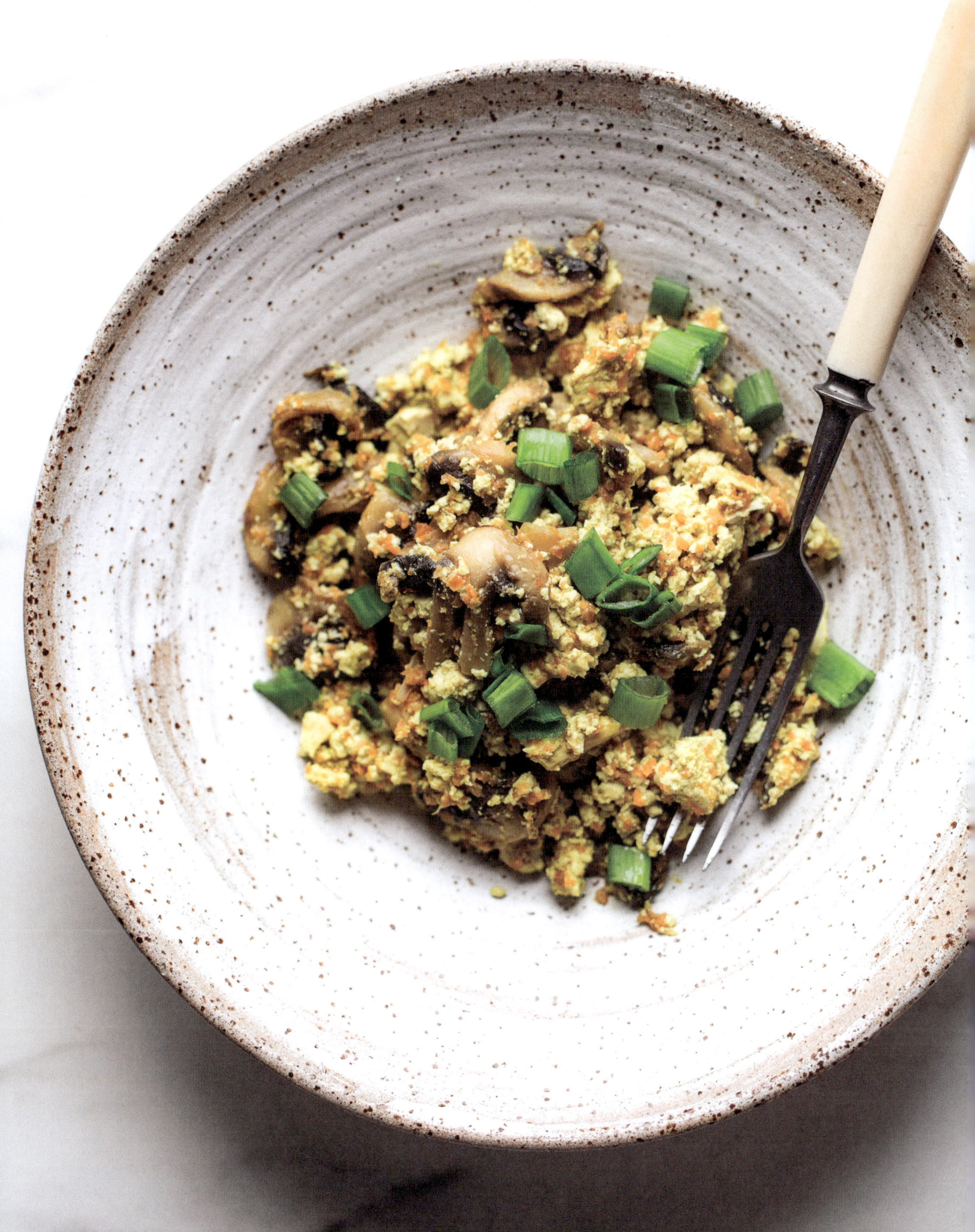

Mini Ham, Pea and Corn Frittatas

6 large eggs

2 tbsps milk or cream

Salt and pepper to taste

100g thick-cut ham, chopped

½ cup (80g) peas

½ cup (85g) corn kernels

½ cup (60g) Cheddar cheese, shredded

¼ cup (30g) mozzarella cheese, shredded

Muffin tray or silicone moulds

Place eggs in a large bowl with milk or cream. Season with salt and pepper and whisk to combine.

Add remaining ingredients into the bowl and stir well.

Place 6 silicone muffin moulds or an air fryer muffin tray filled with paper liners into air fryer basket.

Pour egg mixture into each of the moulds.

Cook for 12-15 minutes at 175°C until egg is set.

MAKES 6

Banana Muffins

2 large bananas

2 large eggs

1 cup (250ml) Greek yoghurt

2 cups (175g) oats

1½ tsps baking powder

4 tbsps honey

1 tsp vanilla extract

¼ cup (30g) flaked almonds

Muffin tray or silicone moulds

Preheat air fryer to 180°C.

Place bananas, eggs, yoghurt, oats, baking powder, honey and vanilla in a food processor and blend until smooth.

Pour into silicone moulds or paper liners inside an air fryer muffin tray.

Working in batches place in air fryer basket and cook for 10 minutes. Scatter with flaked almonds then cook for 3-5 minutes until an inserted skewer comes out clean.

MAKES 10

Cottage Cheese Pancakes

400g cottage cheese

4 eggs

2 tbsps melted butter

1 tsp vanilla extract

1 cup (125g) flour

1 tbsp baking powder

2 tbsps maple syrup

Avocado oil cooking spray

Combine cottage cheese, eggs, butter and vanilla extract in a large bowl. Mix well to combine. Add flour, baking powder and syrup and beat thoroughly.

Preheat air fryer to 160°C.

Line air fryer basket with greaseproof paper and spray with avocado oil. Cooking in batches, spoon half ladlefuls at a time of batter onto the paper.

Cook for 5-7 minutes without flipping until browned. Repeat with remaining batter, spraying each batch.

SERVES 8

Spinach and Feta Muffins

350g frozen chopped spinach, thawed and squeezed to remove moisture

2 large eggs

¼ cup (60ml) olive oil

1 cup (250ml) milk

¼ cup (60ml) Greek yoghurt

2 cups (250g) plain flour

2 tsps baking powder

150g feta cheese, diced

Muffin tray or silicone moulds

Place spinach, eggs, olive oil, milk and yoghurt in a large bowl. Mix well. Add flour, baking powder and cheese. Stir to combine.

Preheat air fryer to 175°C. Spoon mixture into silicone moulds or muffin tray filled with paper liners.

Cook in batches or use a double layer accessory for 15-20 minutes, until an inserted skewer comes out clean.

SERVES 12

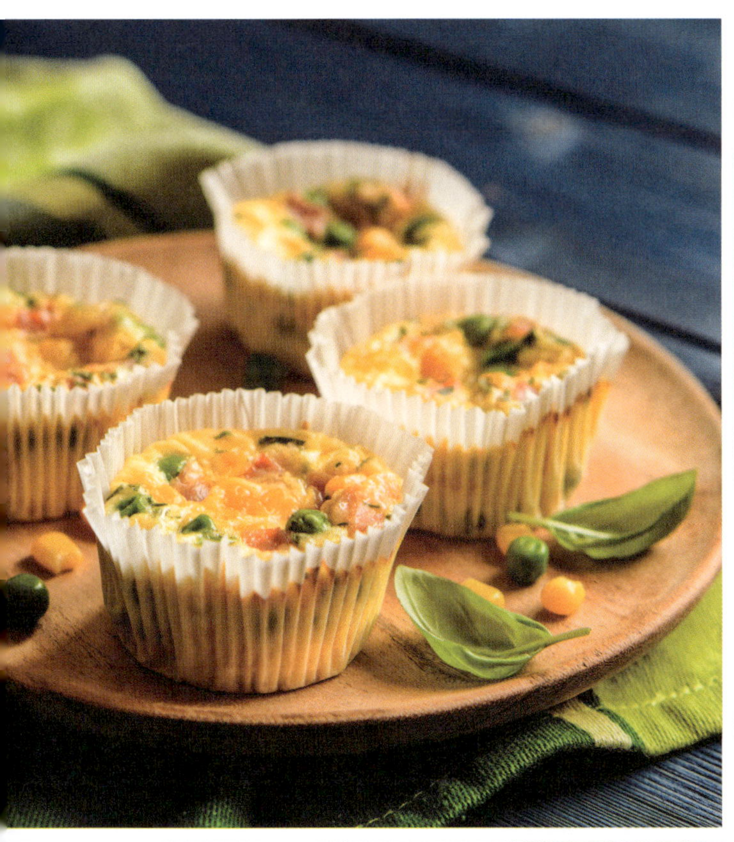
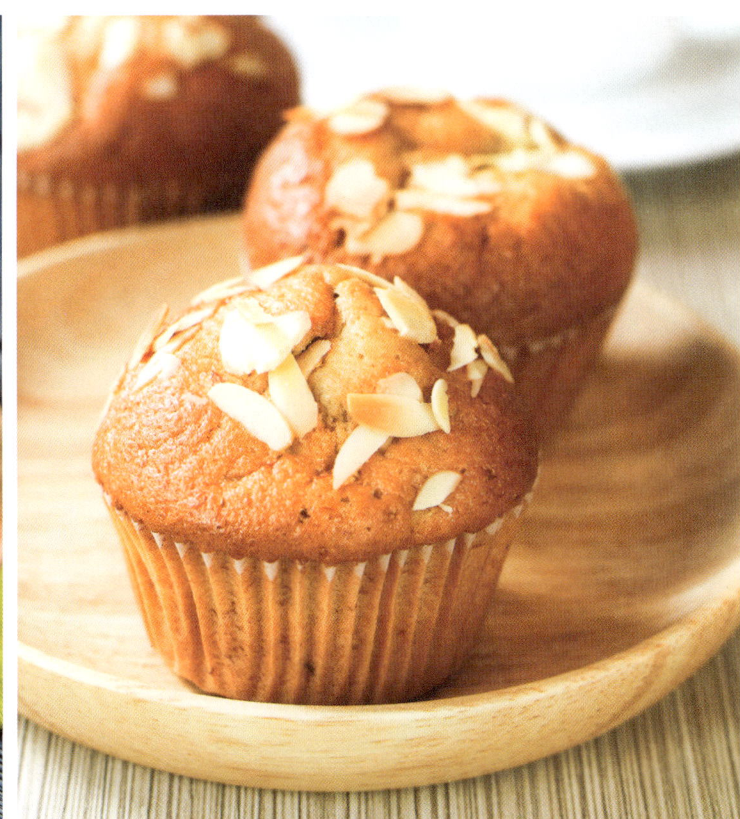
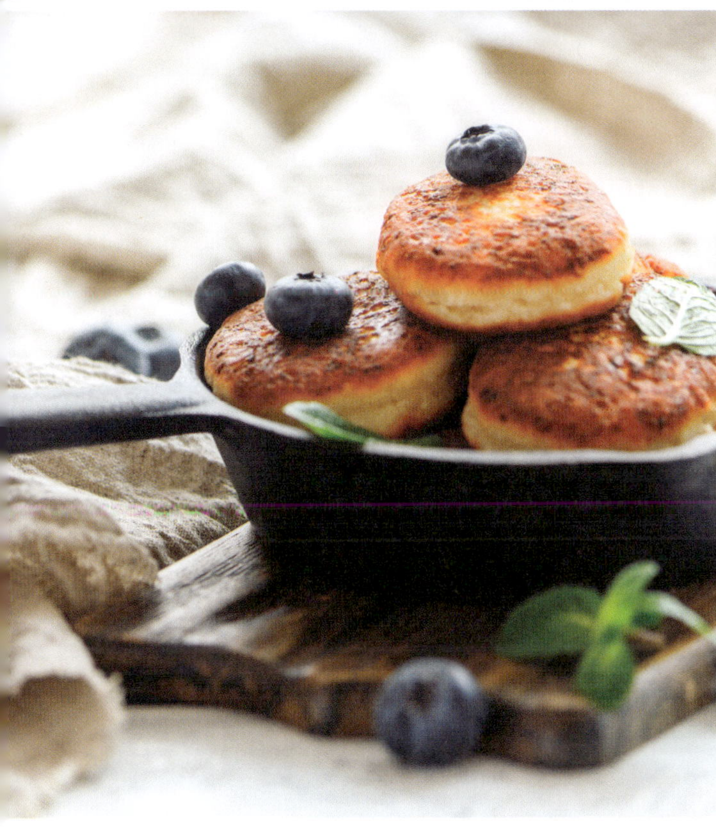
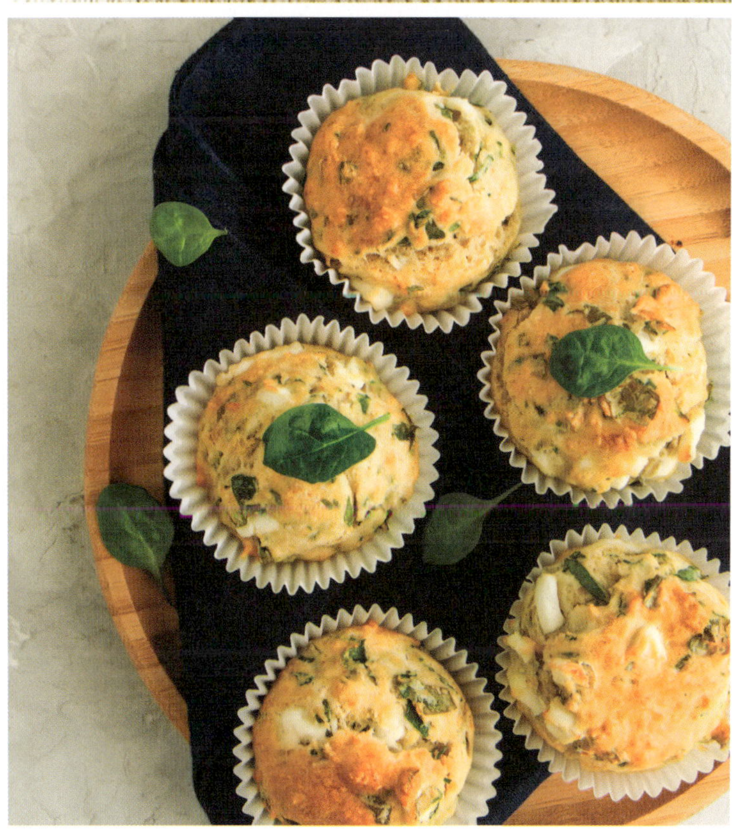

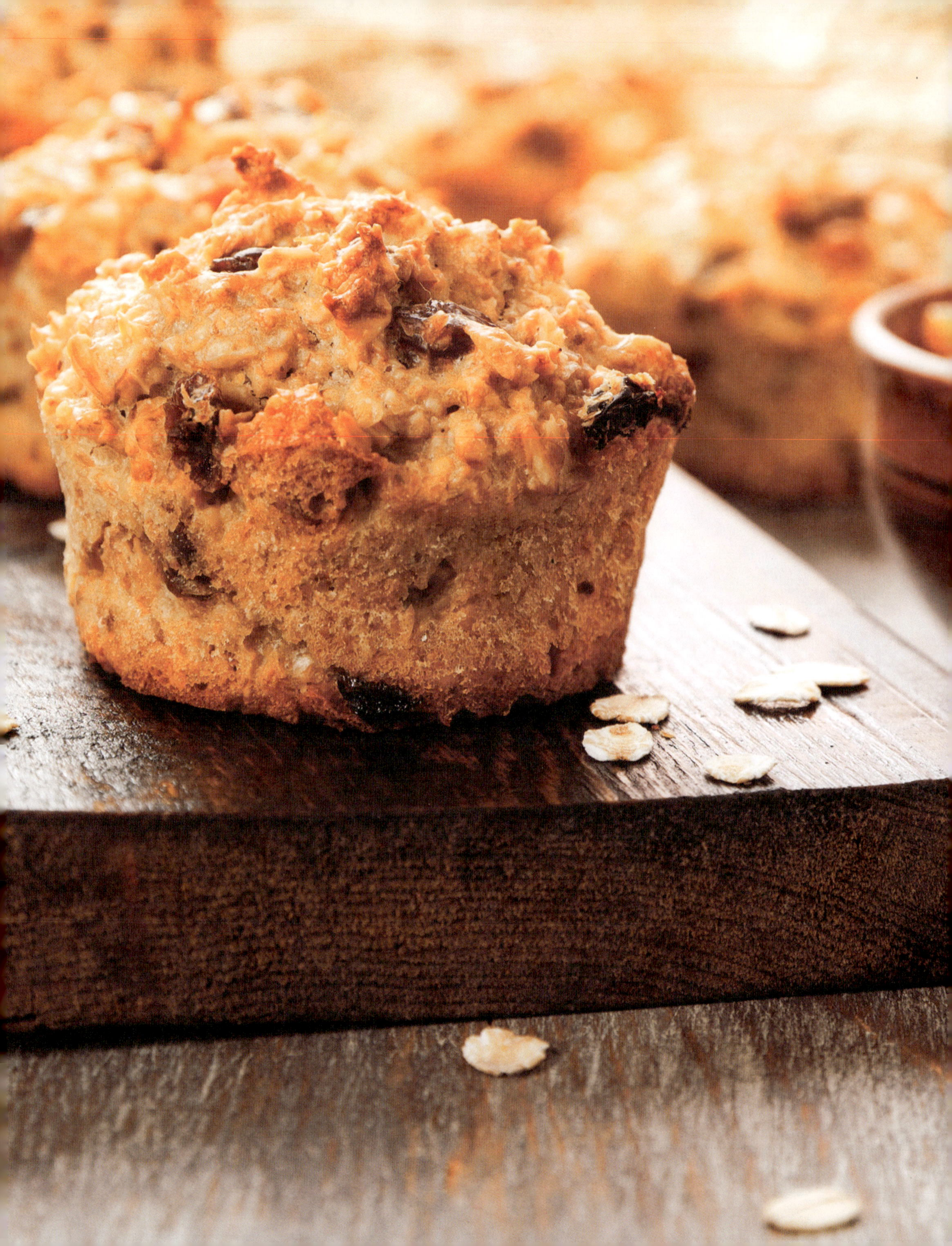

Diet Oat and Raisin Muffins

1 cup (125g) wholemeal flour

¼ cup (40g) brown sugar

1 tbsp baking powder

¾ tsp salt

½ tsp cinnamon

1 cup (90g) rolled oats

½ cup (80g) raisins

¼ cup (60ml) olive oil

1 egg, beaten

1 cup (250ml) milk

Muffin tray or silicone moulds

Mix together flour, sugar, baking powder, salt and cinnamon in a large bowl. Stir in oats and raisins.

In a small bowl whisk together olive oil, egg and milk. Pour into the dry ingredients and stir well to combine.

Working in batches, place silicone moulds or muffin tray filled with paper liners into air fryer basket. Fill moulds or liners two-thirds of the way with batter.

Cook at 200°C for 12 minutes until golden brown and an inserted skewer comes out clean.

Repeat with remaining batter.

MAKES 12

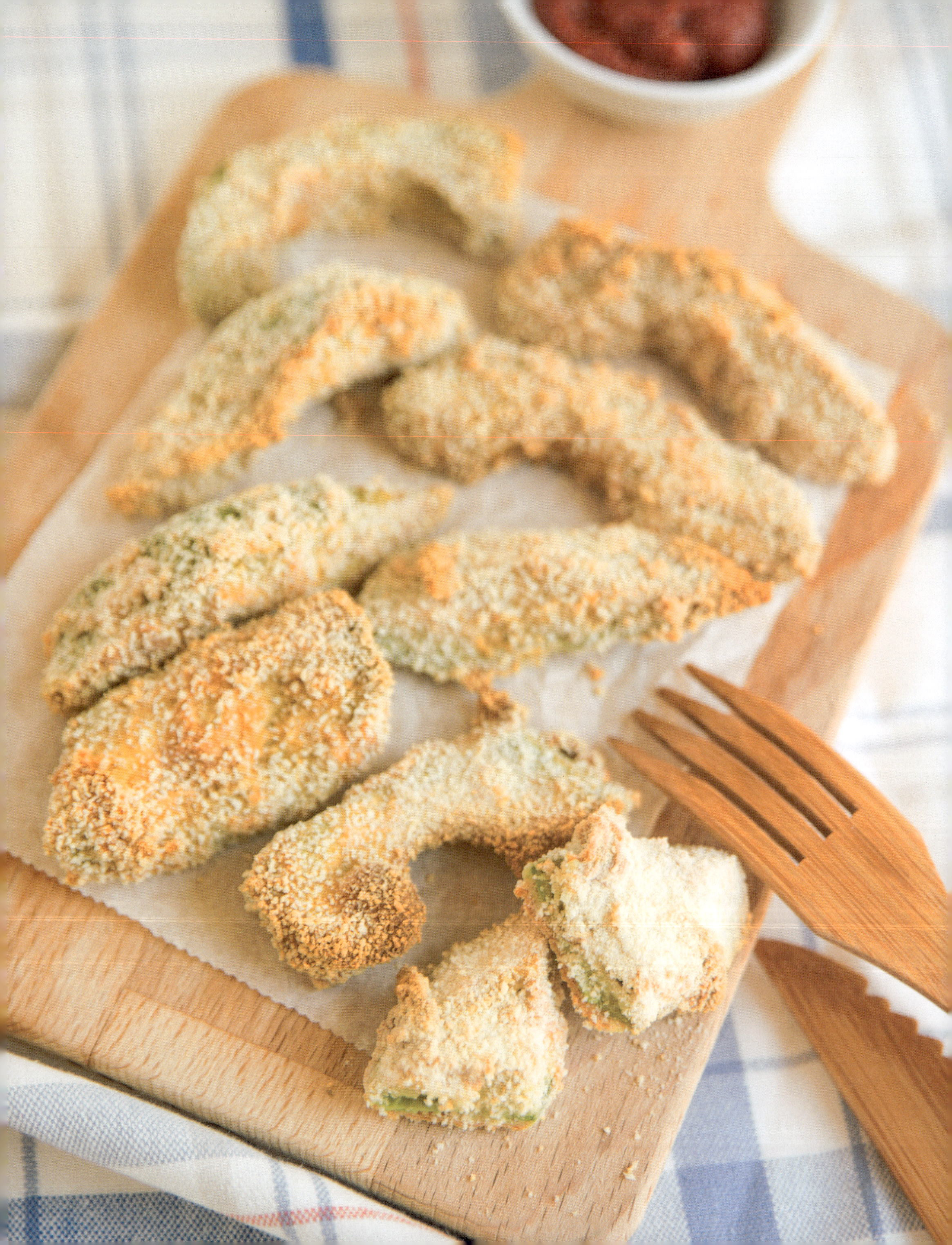

Snacks

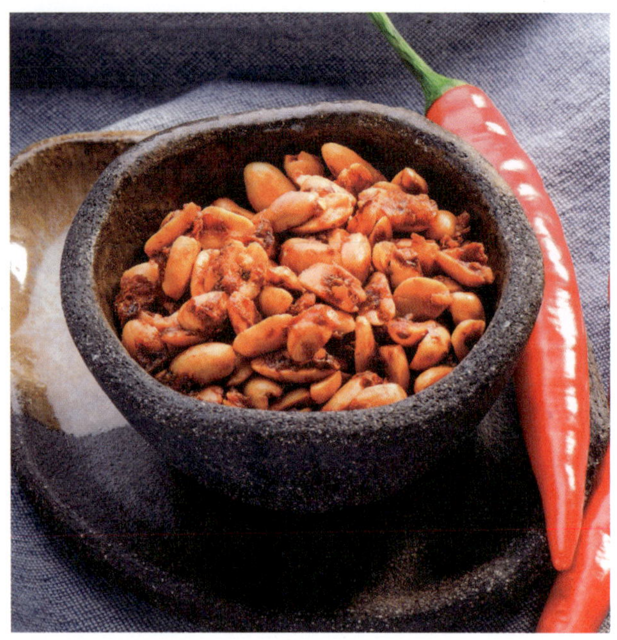

Roasted Spicy Peanuts

2 cups (250g) raw peanuts

1 tbsp olive oil

2 tsps chilli paste

¼ tsp cayenne pepper

Salt to taste

Preheat the air fryer to 160°C.

Place the peanuts in a large bowl and drizzle with olive oil. Add chilli paste and cayenne pepper and toss to coat.

Transfer to air fryer basket and cook for 10 minutes. Toss well then cook for a further 10 minutes.

Remove and salt to taste. Toss to combine then cook for a further 5 minutes.

Allow to cool slightly before serving.

MAKES 2 CUPS

Roasted Spicy Pumpkin Seeds with Chilli and Paprika

1½ cups (170g) whole pumpkin seeds

1 tsp olive oil

1½ tsps salt

1 tsp smoked paprika

½ tsp chilli powder

Bring a large pan of well-salted water to a boil. Add the pumpkin seeds to the boiling water and boil for 10 minutes. Drain the seeds and spread out on a clean tea towel to dry for at least 20 minutes.

Preheat the air fryer to 180°C.

Place the dry seeds in a large bowl with olive oil, salt and spices. Toss well to coat. Transfer to the air fryer basket. Air fry for 35 minutes, shaking the basket every few minutes, until pumpkin seeds are crispy and slightly browned.

Allow the seeds to cool before serving.

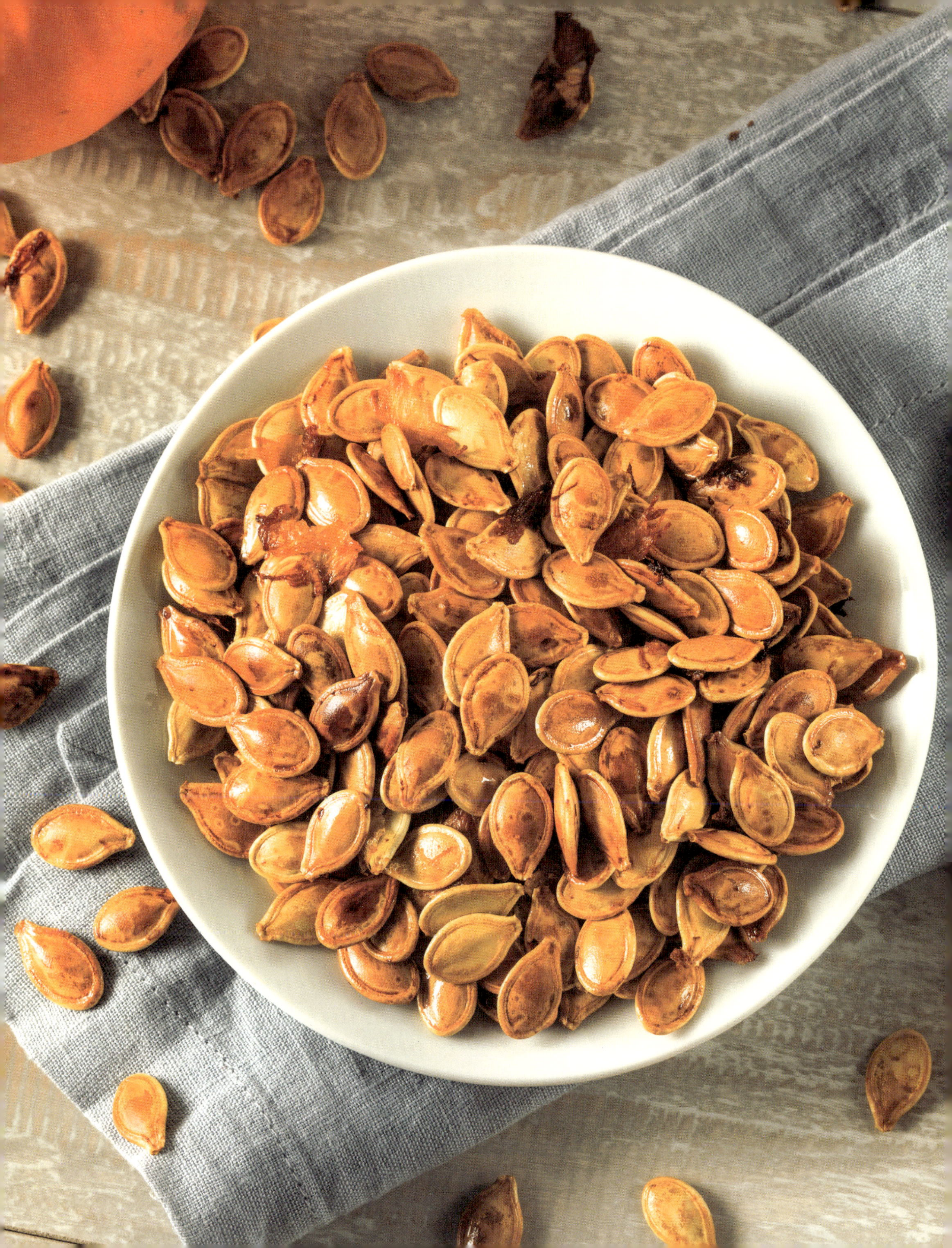

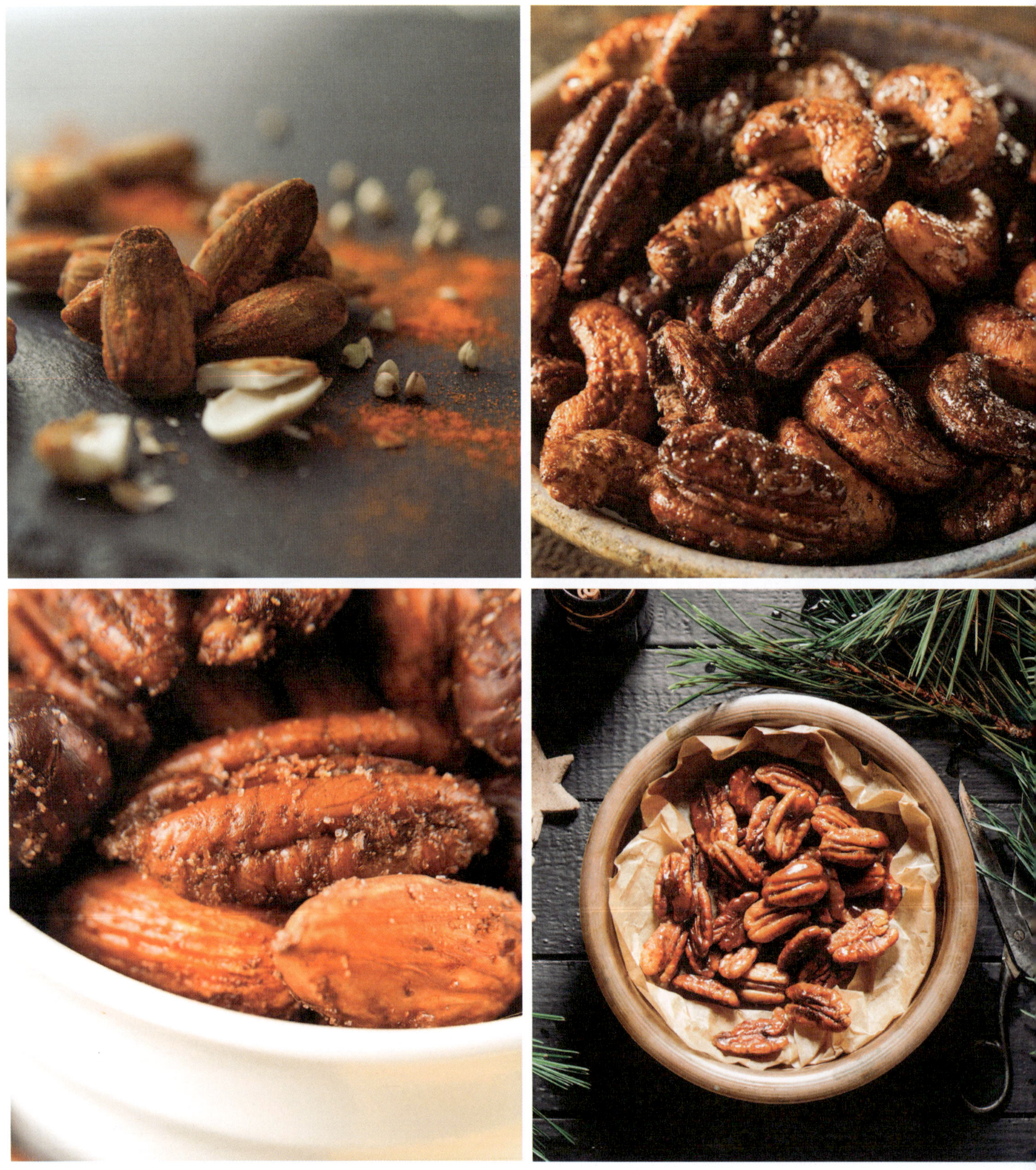

Spiced Almonds

2 cups (250g) whole almonds

1 tsp ground cumin

1 tsp paprika

¼ tsp garlic powder

¼ tsp cayenne pepper

2 tbsps egg white, whisked

½ tsp salt

Preheat air fryer to 160°C.

Place almonds and spices in a large bowl. Add egg white and stir well to coat thoroughly.

Transfer to air fryer basket and cook for 6 minutes. Toss well then cook for a further 2 minutes.

Salt to taste. Toss to combine then cook for a further 3-5 minutes until crispy.

Allow to cool slightly before serving.

MAKES 2 CUPS

Moroccan Spiced Nuts

¾ cup (100g) almonds

¾ cup (100g) pecans

¾ cup (100g) cashews

1 egg white, whisked

1 tsp ground cumin

1 tsp ground coriander

Pinch of cayenne pepper

1 tsp honey

2 tsps salt

Preheat air fryer to 150°C.

Combine the nuts and the egg white in a large bowl.

Add the spices, honey and salt. Stir to combine.

Place in air fryer basket and cook for 10 minutes. Stir well then cook for a further 10 minutes until crispy.

Allow nuts to cool before eating.

MAKES 2¼ CUPS

Roasted Salted Nuts

¾ cup (100g) pecans

¾ cup (100g) almonds

1 tsp melted ghee or avocado oil

⅓ tsp salt

Pepper to taste

Preheat air fryer to 180°C.

Place nuts in a large bowl with melted ghee or oil.

Toss well to coat. Place in air fryer basket and cook for 4 minutes. Shake basket then return to air fryer and cook for a further 2-4 minutes until dark brown and crispy.

Remove from air fryer into a large bowl and season with salt and pepper. Toss well and serve.

MAKES 1½ CUPS

Cinnamon Pecans

2 cups (250g) pecans

2 tbsps peanut oil or melted ghee

¼ tsp salt

2 tsps cinnamon

2 tbsps maple syrup

Place the pecans in a large bowl. Drizzle with peanut oil or ghee. Sprinkle with salt and cinnamon and toss to combine.

Transfer to the air fryer basket and cook at 160°C for 18-20 minutes, stirring every 5 minutes.

When crispy remove from the air fryer and drizzle with maple syrup.

Allow to cool slightly, then serve warm.

MAKES 2 CUPS

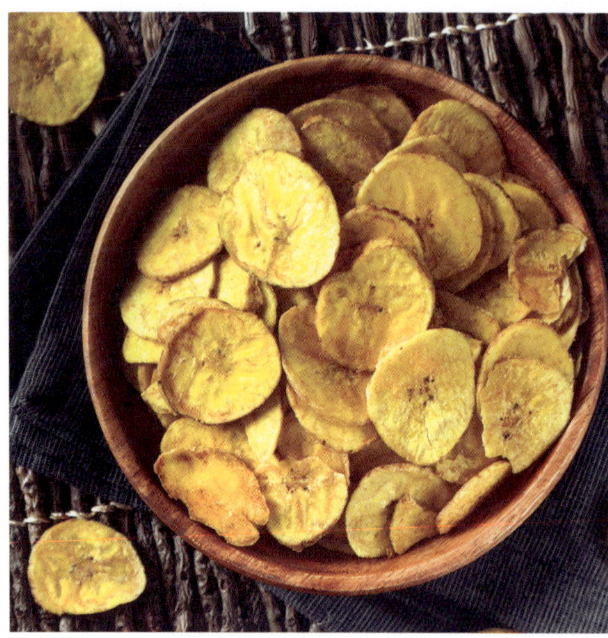

Banana Chips

3 bananas

2 tsps avocado oil or olive oil

¼ tsp salt

Preheat air fryer to 180°C.

Use a mandoline or sharp knife to thinly slice the bananas.

Place banana slices in a large bowl with the oil and salt. Toss very gently to coat.

Place the sliced bananas in one layer, overlapping slightly, in the air fryer basket. Cook in batches or use a double layer accessory if necessary.

Cook for about 10-12 minutes until crisp and golden.

Transfer to a wire rack to cool before serving.

SERVES 4

Seed Crackers

2 cups (500g) cold water

3 tbsps psyllium husk powder

¼ tsp salt

¾ cup (90g) sunflower seeds

¾ cup (120g) sesame seeds

¼ cup (30g) pepitas (pumpkin seeds)

¼ cup (35g) flaxseed

Cake tin

Pour water into a large mixing bowl, add the psyllium husk a little at a time, whisking continuously to dissolve lumps.

Add salt and seeds. Stir well.

Set aside to rest for 10-15 minutes.

Line cake tin with greaseproof paper. Preheat air fryer to 160°C.

Once the mixture has gelled, spread it thinly and evenly in the cake tin.

Place cake tin in air fryer and cook for 20-25 minutes.

Use a pizza cutter or a sharp knife to score cracker shapes into the mixture.

Cook for a further 12 -15 minutes until crisp.

When cooked allow to cool slightly then remove from the tin and break along the scored lines.

MAKES 12

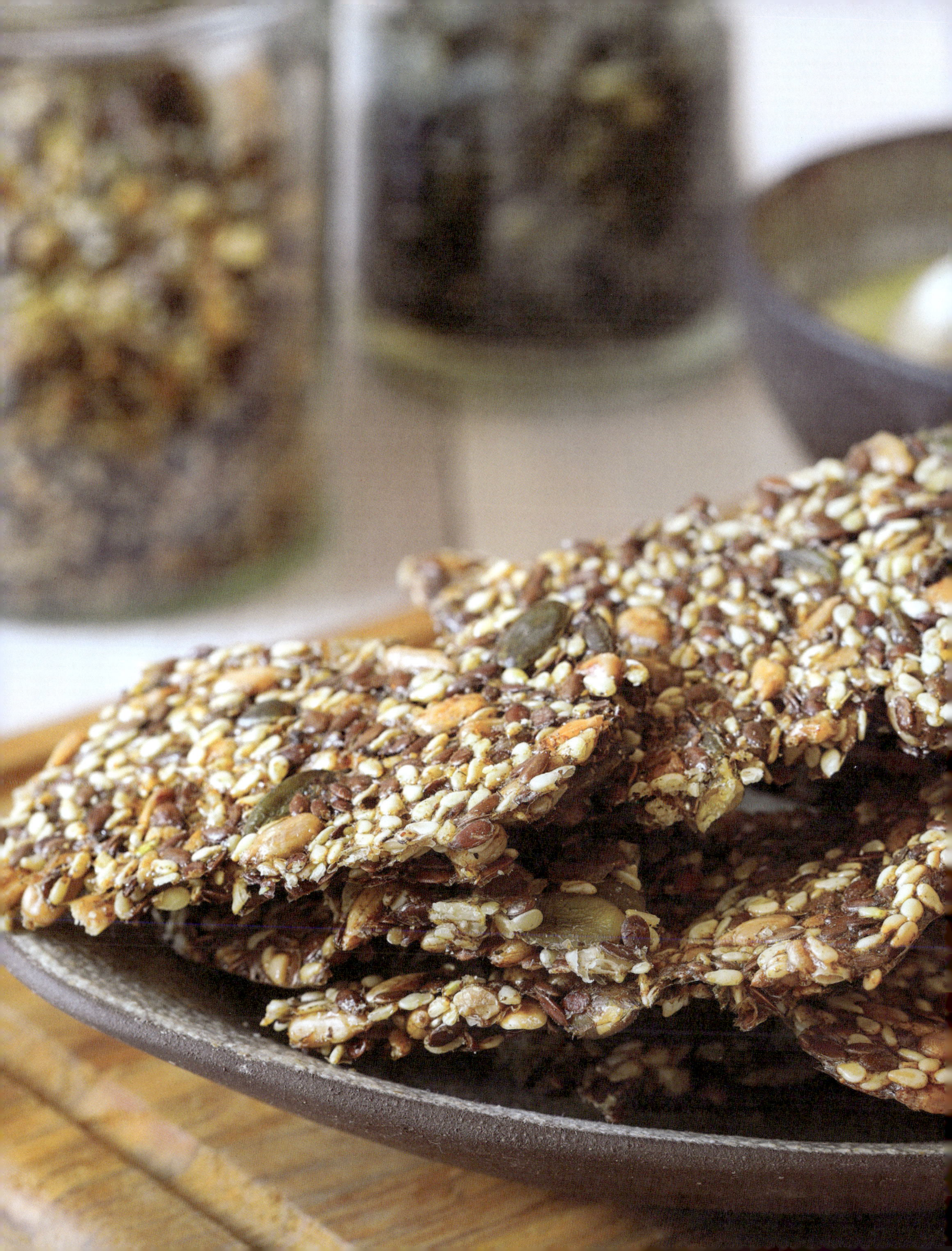

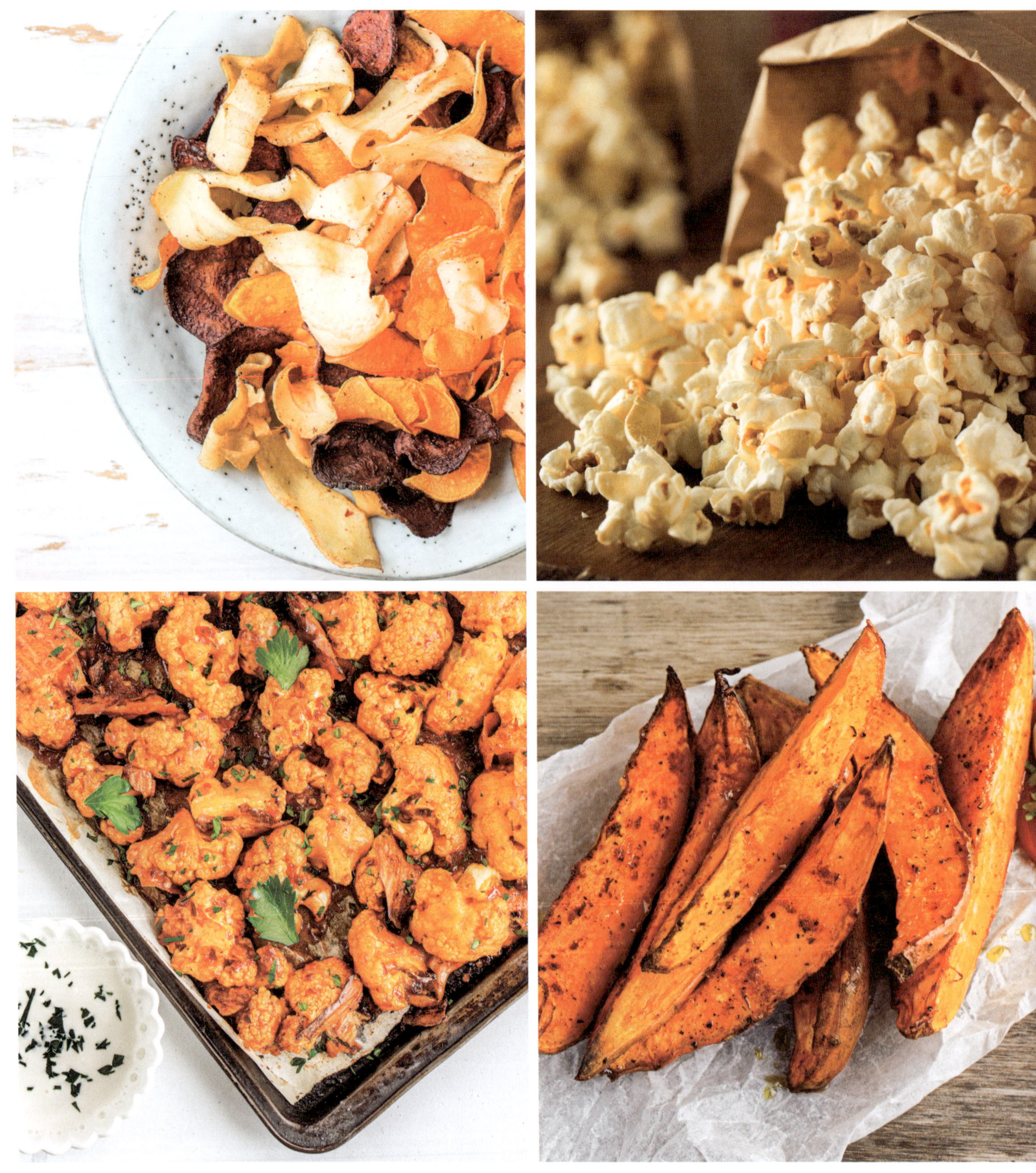

Vegetable Chips

1 parsnip, peeled

1 large carrot, peeled

1 medium beetroot, peeled

1 small sweet potato

2 tbsps olive oil

¼ tsp salt

¼ tsp pepper

Use a mandoline or sharp knife to thinly slice the vegetables, slicing the parsnips and carrots lengthways.

Place in a large bowl and drizzle with oil. Sprinkle with salt and pepper and toss to coat.

Arrange in a single layer in the air fryer. Cook in batches or use a double layer accessory if necessary.

Air fry at 180°C for 12-15 minutes.

Shake the basket halfway through cooking and check after 12 minutes to ensure the chips are not burning.

Remove the chips with tongs and place on a cooling rack to cool slightly before serving.

SERVES 4

Popcorn

¼ cup (50g) popcorn kernels

1 tbsp oil

½ tsp salt

Line the air fryer with foil or create a foil pouch.

Place the corn kernels in a bowl and toss with the oil.

Place on the foil or in the pouch inside the air fryer.

Cook at 200°C for 8-10 minutes or until the popcorn stops popping.

Remove from the air fryer and season with salt.

SERVES 2

Buffalo Cauliflower Bites

2 cups (200g) cauliflower florets

½ red onion, sliced

2 tbsps peanut oil

Salt and pepper to taste

2 tsps garlic powder

1 tsp cumin

1 tsp paprika

1 cup (250ml) hot sauce

1 tbsp melted butter

Preheat air fryer to 200°C.

Place cauliflower and onion in a large bowl with oil, salt and pepper. Toss to coat. Arrange in air fryer basket.

Cook for 8 minutes, shaking halfway through cooking.

Combine remaining ingredients in a bowl, mix well, then baste cauliflower with sauce. Cook basted cauliflower for 7 minutes, shaking once more during cooking.

SERVES 2

Spicy Sweet Potato Chips

2 medium sweet potatoes

2 tbsps avocado or olive oil

Salt and pepper to taste

1 tsp ground coriander

1 tsp garlic powder

½ tsp oregano

½ tsp chilli powder

Preheat air fryer to 180°C.

Cut the sweet potatoes into evenly sized chips. Place in a large bowl.

Drizzle with oil and sprinkle with salt, pepper and spices. Toss to coat evenly.

Transfer to the air fryer and cook for about 20 minutes shaking the basket every 5 minutes.

When crispy and tender remove from the fryer and serve.

SERVES 4

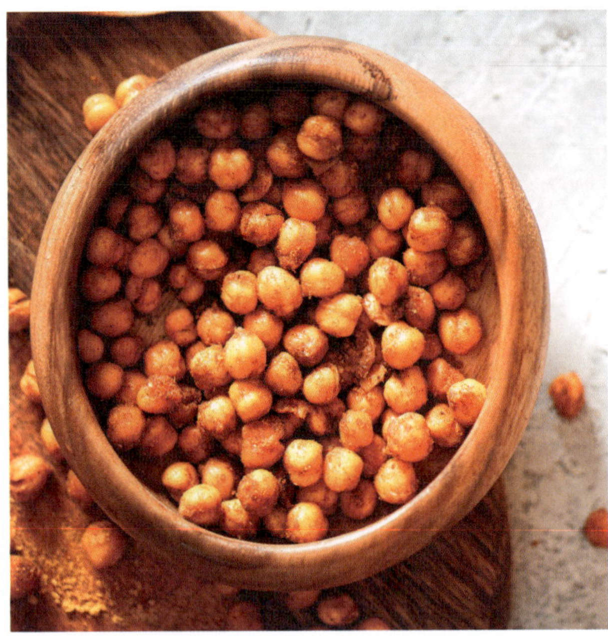

Spiced Chickpeas

1 x 400g can chickpeas

1 tbsp olive oil

¼ tsp salt

3 tsps ground cumin

1 tsp garlic powder

2 tsps paprika

Preheat the air fryer to 190°C.

Drain and rinse the chickpeas. Transfer to a large mixing bowl. Add olive oil, salt and spices. Toss well to coat.

Place chickpeas in the air fryer basket. Cook for 15 minutes, shaking the basket once or twice during cooking.

When crispy remove from the air fryer and allow to cool slightly before serving,

SERVES 2

Brussels Sprouts Chips

500g Brussels sprouts, trimmed and sliced

1 tbsp sesame oil

½ tsp salt

¼ tsp pepper

2 tbsps ponzu sauce

1 nori sheet, cut into small pieces

2 tbsps Kewpie mayonnaise

1 tbsp black and white sesame seeds

Mix Brussels sprouts, oil, salt and pepper together in a bowl.

Place Brussels sprouts in air fryer basket.

Cook for 9-12 minutes on 200°C until brown and crispy.

Transfer Brussels sprouts to a serving bowl. Toss with ponzu sauce, then sprinkle with nori pieces. Drizzle with Kewpie mayonnaise and sprinkle with sesame seeds. Serve immediately.

SERVES 4

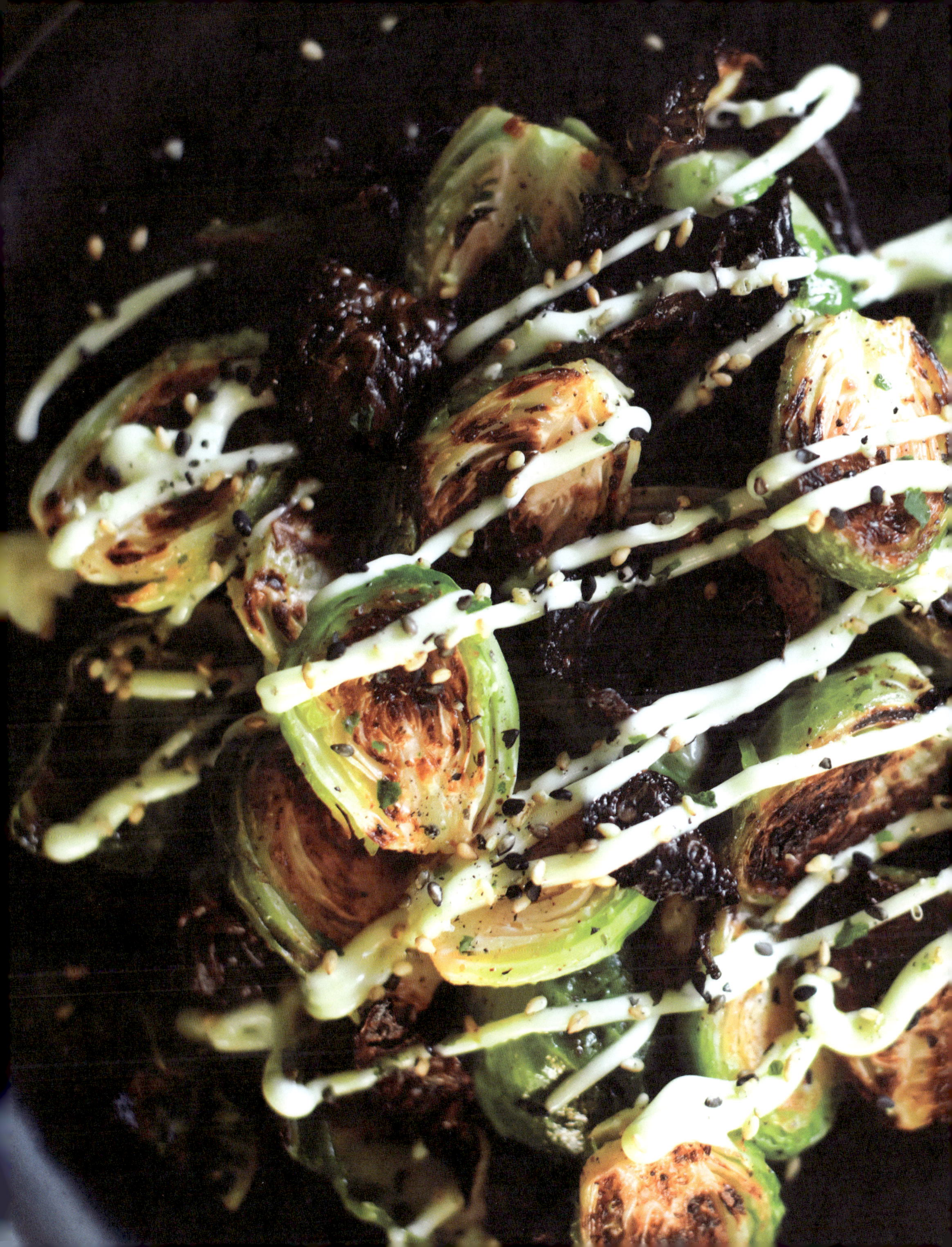

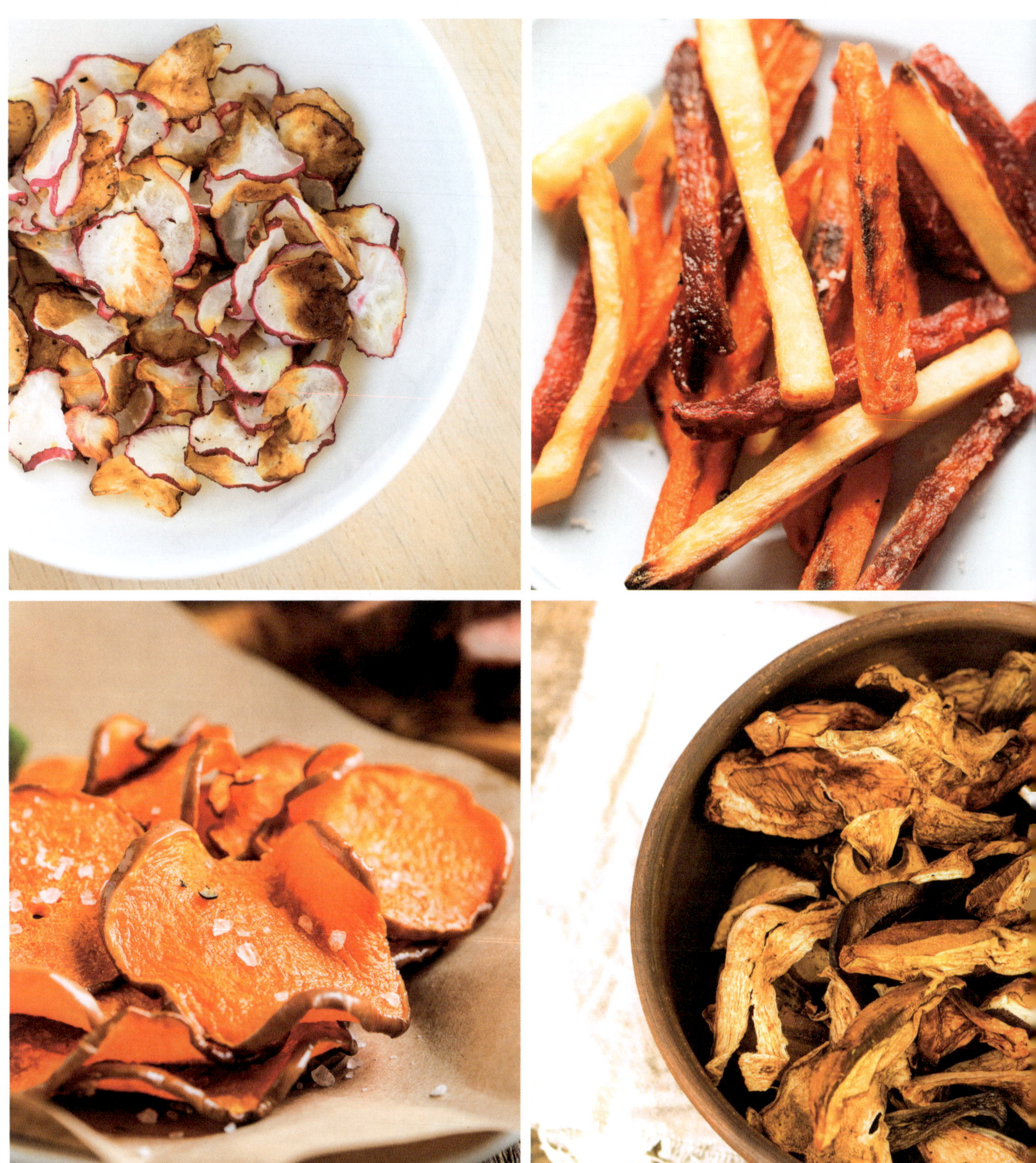

Radish Chips

6 radishes

1 tbsp balsamic vinegar

½ tsp salt

Olive oil spray

Wash and dry the radishes. Use a sharp knife or mandoline to slice thinly.

Place the radishes in a bowl with the vinegar and salt. Toss to coat.

Arrange the radishes in an even layer in the air fryer basket. Take care not to overcrowd the basket; cook in batches or use a double layer accessory if necessary.

Spray the radishes with olive oil.

Cook in the air fryer for 10 minutes at 190°C, shaking the basket halfway through.

Spray with a little more oil then continue to cook for a further 6 minutes, again, shaking halfway through.

SERVES 2

Beetroot, Carrot and Parsnip Fries

1 large beetroot, peeled

2 carrots, peeled

2 parsnips, peeled

1 tbsp olive oil

¼ tsp salt

¼ tsp pepper

Preheat air fryer to 190°C.

Cut vegetables into 2cm-thick, 5cm lengths. Place the beetroot and carrot in one bowl and the parsnips in another. Drizzle vegetables with olive oil and toss to coat.

Place carrots and beetroot in the air fryer and cook for 10-15 minutes until crispy.

Transfer to a wire rack and sprinkle with salt and pepper while still hot.

Cook parsnips for 3-4 minutes until brown and crispy. Toss vegetables together and season further to taste. Serve immediately.

SERVES 4

Sweet Potato Chips

1 medium sweet potato, unpeeled

1 tbsp olive oil

¼ tsp salt

¼ tsp pepper

Use a mandoline or sharp knife to thinly slice the sweet potatoes.

Place in a large bowl and drizzle with oil. Toss to coat.

Sprinkle with salt and pepper and toss once more.

Arrange in a single layer in the air fryer. Cook in batches or use a double layer accessory if necessary.

Air fry at 180°C for 6-9 minutes.

Shake the basket halfway through cooking and check after 6 minutes to ensure the chips are not burning.

Remove the chips with tongs and place on a cooling rack to cool slightly and crisp further.

Serve warm or cold.

SERVES 4

Shiitake Mushroom Chips

250g shiitake mushrooms

¼ tsp salt

Preheat the air fryer to 180°C.

Slice the mushrooms into 1cm-thick slices.

Place in the air fryer basket and cook for 8-12 minutes, shaking the basket halfway through, or until the mushrooms are completely dry.

Sprinkle with salt and serve.

SERVES 2

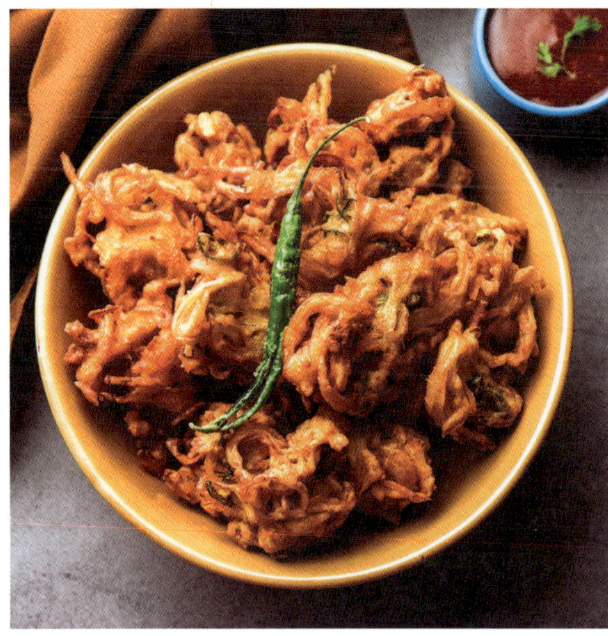

Onion Pakoras

2 cups (190g) chickpea flour (besan)

2 tbsps rice flour

½ tsp ajwain seeds

¼ tsp asafoetida

1 tsp chilli powder

½ tsp ground turmeric

¼ cup (10g) fresh coriander, chopped

Salt to taste

1 large or 2 small onions, sliced

½ cup (125ml) water

2 tbsps peanut or avocado oil

Preheat air fryer to 200°C.

Place the flours, spices, fresh coriander and salt in a bowl. Mix well. Add onion and toss to coat.

Slowly add water and stir gently until it forms a thick and sticky batter. Add 1 teaspoon of oil and mix well.

Spoon small portions of batter into air fryer, taking care not to overcrowd the basket. Brush the pakoras with oil.

Cook for 10 minutes, then flip pakoras and brush once more with oil. Cook for a further 7 minutes until brown and crispy.

Repeat with remaining batter.

SERVES 4

Sesame Ginger and Garlic Edamame

450g frozen whole unshelled edamame

2 tbsps orange juice

2 tbsps tamari

1 tbsp rice wine vinegar

1 tbsp maple syrup

Small piece ginger, grated

2 tsps sesame seeds

2 cloves garlic, minced

½ tsp salt

Place the edamame in a bowl with the rest of the ingredients. Toss together until the edamame are well coated.

Use a slotted spoon to transfer the edamame to the air fryer basket. Reserve the sauce for later.

Cook at 200°C for 5 minutes, then toss and cook for 5 minutes more, until hot and just starting to brown.

Toss the beans with the reserved sauce, or serve the sauce on the side.

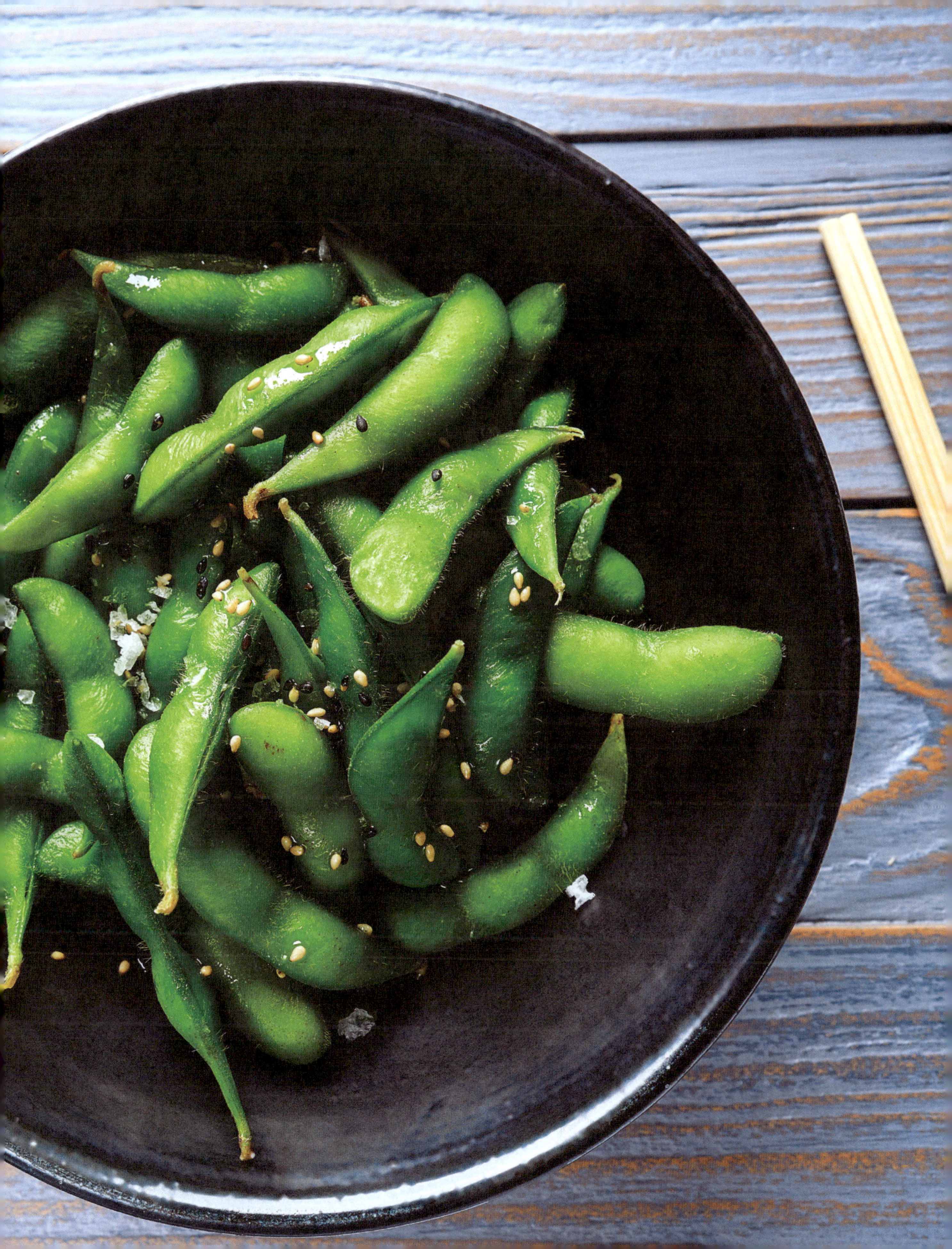

Kale Chips

1 bunch kale (about 5 cups)

1 tbsp olive oil

¼ tsp salt

Remove the stems from the kale and roughly tear into bite-size pieces. Place in a large bowl and massage oil into the leaves. Sprinkle with salt and toss to coat.

Lay kale in a single layer in air fryer basket. Avoid overlapping. Cook in batches or use a double layer accessory if necessary.

Air fry at 190°C for 4-5 minutes until crispy. Shake the basket halfway through cooking.

Serve immediately or store in a paper bag.

SERVES 4

Potato Skins

10 small baking potatoes

2 tbsps peanut or avocado oil

Salt and pepper to taste

Avocado or olive oil cooking spray

Rub potatoes with oil and salt. Place in air fryer basket and cook at 200°C for 1 hour until tender.

Once the potatoes are done and cool enough to handle, slice each one in half. Scoop out most of the flesh from the inside of the potato (this can be used to make mashed potato or gnocchi).

Place skins in a single layer back in air fryer. Spray with cooking spray and season with salt and pepper. Cook for 5-7 minutes until crispy.

Serve immediately.

SERVES 2

Beetroot Chips

2 large beetroots, peeled

1 tbsp olive oil

¼ tsp salt

¼ tsp pepper

Use a mandoline or sharp knife to thinly slice the beetroot.

Place in a large bowl and drizzle with oil. Toss to coat.

Sprinkle with salt and pepper and toss once more.

Arrange in a single layer in the air fryer. Cook in batches or use a double layer accessory if necessary.

Air fry at 180°C for 12-15 minutes.

Shake the basket halfway through cooking and check after 12 minutes to ensure the chips are not burning.

Remove the chips with tongs and place on a cooling rack to cool slightly and crisp further.

Serve warm or cold.

SERVES 4

Baked Potatoes

4 medium Coliban or Sebago potatoes, scrubbed and rinsed

Avocado or olive oil cooking spray

½ tsp salt

½ tsp garlic powder (optional)

Preheat air fryer to 200°C.

Spray potatoes all over with cooking spray. Rub with salt and garlic powder, if using.

Place in air fryer basket and cook for 25 minutes.
Use tongs to turn potatoes, then cook for a further 20-25 minutes until tender.

SERVES 4

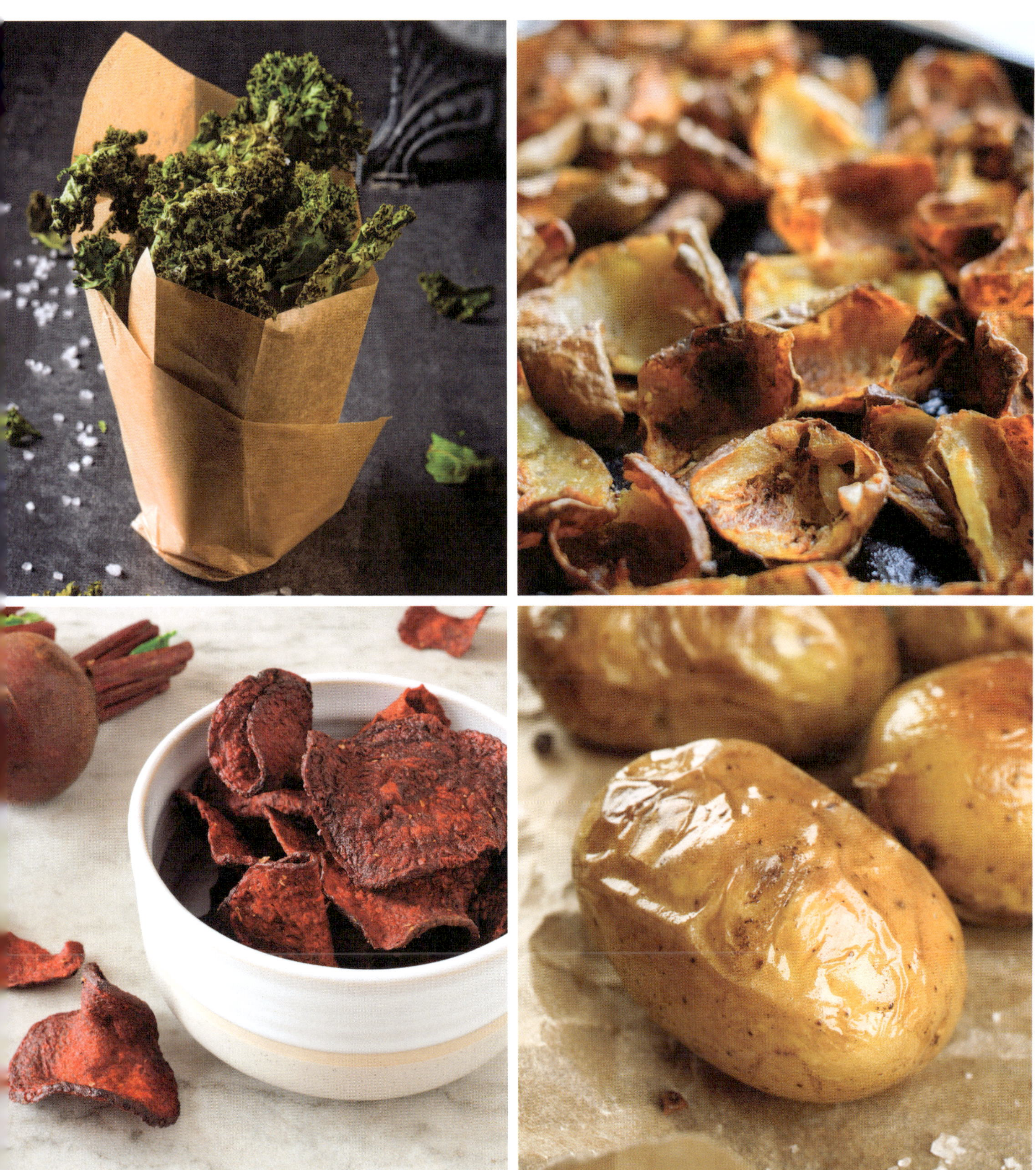

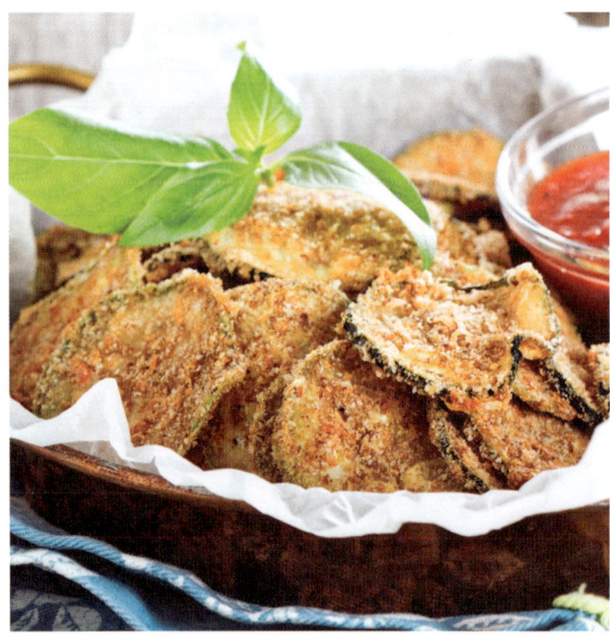

Zucchini Parmesan Chips

1 cup (125g) breadcrumbs

¾ cup (75g) Parmesan cheese, grated

Pinch of salt and pepper

1 large egg

1 medium zucchini, thinly sliced

Cooking spray

Preheat air fryer to 175°C.

Combine breadcrumbs, cheese, salt and pepper on a plate.

Lightly whisk egg in a small bowl.

Dip each zucchini slice firstly into the beaten egg and then into breadcrumb mixture, pressing to coat.

Place in a single layer in the air fryer and spray with cooking spray.

Cook for 10 minutes.

Use tongs to flip, then cook for a further 2 minutes. Remove chips with tongs.

Repeat with remaining zucchini slices.

SERVES 2

Rosemary Potato Wedges

4 medium russet, Coliban or Sebago potatoes

1 tbsp olive oil

1 tsp garlic powder

½ tsp salt

1 tbsp fresh rosemary, finely chopped

Preheat air fryer to 190°C.

Cut the potatoes into 2cm-thick wedges.

Place potatoes in a large bowl and drizzle with olive oil. Sprinkle with garlic powder, salt and rosemary and toss to combine.

Place potatoes in an even layer in basket. Cook in batches or use a double layer accessory if necessary.

Air fry for 10 minutes, flip with tongs and cook for a further 10 minutes until brown and crispy.

SERVES 4

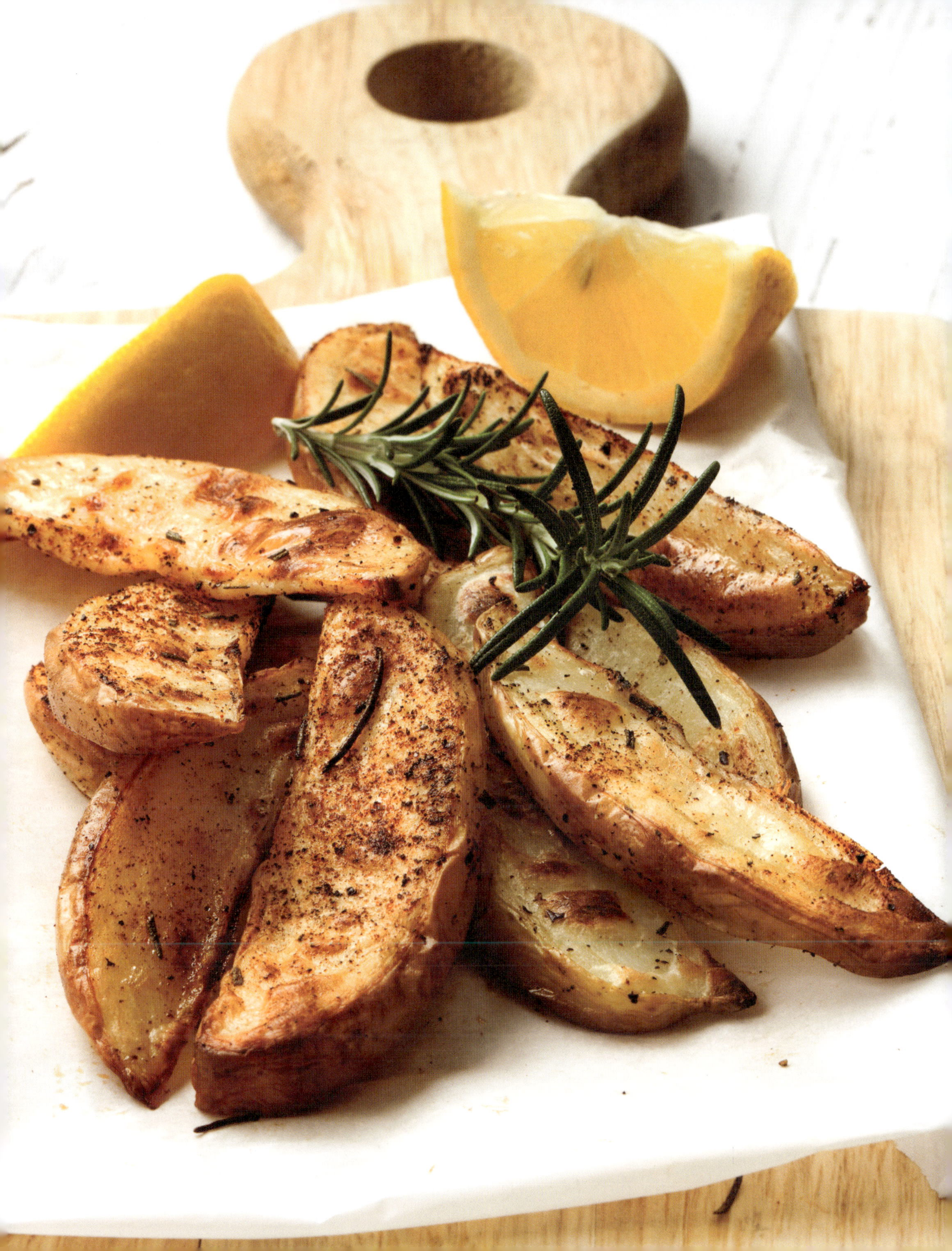

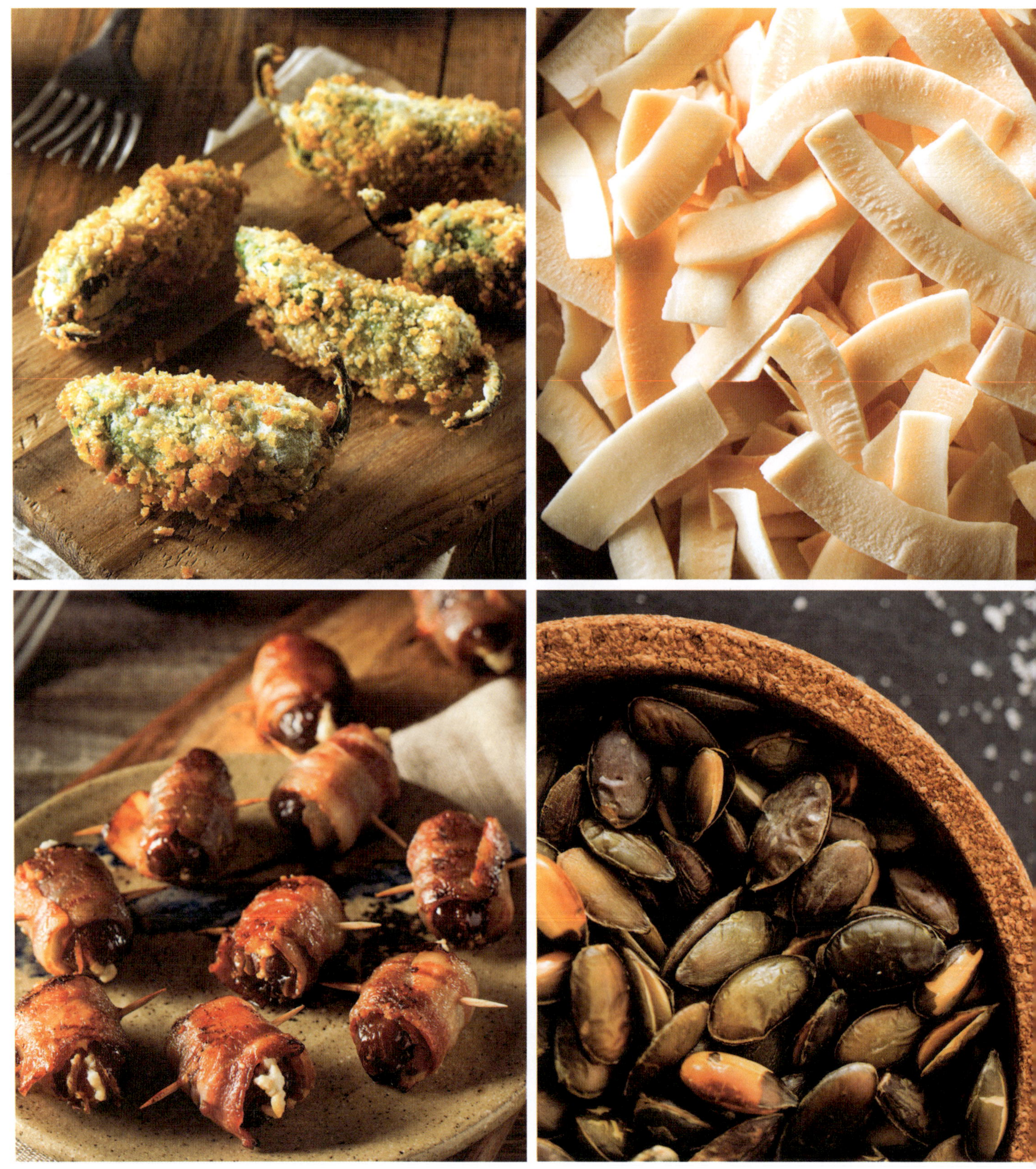

Jalapeno Poppers

8 jalapeno chillies

150g cream cheese, softened

½ cup (50g) Cheddar cheese, grated

2 spring onions, chopped

Salt and pepper to taste

2 large eggs, beaten

1½ cups (185g) panko breadcrumbs

Olive oil cooking spray

Make a slit along the side of each jalapeno. Remove seeds.

Combine cream cheese, Cheddar, spring onion, salt and pepper in a medium bowl; stir until well combined.

Evenly stuff jalapenos with the cream cheese mixture.

Dip each jalapeno into a dish of beaten egg, then in a dish of panko breadcrumbs.

Place the jalapenos in the air fryer basket. Spray with cooking spray. Cook at 190°C for 10-12 minutes, turning halfway through, until brown and tender.

MAKES 8

Toasted Coconut Chips

1 cup (90g) raw coconut flakes

Place coconut flakes into the air fryer basket in one even layer.

Cook for 8-10 minutes at 180°C. Shake the basket halfway through cooking to ensure even toasting.

Transfer to a plate and allow to cool and crisp up.

MAKES 1 CUP

Dates Wrapped in Bacon

10 fresh Medjool dates

80g goat's cheese

5 rashers shortcut bacon, halved

Cut down one side of each date and remove the stones. Use a teaspoon to fill each cut with goat's cheese, using equal amounts in each.

Wrap each date in bacon and secure with a toothpick.

Arrange in the air fryer basket and cook for 12 minutes at 160°C until bacon is crispy.

Serve warm.

SERVES 2

Toasted Pepitas

1 cup (110g) pepitas (pumpkin seeds)

1 tsp avocado oil or olive oil

½ tsp salt

½ tsp smoked paprika (optional)

Rinse pepitas, then allow to dry on a tea towel or paper towels.

Preheat the air fryer to 180°C.

Place pepitas in a large bowl. Add oil, salt and paprika, if using. Mix well.

Place pepitas in the air fryer basket and cook for 25-30 minutes, shaking the basket frequently.

Watch carefully during the last 5 minutes to ensure the pepitas don't burn.

Transfer to a plate and allow to cool.

MAKES 1 CUP

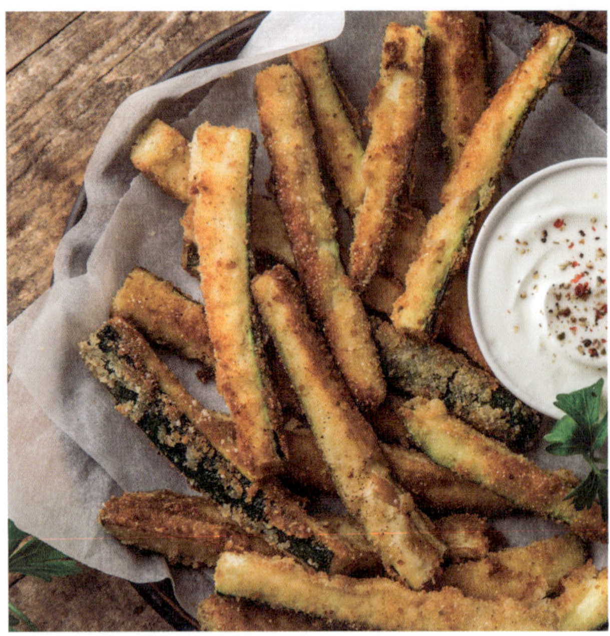

Zucchini Fries

¼ cup (30g) breadcrumbs

¼ cup (25g) Parmesan cheese, grated

½ tsp garlic powder

¼ tsp paprika

Salt and pepper to taste

1 egg

3 large zucchinis, cut into 2cm-thick, 7cm lengths

Olive oil cooking spray

Combine breadcrumbs, Parmesan and seasonings in a shallow dish. Beat the egg in a small bowl.

Dip each zucchini piece first into the egg, then into the breadcrumb mix.

Preheat air fryer to 200°C.

Spray air fryer basket and zucchini with cooking spray.

Arrange fries in a single layer. Cook in batches or use a double layer accessory for 5-6 minutes until golden and crispy.

Serve with dip of choice.

SERVES 4

Mexican Roasted Corn

4 corn cobs

Olive oil cooking spray

2 tbsps butter

2 tsps garlic, chopped

1 lime, zested and juiced

½ tsp salt

½ tsp pepper

2 tbsps fresh coriander, chopped

Lightly coat corn with olive oil cooking spray. Place in a single layer in air fryer basket.

Cook at 200°C for 12-14 minutes until tender and slightly charred, turning halfway through cooking.

Meanwhile, place the butter, garlic, lime juice and 1 teaspoon zest in a small pan. Place over a low heat and stir for 1-2 minutes until the butter is melted and the garlic is fragrant.

Arrange corn on a large serving plate and pour over butter mixture. Sprinkle with salt, pepper and chopped coriander.

SERVES 4

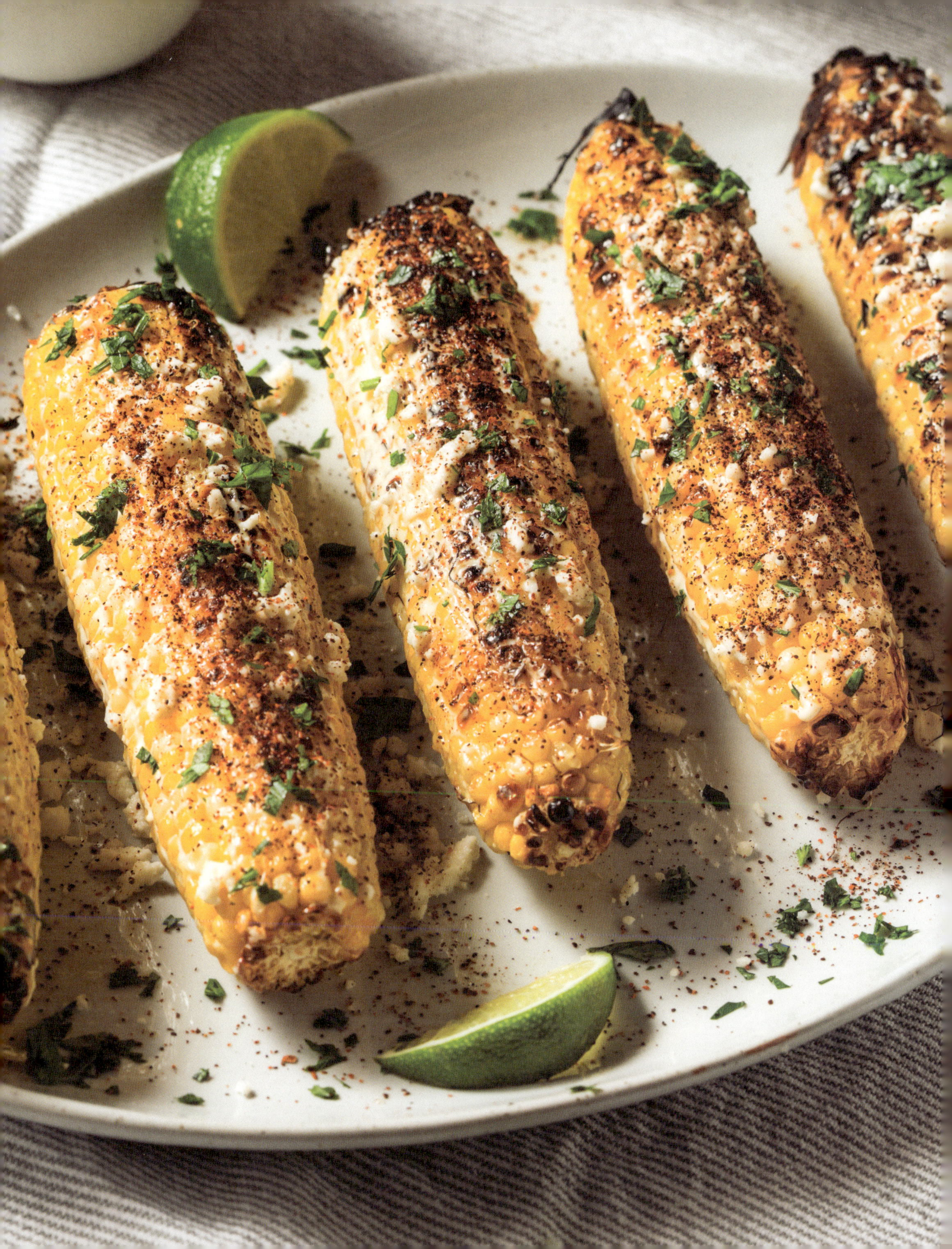

Corn Chips

10 corn tortillas

5 tsps olive oil

¼ tsp salt

⅛ tsp sweet paprika

½ cup (115g) tomato salsa to serve (optional)

Cut each tortilla in half then slice each half into three evenly sized pieces. Brush with olive oil and sprinkle with salt and paprika.

Place in a single layer, overlapping slightly, in the air fryer basket. Cook in batches or use a double layer accessory if necessary.

Cook for 8 minutes or until crisp.

Remove from the air fryer with tongs and repeat with remaining tortilla pieces.

Serve with tomato salsa or the dip of your choice

SERVES 4

Avocado Fries

½ cup (60g) flour

½ tsp salt

1 egg

½ cup (125ml) milk

½ cup (60g) almond meal

½ tsp garlic powder

3 large avocados, peeled and cut into 2cm-thick slices

Cooking spray

Preheat air fryer to 200°C.

Combine flour and ¼ teaspoon salt in a shallow dish. Beat together egg and milk in a bowl. Combine almond meal, garlic powder and remaining salt in another dish.

Dip each avocado slice first into seasoned flour, then egg mix, and finally almond meal mix, pressing gently to coat.

Spray basket and avocados with cooking spray. Arrange avocados in a single layer. Cook in batches if necessary.

Cook for 8-10 minutes until crispy. Serve with dip of choice.

SERVES 4

Hasselback Potatoes

4 medium waxy potatoes such as Bintje

3 tbsps butter

1 tbsp olive oil

3 cloves garlic, crushed

½ tsp paprika

1 sprig rosemary

Salt and pepper to taste

Preheat air fryer to 175°C.

Slice evenly every ½ cm across entire length of each potato keeping the bottom of the potato intact.

Combine butter, olive oil, garlic, paprika and rosemary in a small pan. Heat over low heat for 3 minutes.

Brush potatoes with butter mixture allowing some to go into the slices.

Place potatoes in air fryer basket and cook for 15 minutes. Brush again with butter mixture, and cook for a further 15 minutes until potatoes are cooked through.

SERVES 4

Parmesan Chips

½ cup (50g) Parmesan cheese

1 tsp dried thyme or dried rosemary

Baking tray (optional)

Preheat air fryer to 200°C and the line the air fryer basket (or ovenproof baking tray) with baking paper.

Cut the cheese into very thin slices and sprinkle over a few dried herbs.

Place on the prepared tray.

Cook at 190°C for about 5 minutes until crisp and slightly golden brown.

SERVES 2

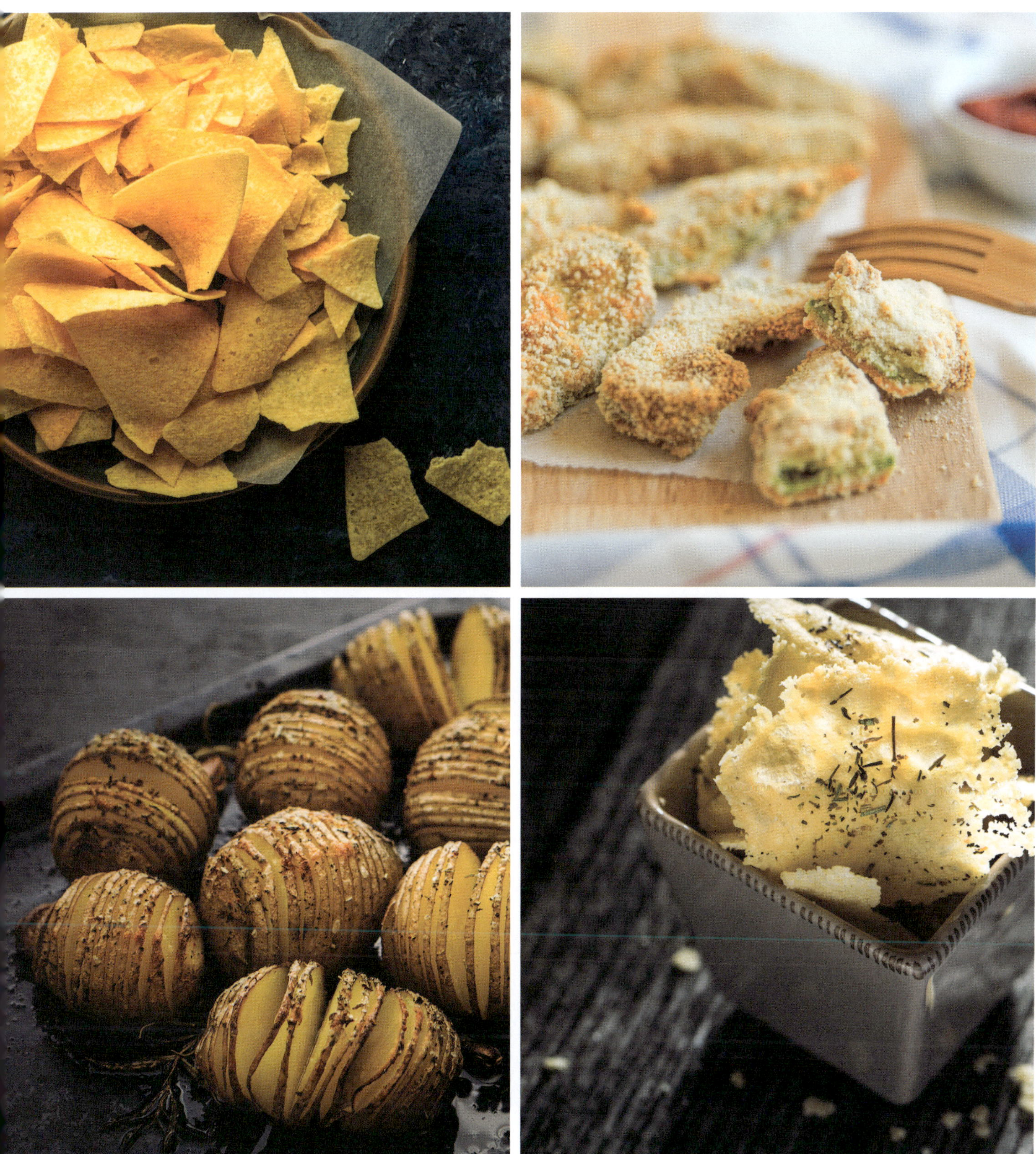

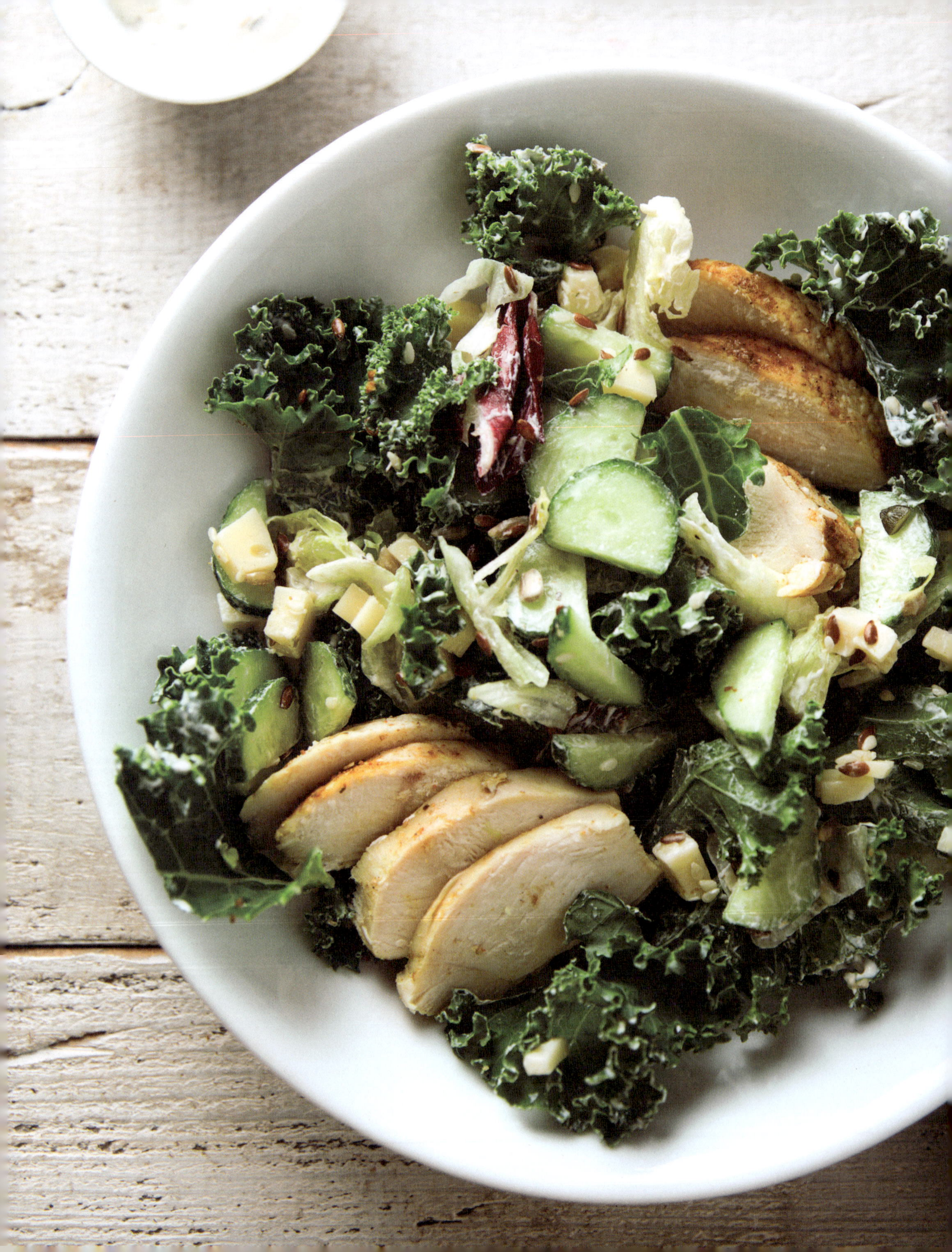

Lite Meals

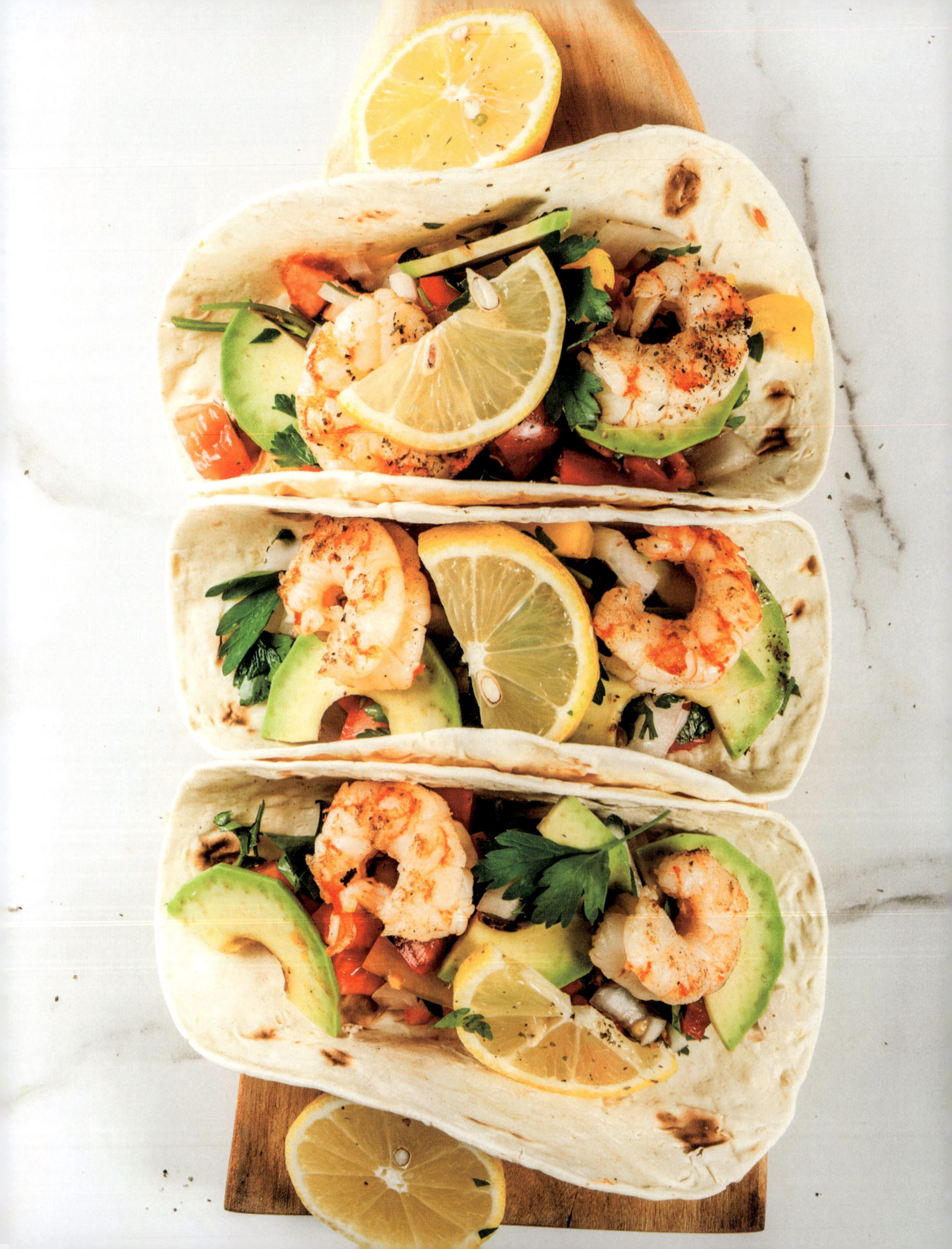

Prawn Tacos

500g peeled, deveined prawns

2 tbsps olive oil

½ tsp garlic powder

¼ tsp ground cumin

¼ tsp onion powder

Salt and pepper to taste

4 flour tortillas, warmed

1 cup (225g) cherry tomatoes, chopped

½ yellow capsicum, diced

1 avocado, sliced

½ red onion, diced

¼ cup (5g) fresh coriander leaves

Juice of 1 lemon

Lemon slices, to serve

Toss prawns with oil, garlic powder, cumin, onion powder, salt and pepper. Transfer to greased air fryer basket.

Cook at 200°C for 5-6 minutes or until cooked through.

Assemble tortillas filled with prawns, tomatoes, capsicum, avocado, red onion and coriander. Squeeze over lemon juice and add lemon slices to serve.

SERVES 2

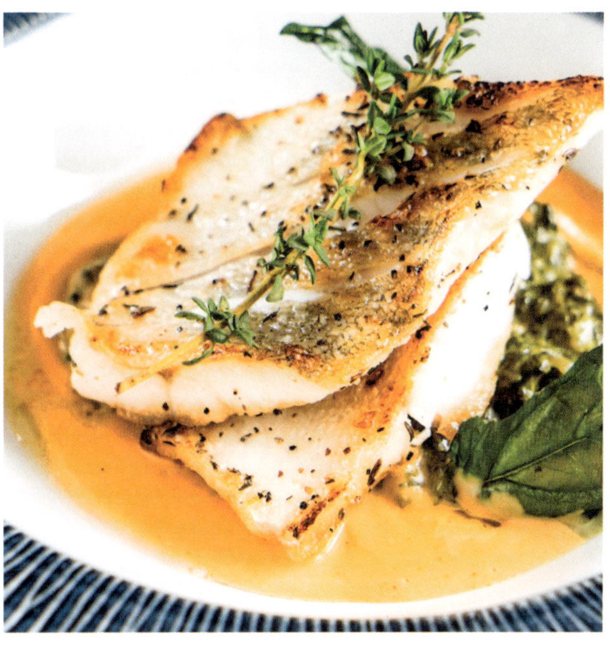

Fish with Mustard Cream Sauce

500g firm white fish fillets

2 tbsps olive oil

Salt and pepper to taste

1 tbsp lemon juice

½ cup (125ml) thickened cream

1 tbsp butter

3 tbsps Dijon mustard

Rub fish with olive oil. Season with salt, pepper and lemon juice. Transfer to greased air fryer basket.

Cook fish for 5 minutes at 175°C, then increase temperature to 200°C and cook for a further 5 minutes.

Meanwhile place cream, butter and mustard in a small pan over medium-low heat. Season with salt and pepper. Mix well and simmer for 3-4 minutes until sauce starts to thicken. Remove from heat.

Spoon sauce into bowls and top with fish fillets to serve.

SERVES 2

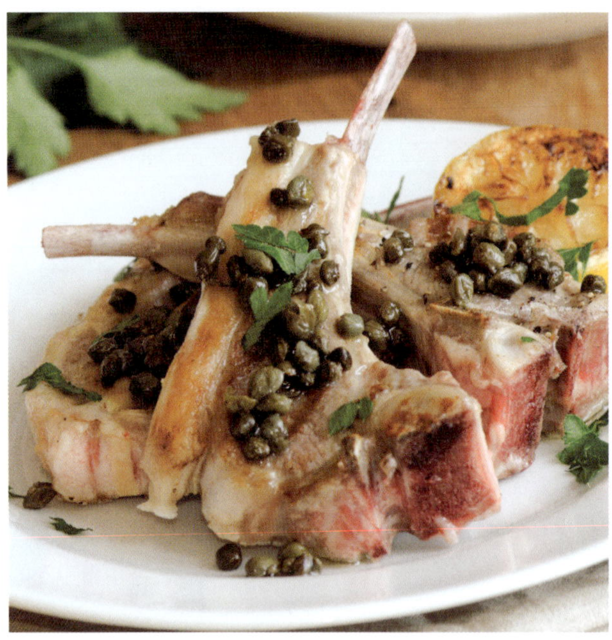

Lamb Chops with Anchovies and Capers

6 small lamb chops

Salt and pepper to taste

3 tbsps olive oil

3 anchovy fillets

½ lemon, thickly sliced

3 tbsps capers, drained

2 cloves garlic, minced

1 tbsp parsley, chopped

Baking pan

Season lamb chops with salt and pepper.

Place olive oil, anchovies, lemon and capers in pan and place in air fryer. Cook for 8-10 minutes at 200°C, stirring every few minutes, until anchovies break down.

Remove dish from air fryer and stir in garlic and parsley.

Baste lamb chops with anchovy mixture. Place lamb chops in air fryer. Cook for 12 minutes at 200°C, turning and basting halfway through cooking. Rest for 5 minutes.

SERVES 2

Lamb Koftas with Yoghurt Sauce

500g lamb mince

½ onion, grated

2 cloves garlic, crushed

2 tbsps fresh coriander, chopped

2 tsps cumin

2 tsps coriander

1 tsp salt

½ tsp pepper

2 tsps paprika

½ tsp ground cinnamon

1 tsp cayenne pepper (optional)

Olive oil cooking spray

Skewers

YOGHURT SAUCE

1 cup (250ml) Greek yoghurt

1 tbsp olive oil

1 clove garlic, crushed

1 tsp cumin

1 tbsp fresh coriander, chopped

1 tbsp lemon juice

¼ tsp salt

¼ tsp pepper

Combine the ingredients for the yoghurt sauce in a small bowl. Mix well to combine and refrigerate for at least 30 minutes or overnight.

Place the lamb mince in a large bowl with the grated onion, garlic, fresh coriander and salt and pepper.

Mix well with hands then divide into eight equal portions. Push and shape the meat onto eight skewers. Spray with olive oil cooking spray.

Place the skewers in the air fryer basket ensuring there is space between each skewer. Cook in batches or use a double layer accessory if necessary.

Cook at 190°C for 10-12 minutes turning halfway through.

Remove from air fryer and serve with prepared yoghurt sauce.

SERVES 4

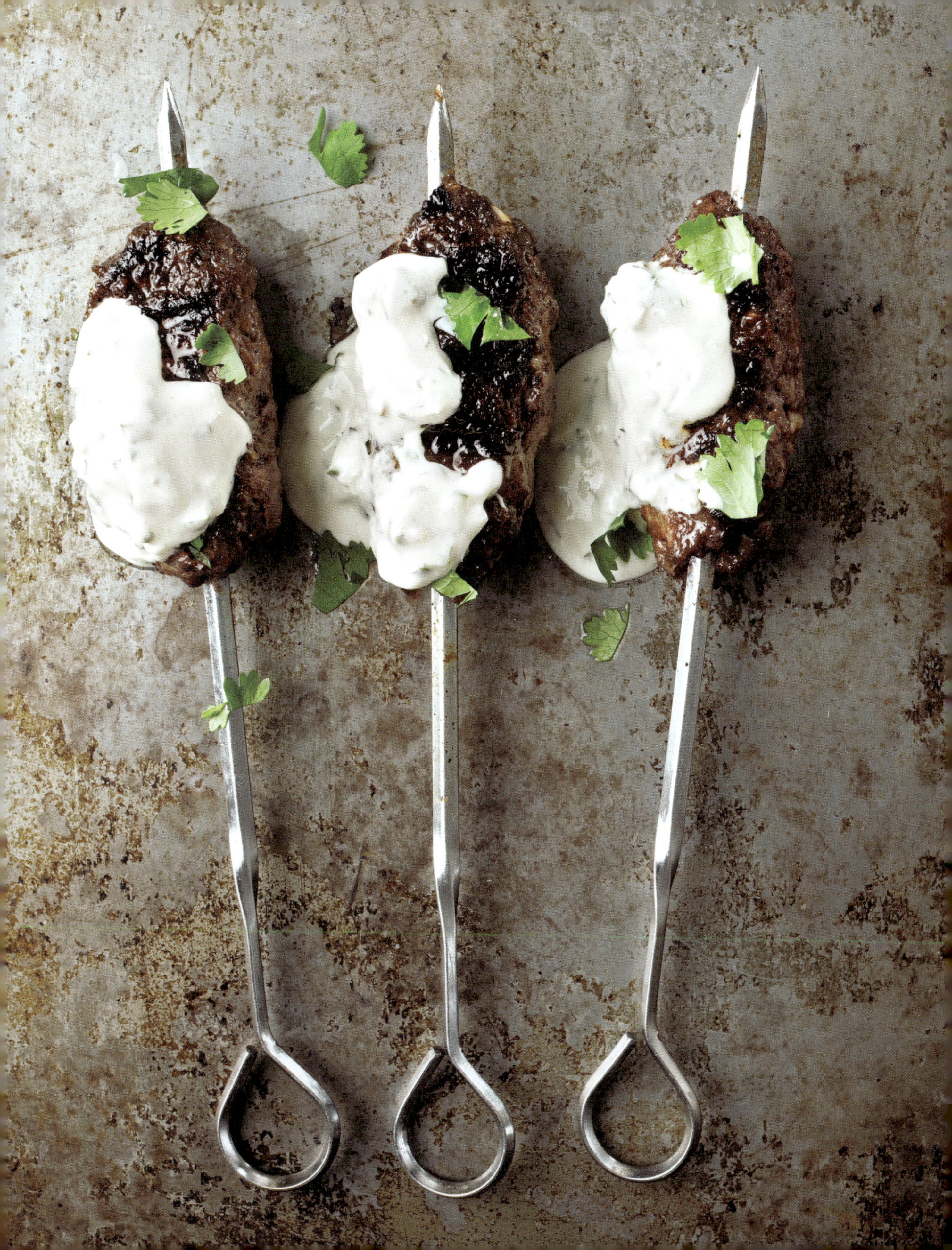

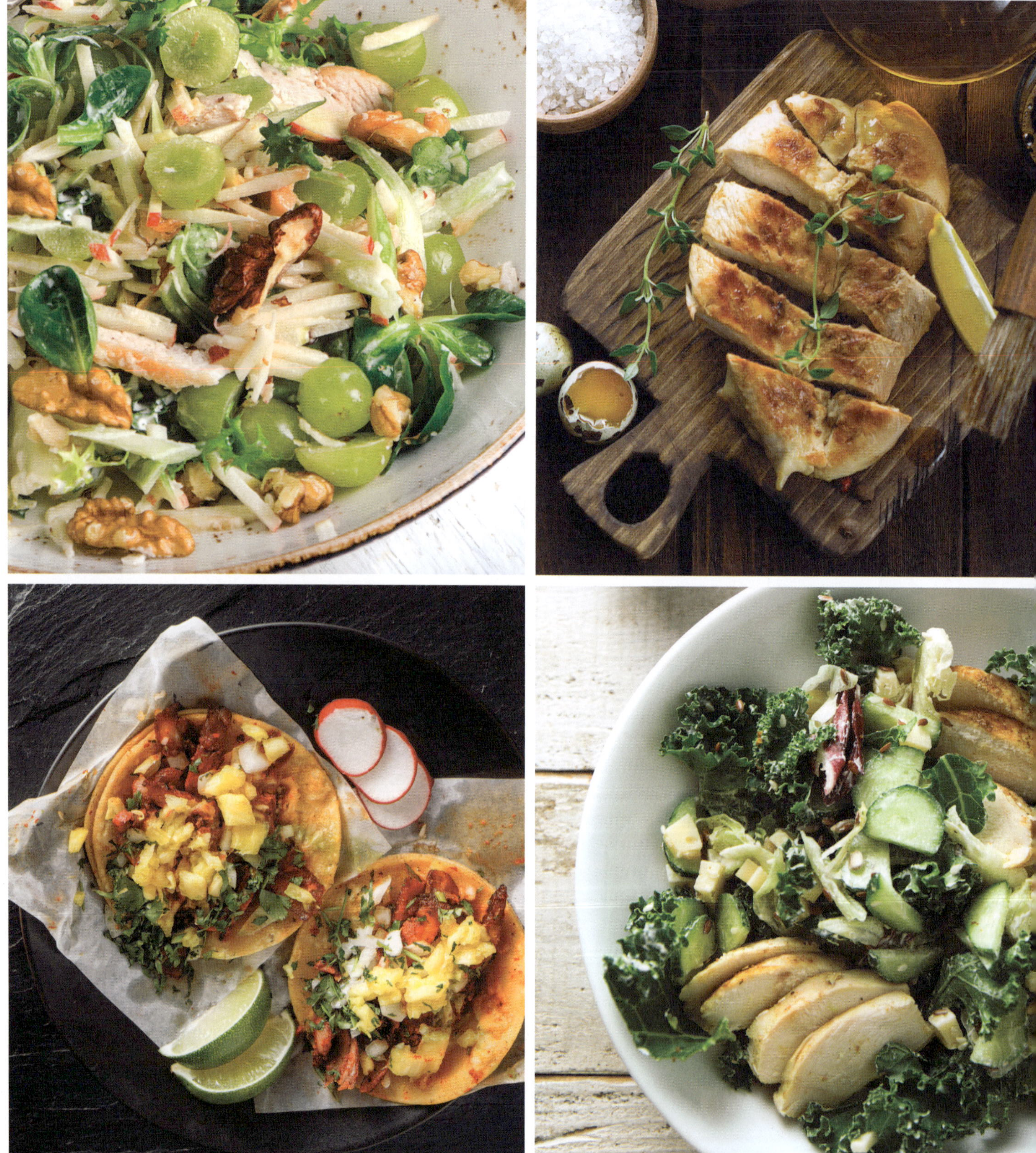

Chicken Waldorf Salad

500g chicken breast

Olive oil cooking spray

Salt and pepper

6 tbsps Greek yoghurt

1 tbsp lemon juice

200g mixed salad leaves

¼ cup (30g) walnut pieces

1 apple, julienned

2 stalks celery, chopped

1 spring onion, chopped

Place chicken breasts in air fryer. Spray with cooking spray. Season with salt and pepper. Cook for 7 minutes at 190°C. Flip over, spray once more and cook for a further 7 minutes until cooked through. Set aside to rest.

Place yoghurt and lemon juice in a bowl. Stir to combine.

Place remaining ingredients in a serving bowl. Slice chicken and add to bowl along with yoghurt dressing. Toss to combine and serve immediately.

SERVES 2

Lemon Chicken Breasts

2 chicken breasts, boneless and skinless

2 tsps olive oil

Juice of ½ lemon

½ tsp salt

¼ tsp pepper

Brush chicken with olive oil, squeeze over lemon juice and season with salt and pepper on both sides.

Place the chicken breasts in a single layer in the air fryer basket.

Cook at 200°C for 12-16 minutes, depending on the size of the chicken breast, until juices run clear and internal temperature reaches 74°C.

Remove from air fryer and transfer to a cutting board. Allow to rest for 2-3 minutes before cutting or serving.

SERVES 2

Bacon and Pineapple Tacos

4 corn tortillas, warmed through

8 rashers middle bacon

2 tbsps sweet chilli sauce

¼ small pineapple, coarsely chopped

¼ cup (60g) shop bought tomato salsa

½ cup (20g) coriander, coarsely chopped

½ red onion, finely chopped

Lime wedges, to garnish

Preheat air fryer to 200°C.

Lay bacon in the air fryer basket in a single layer overlapping slightly.

Cook for 8 minutes. Flip and continue cooking for about 6 minutes until bacon is just crisp. Brush both sides of bacon with sweet chilli sauce. Cook for 2 minutes more.

Serve tortillas filled with bacon, pineapple, tomato salsa, coriander and onion and garnished with lime wedges.

SERVES 4

Kale and Chicken Salad

500g chicken breast

Olive oil cooking spray

Salt and pepper

¼ cup (60ml) olive oil

1½ tbsps red or white wine vinegar

1 tbsp wholegrain mustard

1 tbsp honey

150g kale, washed and roughly torn

1 cucumber, sliced

1 avocado, diced

¼ cup (25g) red cabbage, chopped

½ bulb fennel, sliced

Place chicken breasts in air fryer. Spray with cooking spray. Season with salt and pepper. Cook for 14 minutes at 190°C, turning and spraying halfway through. Rest.

Whisk together olive oil, vinegar, mustard and honey.

Slice chicken and arrange with remaining ingredients in serving bowls. Drizzle with dressing and toss to coat.

SERVES 2

Turmeric Fish Burger

4 tbsps plain flour

1 tsp ground turmeric

1 lemon, zested

Pinch of chilli flakes

Salt and pepper to taste

4 firm white fish fillets

Olive oil cooking spray

4 brioche buns, halved and toasted

4 tbsps mayonnaise

Handful of rocket leaves

1 large beef tomato, sliced

½ white onion, thinly sliced

½ red chilli, deseeded and sliced

Coriander leaves and micro greens, to serve

Preheat air fryer to 200°C.

Mix the flour, turmeric, lemon zest and chilli flakes on a large plate and season well with salt and pepper. Coat each piece of fish in the seasoned flour.

Spray air fryer basket with cooking spray. Arrange fish fillets in basket and spray each one with cooking spray.

Cook for 4 minutes, then flip and spray once more. Cook for a further 4-6 minutes until fish is cooked through.

Spread brioche bun bases with mayonnaise, then add rocket leaves and slices of tomato and top each with a fish fillet. Sprinkle with sliced onion, chilli, coriander and micro greens. Place the brioche bun tops on to serve.

SERVES 4

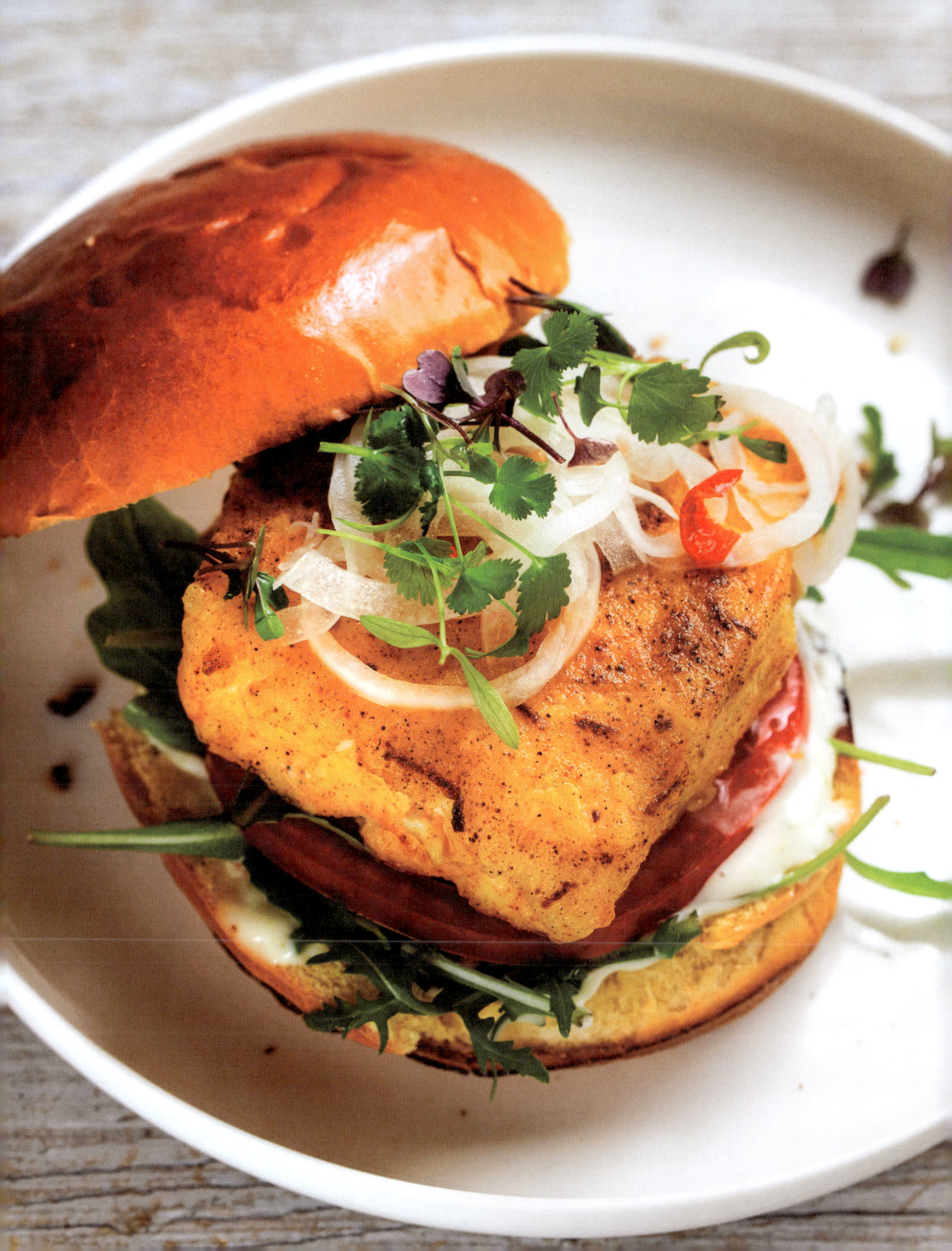

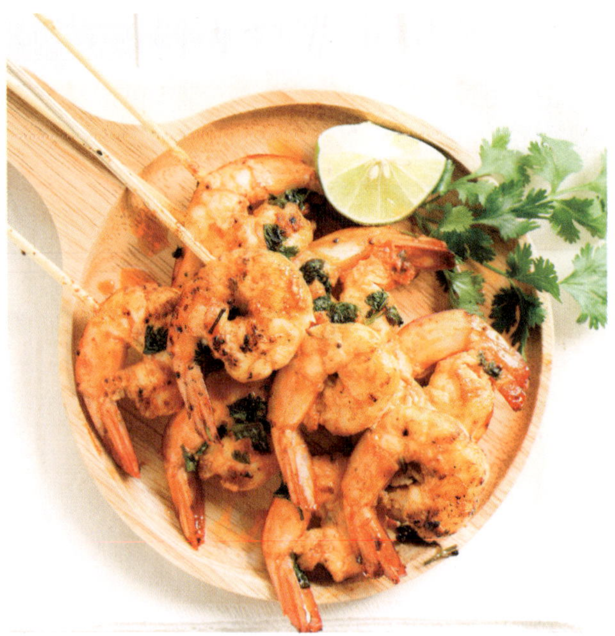

Garlic Prawn Kebabs

500g raw prawns, peeled and deveined

¼ tsp garlic powder

½ chilli, finely chopped

1 tbsp avocado or olive oil

2 tbsps fresh coriander, chopped

Salt and pepper to taste

Juice of 1 lime

Skewers

Place the prawns in a large bowl with garlic, chilli, oil and coriander. Season with salt and pepper and toss to coat.

Thread the prawns onto skewers and arrange in air fryer basket.

Cook for 10-14 minutes at 200°C until just pink.

Squeeze over lime juice to serve.

SERVES 2

Lemon Butter Lobster Tails

2 x 125g lobster tails

4 tbsps butter

1 tsp lemon zest

1 clove garlic, minced

Salt and pepper to taste

Lemon wedges, to serve

Use kitchen scissors to cut lengthways through hard top lobster shells. Cut flesh in half and spread apart.

Melt butter in a small saucepan over medium heat. Add lemon zest and garlic and cook for 30 seconds until fragrant.

Pour half of the melted butter into a bowl and set aside.

Brush lobster tails with remaining lemon garlic butter. Season well with salt and pepper.

Cook lobster tails in air fryer at 195°C for 5-7 minutes until lobster meat is opaque.

Spoon reserved butter over lobster meat. Serve with lemon wedges.

SERVES 1

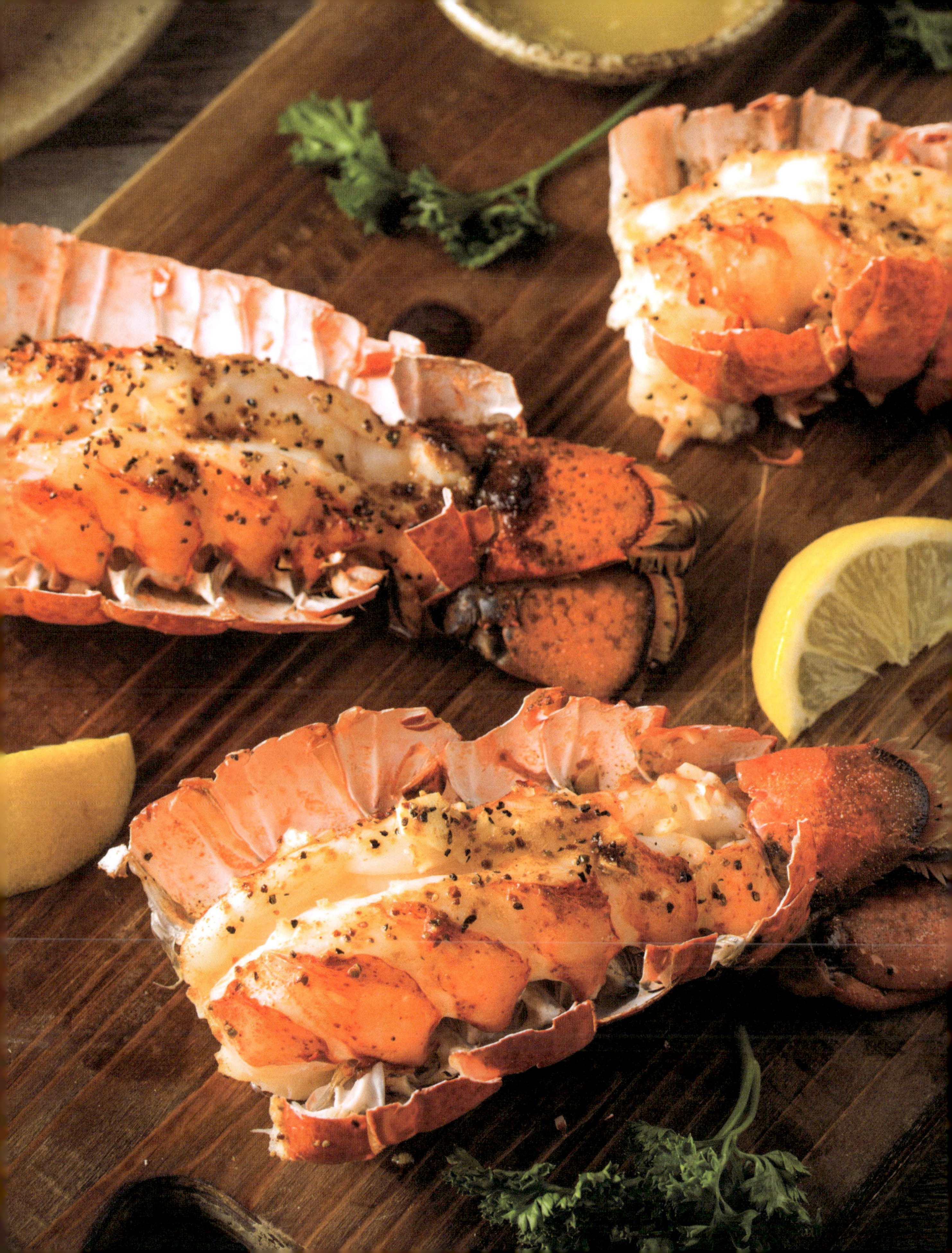

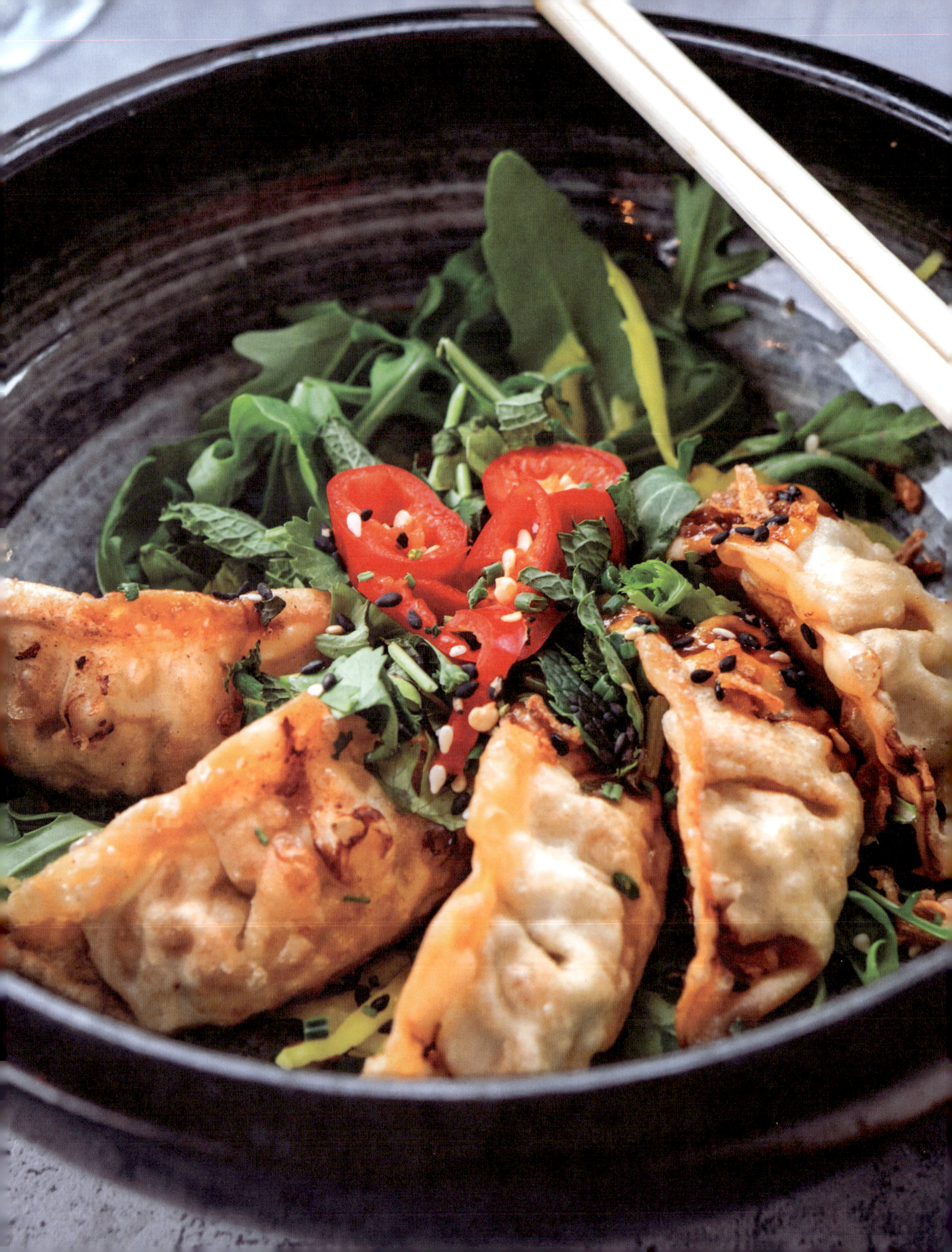

Homemade Gyoza

2 cups (200g) Chinese cabbage (wombok), finely chopped
250g pork mince
Medium piece ginger, grated
2 cloves garlic, minced
2 spring onions, finely chopped
1 tsp cornflour
1 tsp rice wine vinegar
1 tsp soy sauce
1 tsp sesame oil
Salt and pepper to taste
30 dumpling or wonton wrappers
Cooking spray

DIPPING SAUCE

2 tbsps rice wine vinegar
2 tbsps soy sauce

TO SERVE

Mixed salad leaves, sliced red chillies, chopped mint, chopped chives, black and white sesame seeds

Place cabbage in a saucepan of boiling water and cook for 1-2 minutes until soft. Drain well then use a clean tea towel to pat dry. Set aside to cool.

Place pork mince in a large bowl with ginger, garlic, spring onions, cornflour, rice wine vinegar, soy sauce and sesame oil. Season with salt and pepper. Add the cooled cabbage and use your hands to mix well.

Place a dumpling wrapper on a flat work surface. Spoon about 1 tablespoon of filling into centre of wrapper. Lightly moisten edges of wrapper with water. Fold wrapper over to make a half-moon shape, pressing edges to seal. Repeat process with remaining wrappers and filling.

Spray air fryer basket with cooking spray. Place six dumplings in basket, leaving room between each. Spray dumplings with cooking spray. Cook at 190°C for 12 minutes until lightly browned. Repeat with remaining dumplings.

Meanwhile, stir together rice wine vinegar and soy sauce to make dipping sauce.

Serve dumplings on a bed of salad leaves. Top with chillies, mint, chives and sesame seeds. Serve with dipping sauce.

SERVES 5

Teriyaki Salmon

2 skin-on salmon fillets

Salt and pepper to taste

1 tbsp soy sauce

1 tsp soft brown sugar

1 tsp rice wine vinegar

¼ tsp cornflour

Small piece ginger, grated

1 spring onion, thinly sliced

1 tsp sesame seeds

Cooked white rice, to serve

Season salmon fillets salt and pepper.

Combine soy sauce, sugar, vinegar, cornflour and ginger in a bowl. Brush over salmon on all sides.

Arrange the salmon skin-side down in air fryer basket.

Cook at 190°C for 6-8 minutes until salmon is cooked through. Top with spring onion and sesame seeds and serve with rice.

SERVES 2

Baked Trout with Lemon and Herbs

1 whole trout, deboned

Salt and pepper to taste

1 lemon, sliced

3-4 sprigs fresh dill

3-4 sprigs fresh parsley

1 tbsp olive oil

Season the inside of the trout with salt and pepper.

Arrange half the lemon slices in a single layer inside the fish and top with the herbs. Drizzle the outside of the fish with olive oil. Rub all over the skin.

Place trout in air fryer basket. Lay the remaining lemon slices on top of the skin.

Cook for 15 minutes at 170°C or until the flesh flakes easily with a fork.

SERVES 2

Fish Cutlets

400g skinless white fish fillet

1 tbsp capers, rinsed

1 tbsp parsley, chopped

Zest of 1 lemon

2 tbsps plain flour

Salt and pepper to taste

Olive oil cooking spray

Finely chop the fish or place in a food processor and pulse until chopped but still chunky.

Add capers, parsley, lemon zest, flour and seasoning. Squeeze the mixture well in your hands to drain any excess liquid, then shape into three cutlets. Refrigerate for 30 minutes.

Preheat air fryer to 180°C.

Spray cutlets and air fryer basket with cooking spray. Place cutlets in air fryer. Cooking for 8-10 minutes, until cooked through, turning halfway.

SERVES 3

Sesame Salmon

4 skin-on salmon fillets

Salt and pepper to taste

2 tsps soy sauce

1 tbsp honey

2 tsps black and white sesame seeds

Preheat the air fryer to 190°C.

Season each salmon fillet with salt and pepper then brush with soy sauce.

Place the fillets skin-side down into the air fryer basket and cook for 6 minutes.

Brush each salmon fillet with honey and sprinkle with sesame seeds.

Return salmon to air fryer and cook for a further 2 minutes until salmon is opaque and the flesh flakes off easily with a fork.

SERVES 4

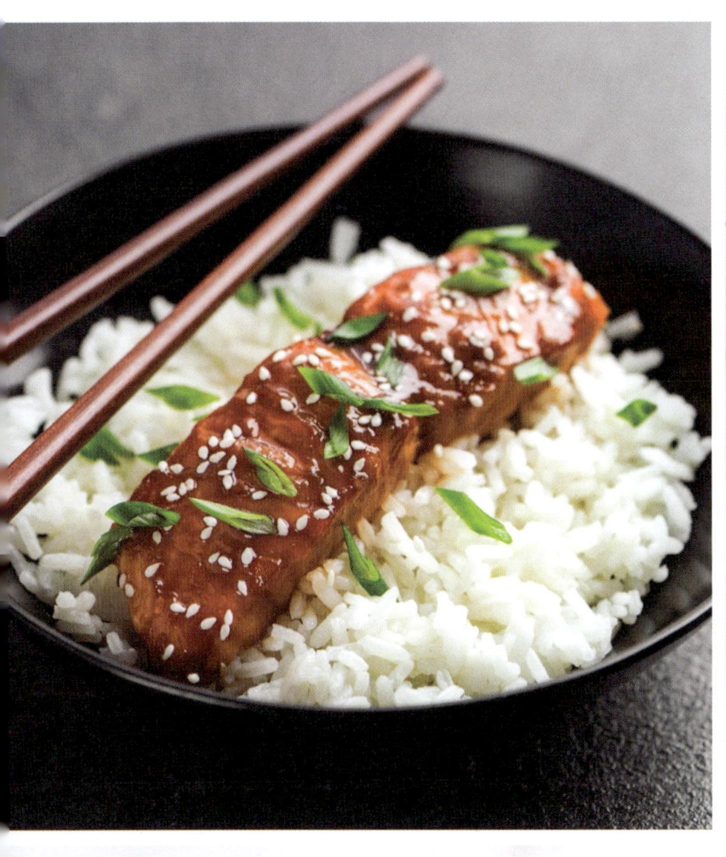
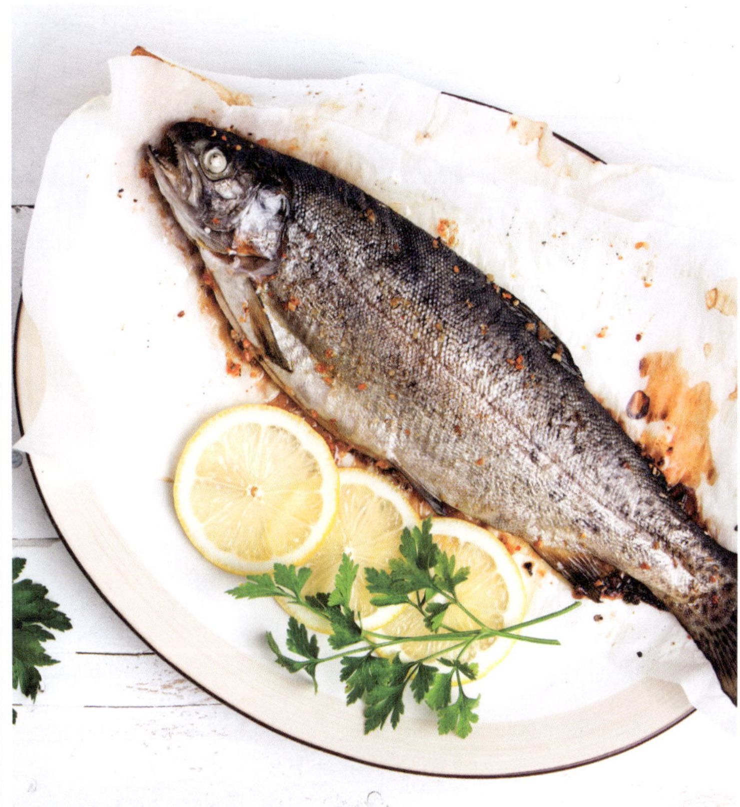
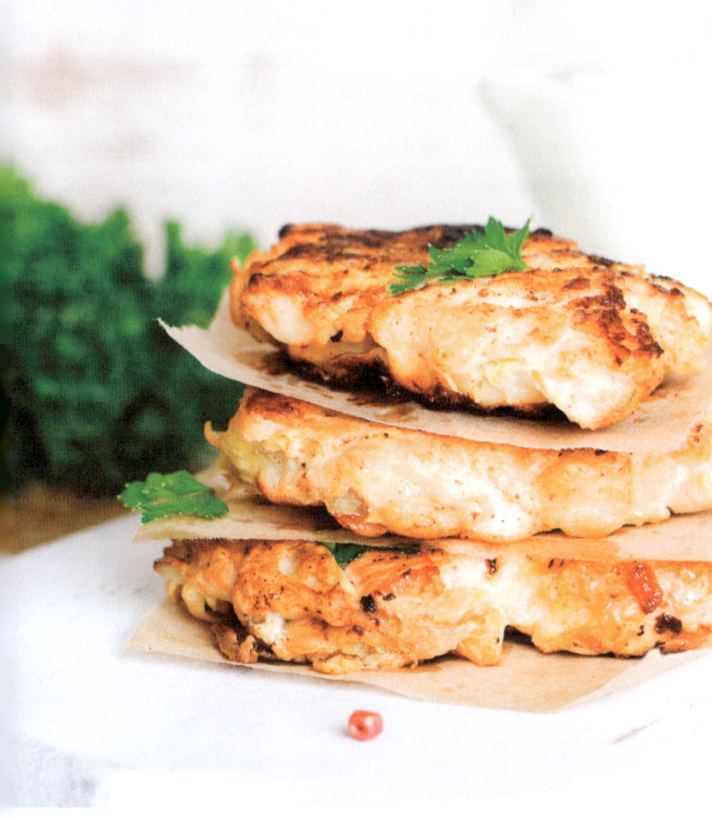
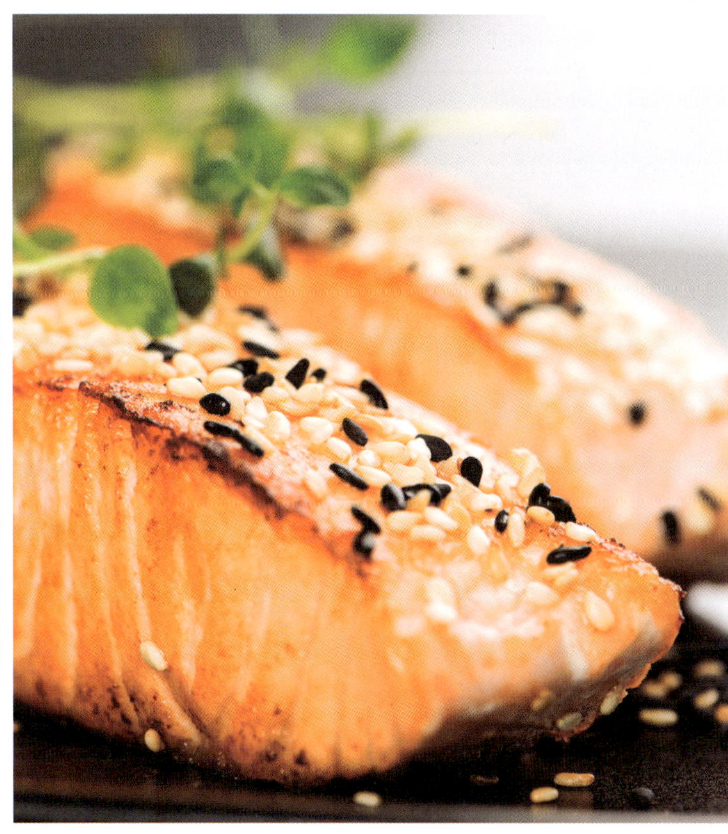

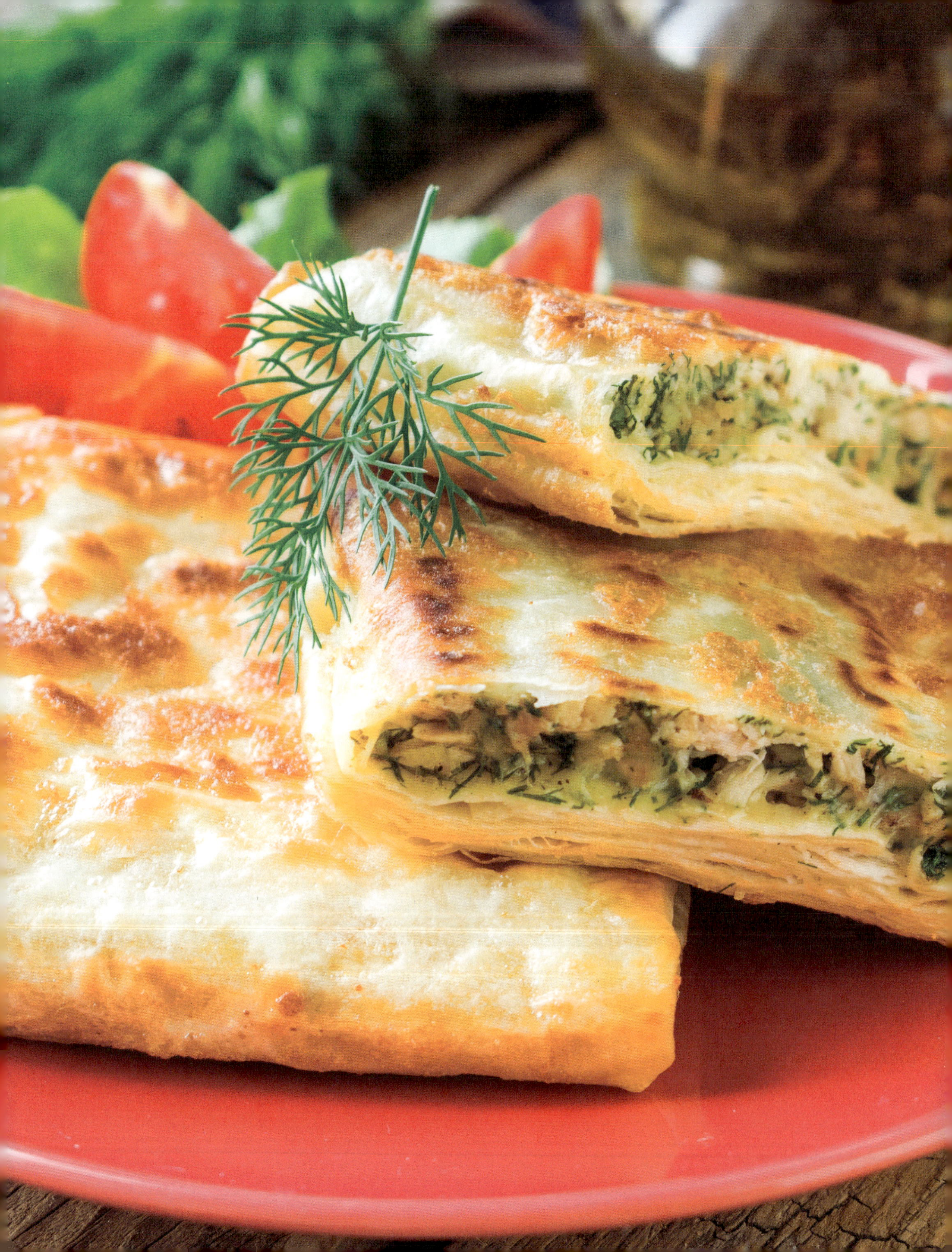

Chicken and Cheese Filo Parcels

350g cooked chicken, diced

1 cup (125g) Cheddar cheese, grated

2 tbsps fresh dill, chopped

Salt and pepper to taste

85g butter, melted

1 clove garlic, minced

12 sheets filo pastry

Place diced chicken, grated cheese and dill in a large bowl. Season with salt and pepper and toss well to combine.

In another small bowl, mix together melted butter and garlic.

Cut the sheets of filo pastry in half lengthways. Place one half sheet on a work surface with a short edge facing you. Brush evenly with butter mixture. take another half sheet and place on top, brush with butter mixture. Repeat with one more half sheet. (Keep the remaining sheets covered with a tea towel or plastic wrap to avoid them drying out.)

Spoon one-quarter of the chicken and cheese mixture onto the short end of the buttered filo pastry. Roll up into a rectangular parcel, tucking in the edges as you roll. Brush once more with garlic butter.

Repeat with remaining pastry and filling.

Place the filo parcels in air fryer basket. Cook at 170°C for 18 20 minutes or until pastry is golden brown.

SERVES 4

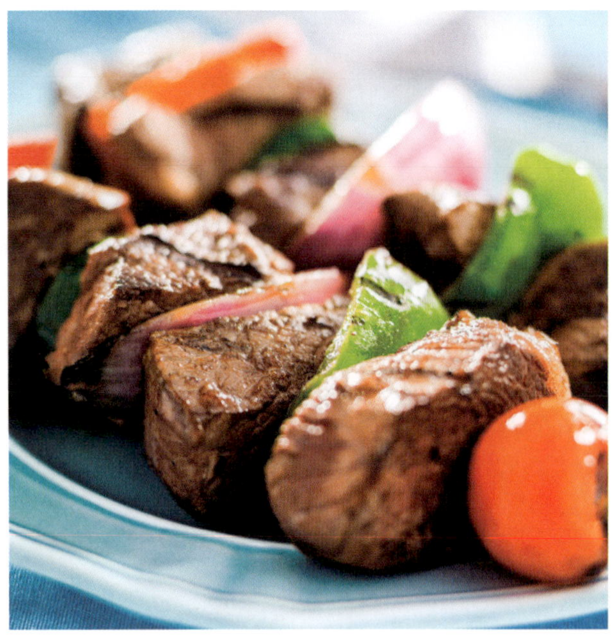

Steak Kebabs

¼ cup (60ml) olive oil

¼ cup (60ml) tamari

3 cloves garlic, minced

1 tsp brown sugar

½ tsp ground cumin

½ tsp salt

¼ tsp pepper

500g sirloin steak, cut into 3cm chunks

1 red onion, chopped into 3cm pieces

1 green capsicum, chopped into 3cm pieces

½ cup (110g) cherry tomatoes

Skewers

Combine olive oil, tamari, garlic, sugar, cumin, salt and pepper in a large bowl. Add steak and toss to coat well.

Cover bowl and refrigerate for at least 1 hour or overnight.

Add onion, capsicum and tomatoes to the bowl and toss to coat with marinade. Thread meat and vegetables onto skewers.

Preheat air fryer to 200°C.

Place skewers inside air fryer, taking care not to overcrowd basket. Cook in batches or use a double layer accessory if necessary. Cook for 5 minutes then flip the skewers and cook for a further 5-6 minutes until cooked to your liking.

SERVES 4

Fish with Coriander Pesto

4 white fish fillets

1 tbsp olive oil

1 tsp paprika

Salt and pepper to taste

⅓ cup (40g) raw cashews

½ red chilli, chopped

2 cups (90g) firmly packed fresh coriander leaves

1 clove garlic, quartered

Juice and zest of 1 lime

2 tbsps olive oil

Preheat air fryer to 180°C.

Brush fish fillets with oil and season with paprika, salt and pepper. Place in air fryer basket and cook for 8 minutes, until fish is soft and opaque.

Meanwhile place remaining ingredients in a food processor and pulse until smooth.

Spoon pesto onto fish to serve.

SERVES 4

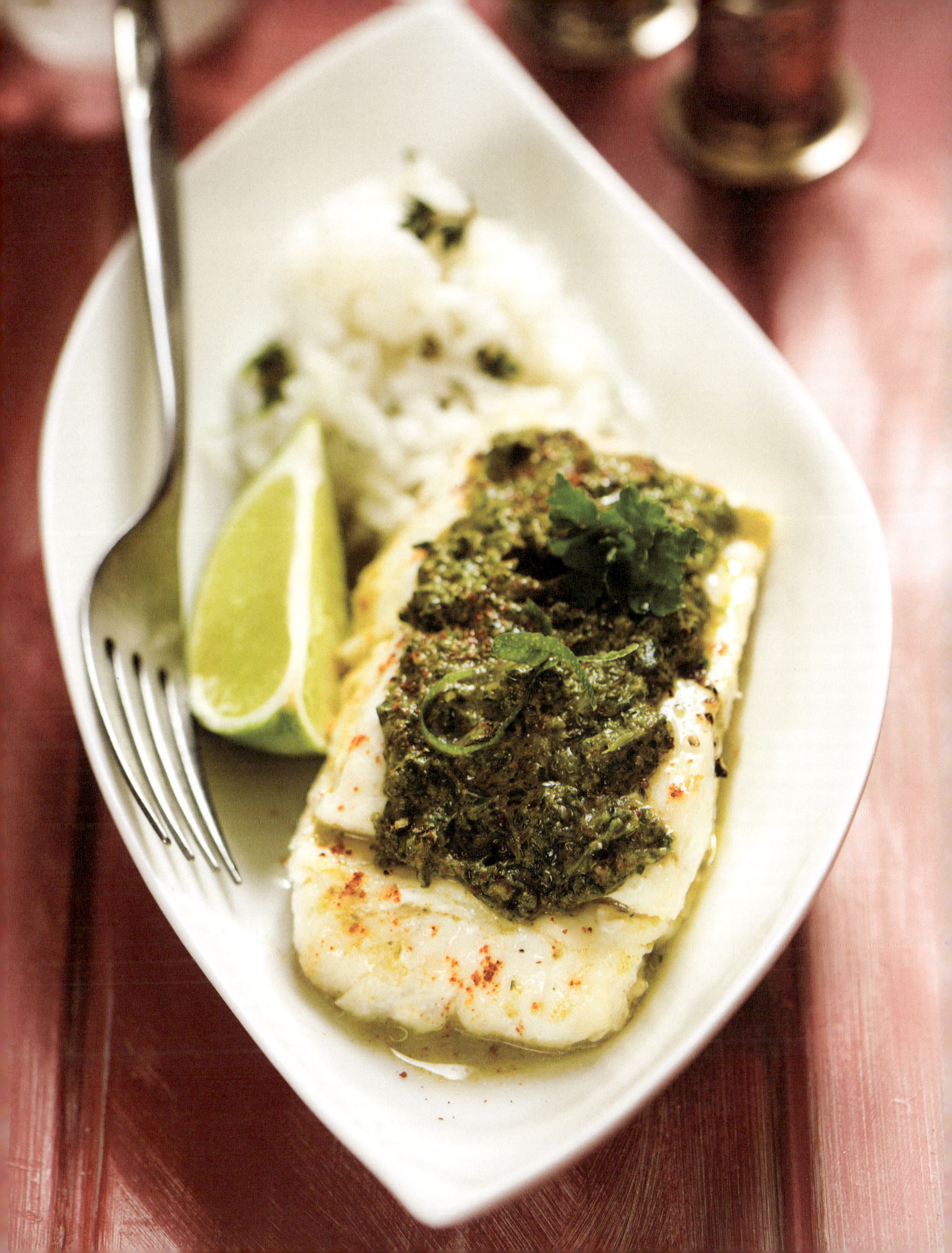

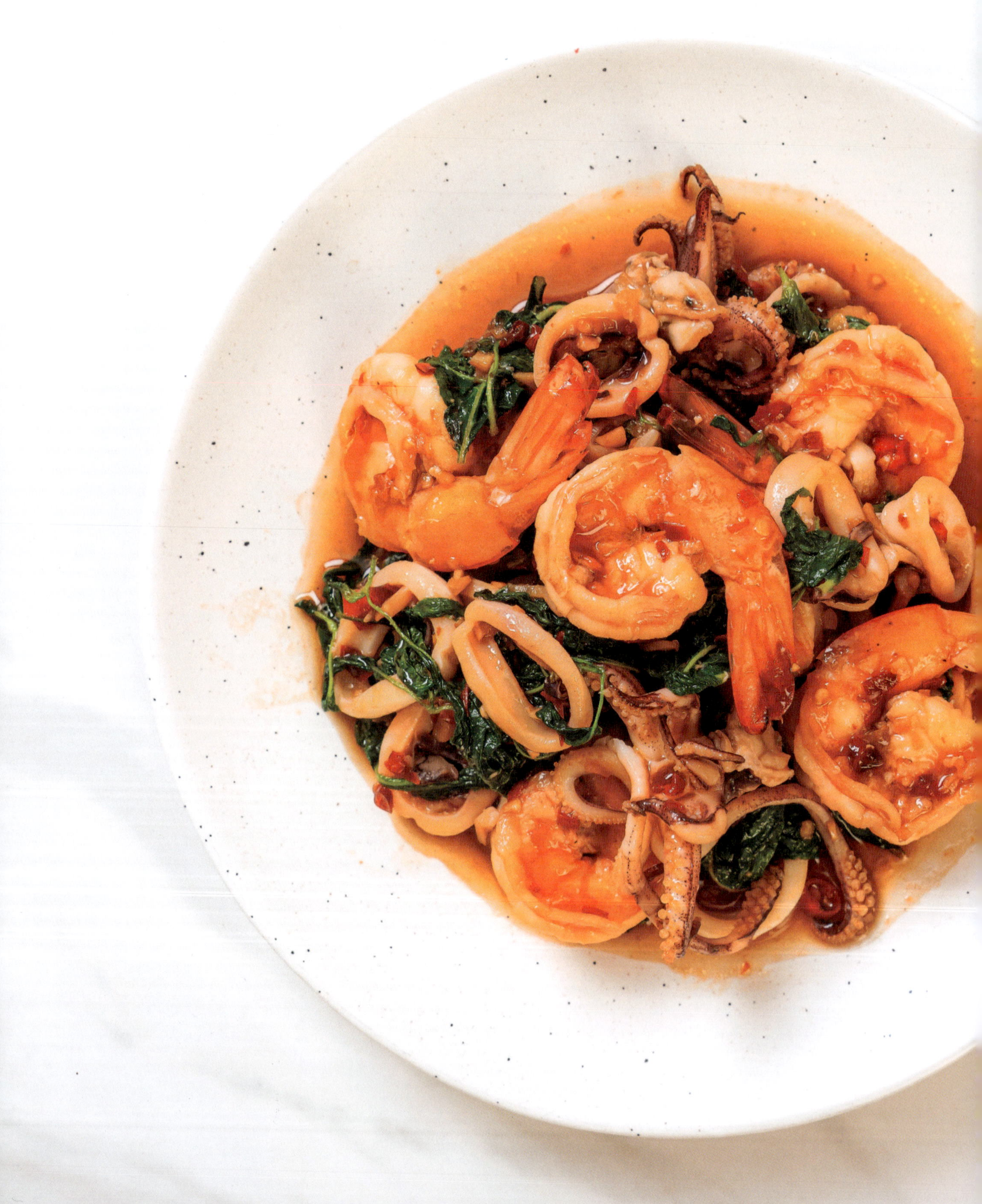

Thai Seafood Stir-Fry

3 tbsps Thai chilli paste (nam prik pao)

1½ tbsps soy sauce

1½ tbsps fish sauce

1 tsp brown sugar

1 tbsp water

2 tbsps peanut or avocado oil

500g prawns, shelled and deveined

500g squid, cleaned and cut into tentacles and rings

4 cloves garlic, minced

Small piece ginger, chopped

1 small chilli, chopped

1 cup (15g) Thai basil

Baking pan

In a small bowl, mix together Thai chilli paste, soy sauce, fish sauce, brown sugar and water. Set aside.

Place oil and prawns in pan. Toss to coat then place pan in air fryer basket. Cook for 5 minutes at 175°C.

Add squid, garlic, ginger and chilli. Stir to combine, then cook for 3 minutes until squid is almost cooked.

Add reserved sauce and Thai basil. Stir to combine and cook for 1-2 more minutes until squid is just cooked and sauce is heated through. Take care not to overcook squid.

Spoon onto plates to serve.

SERVES 4

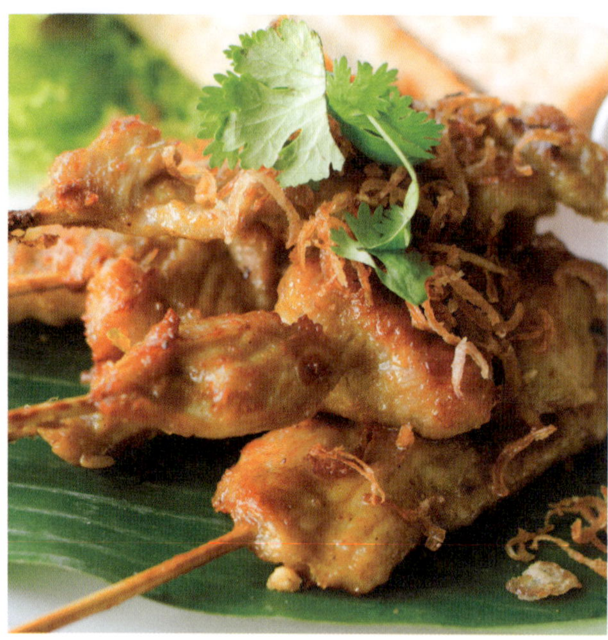

Satay Pork

2 cloves garlic, crushed

Small piece ginger, grated

1 tsp chilli paste

3 tbsps tamari

1 tbsp peanut butter

1 tbsp lime juice

1 tbsp brown sugar

400g pork, cut into 3cm cubes

Crispy shallots and fresh coriander, to serve

Skewers

Combine garlic, ginger, chilli paste, tamari, peanut butter, lime juice and sugar in a large bowl. Add the pork and toss well to coat. Refrigerate for at least 1 hour or overnight.

Preheat the air fryer to 200°C.

Thread meat onto skewers and place in air fryer basket. Cook for 12 minutes, turning once halfway through, until brown and cooked through.

Sprinkle with crispy shallots and fresh coriander to serve.

SERVES 2

Lime and Pepper Chicken

Juice and zest of 2 limes

3 tbsps olive oil

2 cloves garlic, minced

1 tsp salt

½ tsp pepper

⅛ tsp cayenne pepper

4 chicken breasts

Olive oil cooking spray

Combine lime juice, lime zest, olive oil, garlic, salt, pepper and cayenne pepper in a shallow dish.

Add chicken breasts and toss to coat. Cover and refrigerate for at least 1 hour, preferably overnight.

Preheat air fryer to 175°C. Spray air fryer basket with cooking spray.

Arrange chicken in air fryer. Cook for 15 minutes, flip and cook for a further 5-8 minutes until cooked through. Rest for 5 minutes before slicing.

SERVES 4

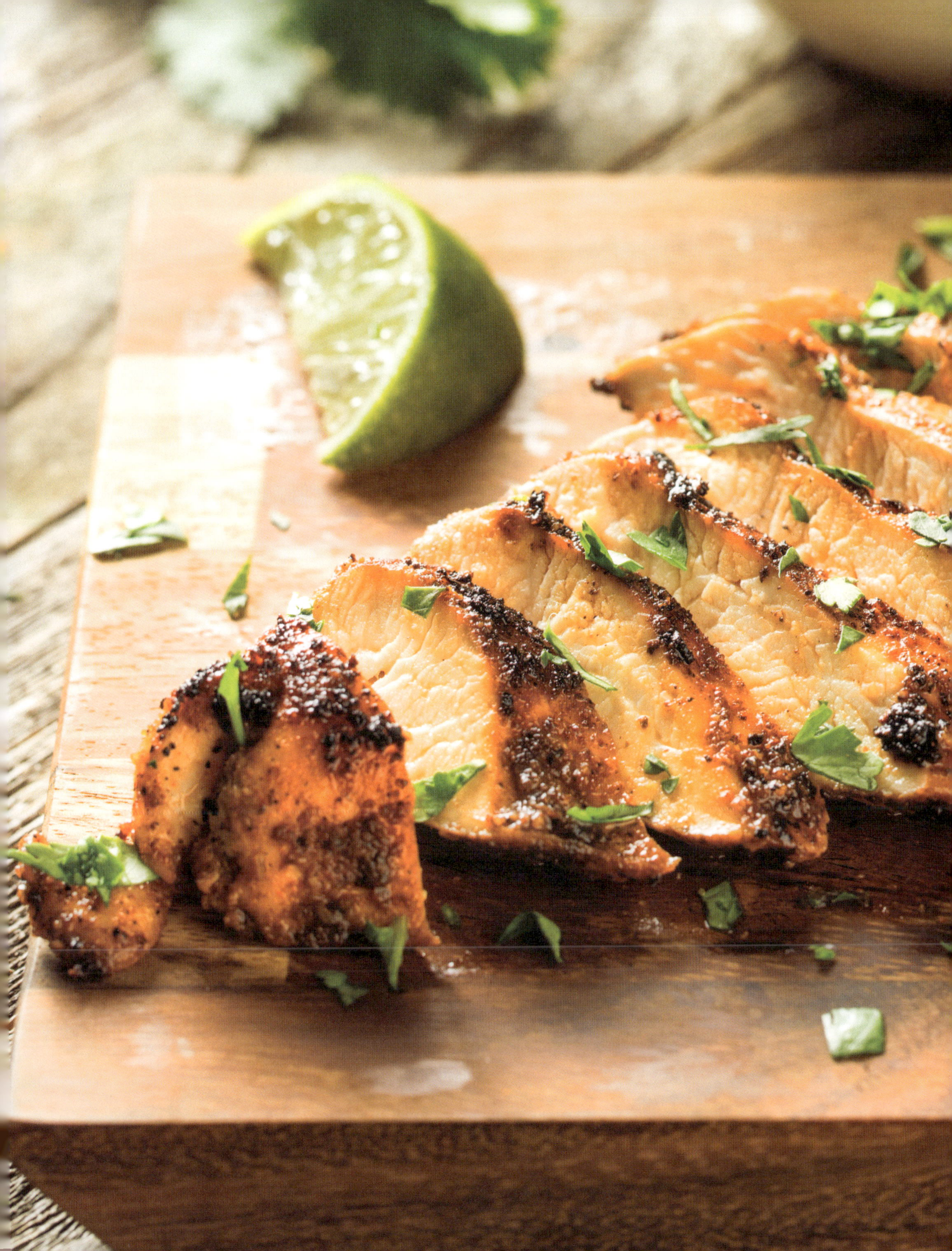

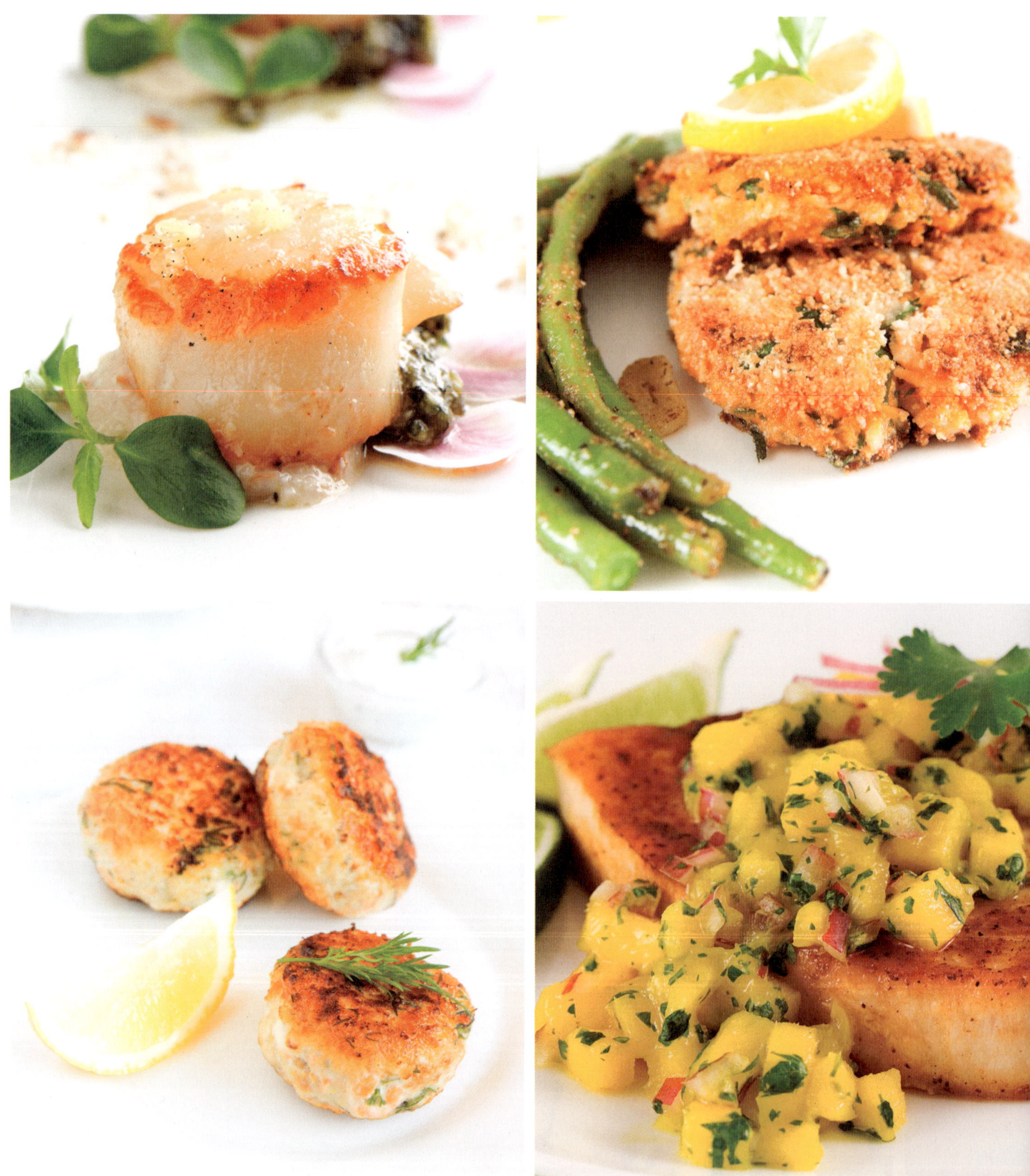

Seared Scallops

8 large scallops, cleaned and patted dry

¼ tsp salt

¼ tsp pepper

Olive oil cooking spray

Lime zest, to serve

Coriander pesto, to serve (see recipe on page 72)

Sprinkle scallops with salt and pepper.

Spray air fryer basket with cooking spray. Place scallops in the basket and spray with cooking spray.

Cook the scallops at 200°C for 6 minutes until opaque and just cooked through.

Grate over lime zest and serve with coriander pesto.

SERVES 2

Salmon and Sweet Potato Cakes

750g sweet potato, cut into 3cm pieces

2 x 180g pieces salmon, skin removed and pin-boned

100g baby spinach, finely chopped

2 cups (100g) breadcrumbs

2 eggs, beaten

Salt and pepper to taste

¼ cup (60ml) olive oil

Cook sweet potato in a saucepan of boiling water for 8 minutes, then place a steamer basket on top with the salmon. Cover and cook for 3-4 minutes until almost cooked. Remove from heat. Drain sweet potato and set aside to cool.

Flake fish into a bowl. Add sweet potato, spinach, half the breadcrumbs, half the egg, salt and pepper and combine.

Shape mixture into patties, then dip each patty into remaining egg, then remaining breadcrumbs.

Spray patties with cooking spray. Place in air fryer basket and cook for 12 minutes at 200°C until browned.

SERVES 4

Crab Cakes

250g crab meat

½ cup (60g) breadcrumbs

2 spring onions, chopped

1 tbsp fresh dill, chopped

1 egg

3 tbsps mayonnaise

2 tsps Dijon mustard

Juice of 1 lemon

Salt and pepper to taste

Olive oil cooking spray

In a large bowl break up the crab meat with a fork. Add breadcrumbs, spring onions, dill, egg, mayonnaise, mustard, lemon juice, salt and pepper. Stir well then use hands to form mixture into eight small or four large patties.

Spray air fryer baskets and crab cakes with cooking spray.

Cook crab cakes in air fryer for 10 minutes at 180°C until golden brown, turning halfway through.

SERVES 4

Swordfish with Mango Salsa

4 swordfish steaks

Salt and pepper to taste

Avocado oil cooking spray

MANGO SALSA

2 mangoes, diced

1 red onion, finely diced

1 jalapeno, finely chopped

½ cup (20g) fresh coriander, chopped

2 tbsps lime juice

Preheat air fryer to 200°C.

Season swordfish steaks with salt and pepper. Spray all over with avocado cooking spray.

Place steaks in air fryer basket and cook for 10-12 minutes, flipping halfway through.

Combine salsa ingredients in a bowl. Stir gently.

Spoon salsa over swordfish steaks to serve.

SERVES 4

Lemon Butter Barramundi with Potatoes and Asparagus

500g chat potatoes

1 tsp olive oil

¼ bunch thyme

Salt and pepper to taste

2 x 200g barramundi fillets

1 bunch asparagus

Olive oil cooking spray

LEMON BUTTER SAUCE

250g unsalted butter

1 clove garlic, chopped

10 black peppercorns

1 bay leaf

½ cup (125ml) white wine

½ cup (125ml) thickened cream

Juice of 1 lemon

Salt and pepper to taste

Preheat air fryer to 200°C.

Place potatoes in a bowl with oil, thyme and salt and pepper, toss to coat then place potatoes in air fryer and cook for 20 minutes.

Place fish fillets on top of par-cooked potatoes, spray with cooking spray and season with salt and pepper. Cook for 10-15 minutes until fish flakes away easily with a fork.

Remove fish and potatoes from air fryer. Cover and set aside to rest.

Add asparagus to basket. Spray with olive oil spray and season with salt and pepper. Cook for 7 minutes at 200°C.

Meanwhile melt 1 tablespoon of the butter in a large pan over medium-low heat. Add garlic, peppercorns and bay leaf. Cook for 30 seconds until fragrant. Add wine and simmer until reduced by three-quarters.

Reduce heat to low and add cream and remaining butter. Allow butter to melt then whisk to combine. Add lemon juice and season with salt and pepper.

Serve potatoes and asparagus in bowls. Top with fish and drizzle with sauce.

SERVES 2

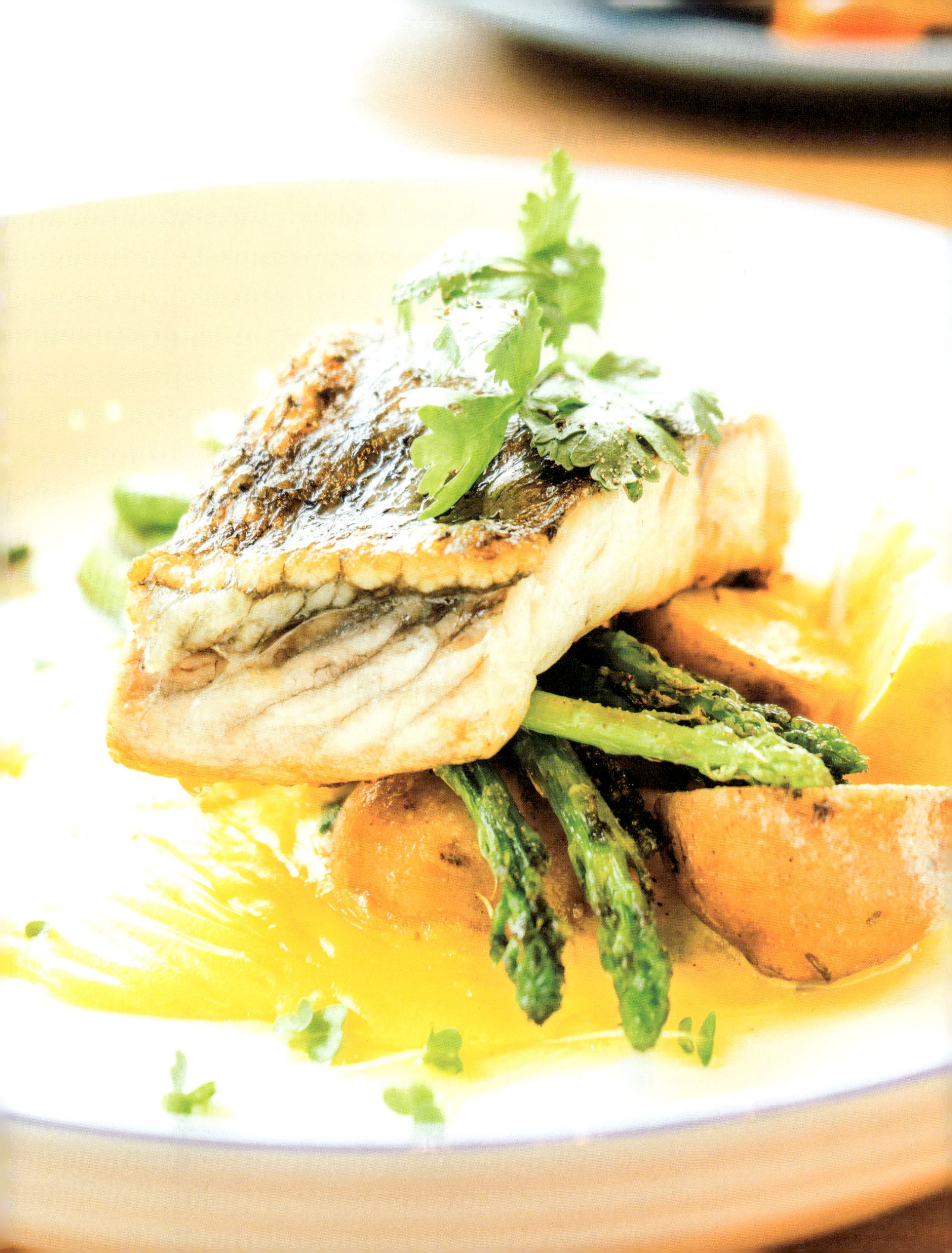

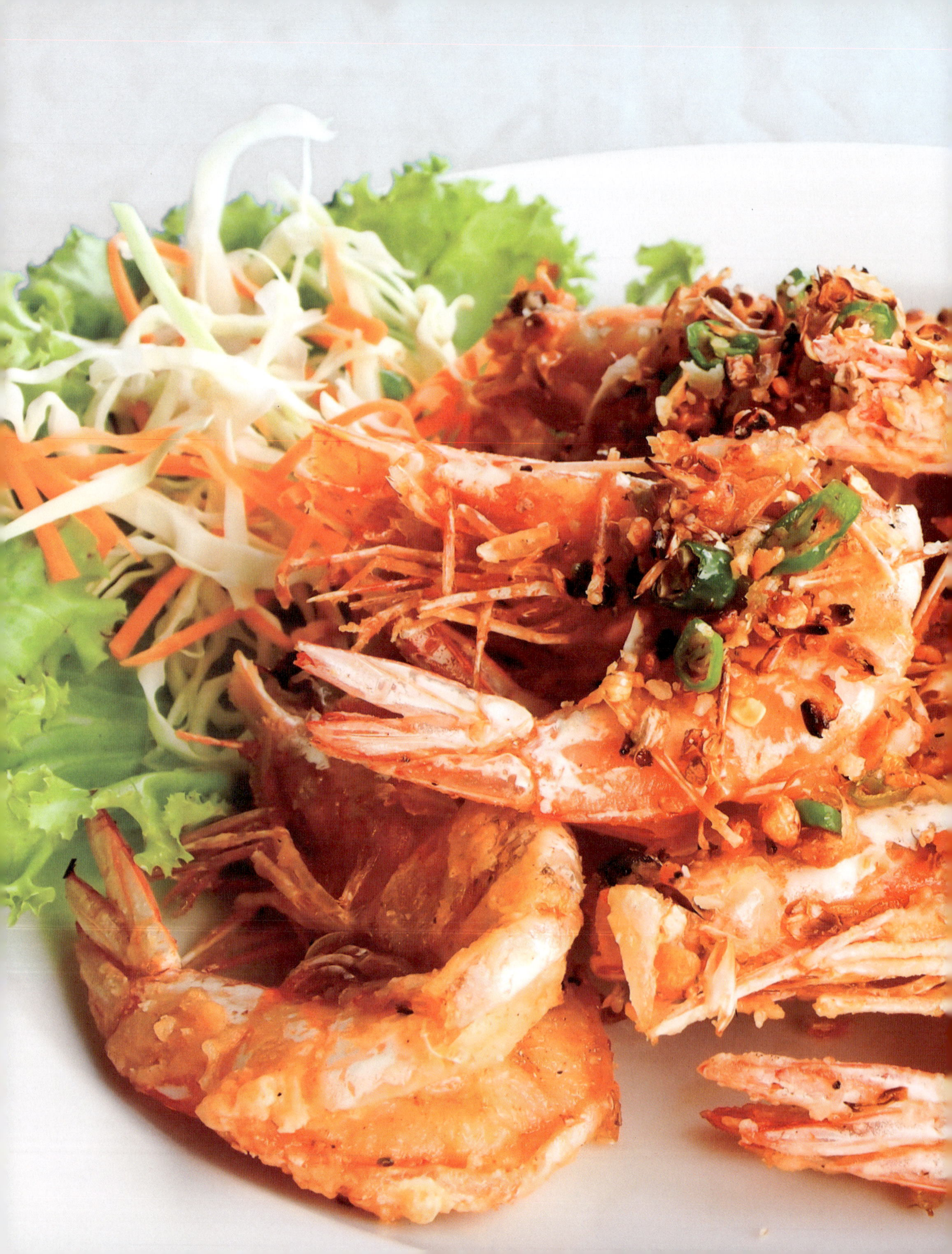

Salt and Pepper Prawns

½ tsp white pepper

½ tsp sugar

¼ tsp salt

2 tsps cornflour

500g shell-on prawns

1½ tsps + 1 tbsp peanut or other neutral oil

1 long red chilli, chopped

5 cloves garlic, chopped

1 spring onion, chopped

Preheat air fryer to 230°C.

In a medium bowl, stir together white pepper, sugar, salt and cornflour. Add prawns and rub in the seasonings. Drizzle on 1½ teaspoons oil and toss to coat.

Cook in air fryer for 2 minutes on each side.

Heat remaining oil in a frying pan over medium-high heat. Add chilli and garlic and cook for 30 seconds, until fragrant. Add prawns, toss to coat and cook for 1 minute. Sprinkle with spring onion to serve.

SERVES 2

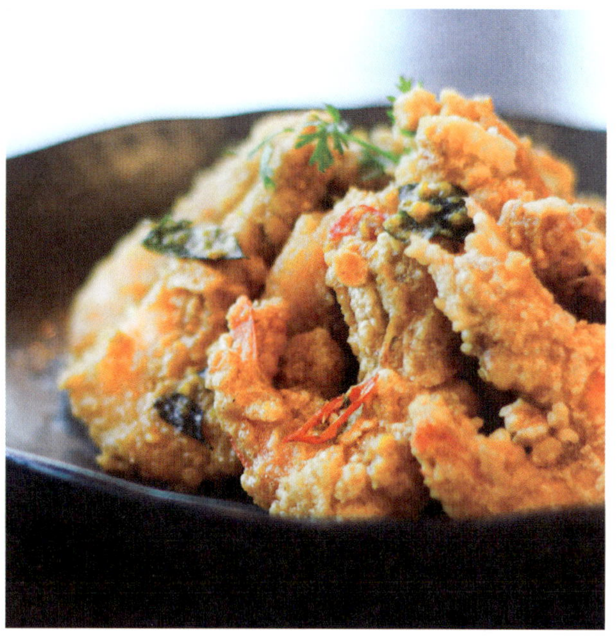

Coconut Prawns

½ cup (60g) plain flour

2 eggs, beaten

½ cup (45g) shredded coconut

¼ cup (30g) panko breadcrumbs

1 red chilli, chopped

1 tbsp coriander leaves, chopped

Salt and pepper to taste

500g raw prawns, peeled and deveined, tails intact

Avocado oil cooking spray

Preheat air fryer to 200°C.

Take three bowls. Place flour in one bowl, beaten egg in second bowl and combine coconut, breadcrumbs, chilli, coriander, salt and pepper in third bowl.

Dip each prawn first in flour, then egg, then coconut mixture, pressing gently to coat.

Spray prawns and air fryer basket with cooking spray.

Arrange prawns in basket and cook for 4 minutes, then flip, spray once more and cook for a further 5 minutes.

SERVES 2

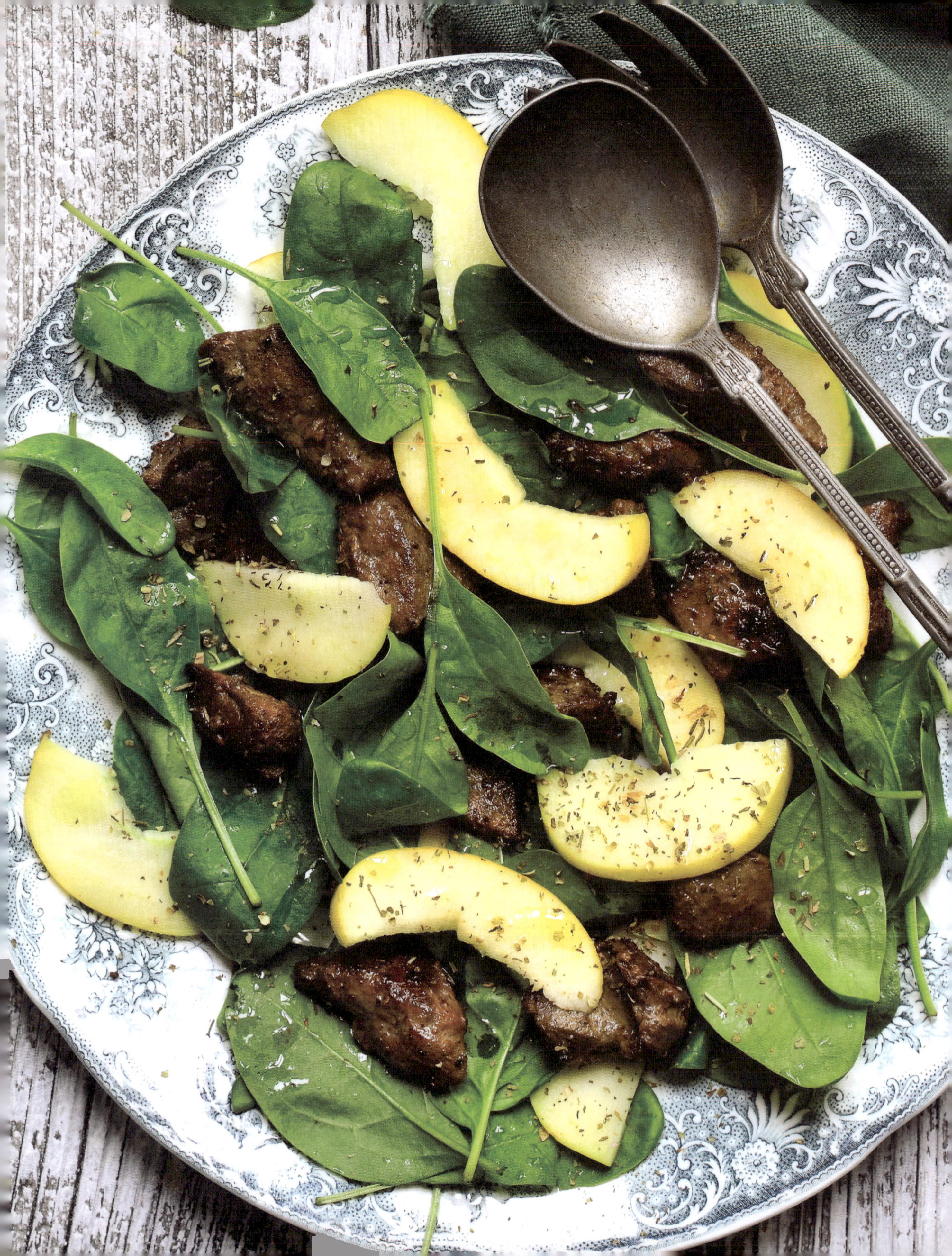

Paleo

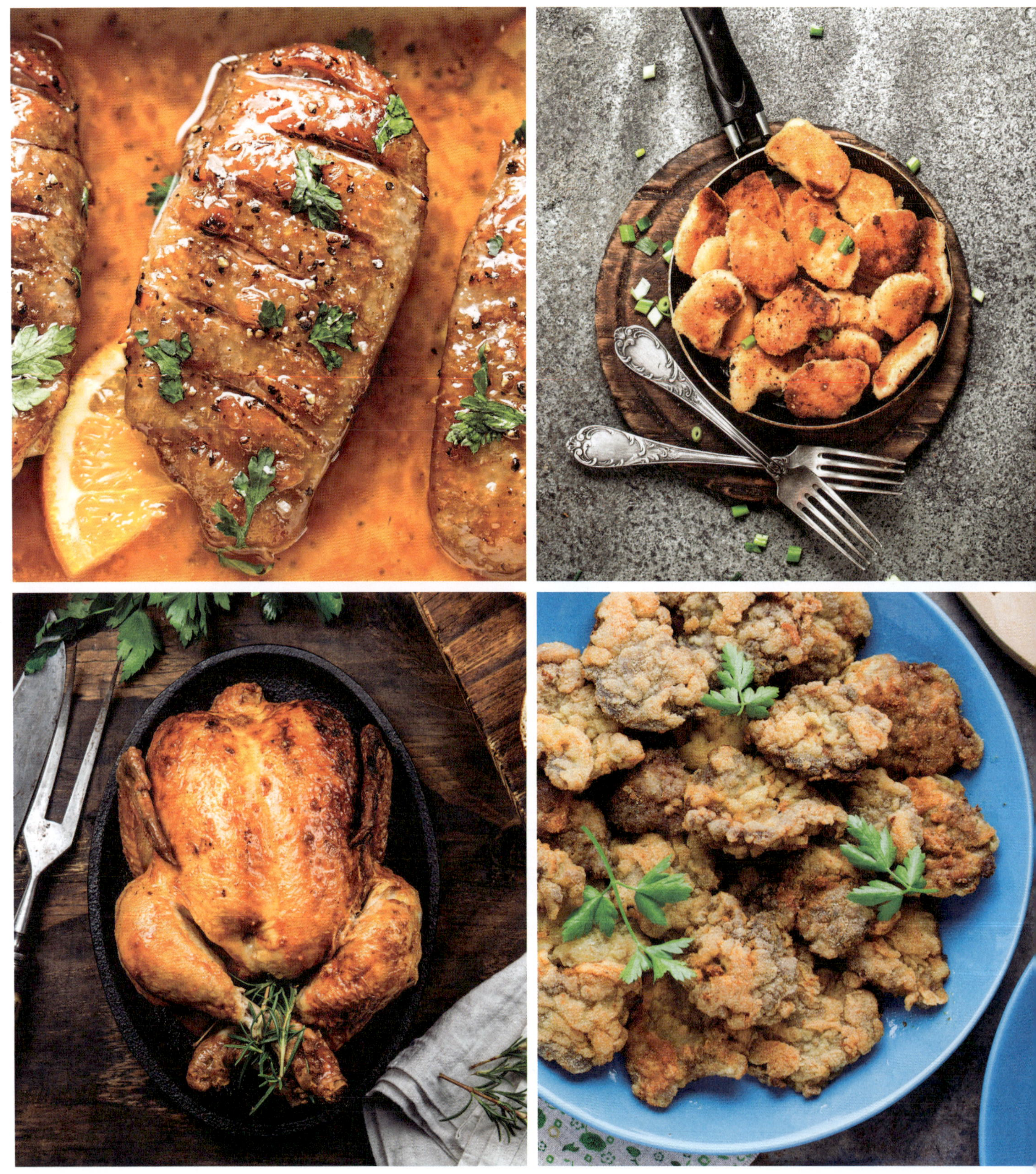

Duck with Orange Sauce

2 duck breasts, skin on

Salt and pepper to taste

⅓ cup (50g) brown sugar

1 tbsp sherry vinegar

Juice and zest of 1 orange

1 tbsp butter

½ cup (125ml) chicken stock

Preheat the air fryer to 200°C.

Score skin several times and rub with salt and pepper.

Place duck in basket skin-side up. Cook for 10 minutes. Flip over and cook for 6-8 minutes. Flip over once more and cook for 1 further minute to crisp skin. Set aside duck to rest.

Meanwhile place sugar, vinegar, orange juice, zest, butter and stock in a small saucepan over medium-high heat. Bring to boil, stirring frequently. Reduce heat to medium-low and gently boil for 10 minutes until thick and syrupy. Pour over duck to serve.

SERVES 2

Paleo Chicken Nuggets

¾ cup (90g) almond meal

¼ cup (35g) ground flaxseed

1 tsp garlic powder

Pinch of paprika

Salt and pepper to taste

2 eggs, beaten

500g chicken breast, cut into bite-sized nugget shapes

Avocado cooking spray

Preheat air fryer to 200°C.

Combine almond meal, flaxseed, garlic powder, paprika, salt and pepper in one bowl. Place beaten egg in another.

Dip chicken pieces first into egg then into almond meal, pressing gently to coat.

Spray air fryer basket and arrange chicken nuggets in one evenly spaced layer. Cook in batches if necessary.

Spray with avocado oil and cook for 10 minutes. Flip nuggets and cook for a further 10 minutes until cooked through.

SERVES 4

Whole Roast Chicken

1 x 1.3kg whole chicken

¼ cup (60ml) melted butter or olive oil

Juice of 1 lemon

4 cloves garlic, minced

Salt and pepper, to taste

2-3 sprigs fresh rosemary

Cooking spray

Preheat air fryer to 170°C.

Rub chicken all over with butter or oil, lemon juice and minced garlic. Season with salt and pepper. Stuff chicken cavity with rosemary. Spray air fryer basket with cooking spray.

Place the chicken in the basket with the legs down and roast for 30 minutes.

Carefully flip the chicken using tongs. Cook for a further 20 minutes, until juices run clear.

Allow to rest for 5 minutes before cutting or serving.

SERVES 4

Crispy Coated Chicken Livers

500g chicken livers

½ cup (125ml) coconut milk

⅓ cup (30g) coconut flour

2 tbsps arrowroot powder

2 tsps paprika

2 tsps garlic powder

½ tbsp ground cumin

2 tsps salt

½ tsp pepper

Cooking spray

Cut chicken livers into 5cm pieces. Place coconut milk in a shallow bowl. Add chicken livers; marinate for 10 minutes.

In a shallow bowl, mix coconut flour, arrowroot powder, spices and seasoning. Add chicken livers, and toss to coat.

Working in batches, spray livers with cooking spray and place in air fryer basket. Cook for 15-20 minutes at 200°C flipping halfway through cooking.

SERVES 4

Herb Spiced Pork Tenderloin

½ cup (125ml) melted butter

1 tbsp fresh rosemary, chopped

1 tbsp fresh thyme, chopped

1 tsp dried oregano

½ tsp chilli powder

3 cloves garlic, minced

Salt and pepper to taste

750g pork tenderloin

1 tbsp olive oil

Preheat air fryer to 200°C.

In a small bowl mix together melted butter with herbs, chilli powder, garlic, salt and pepper.

Brush pork tenderloin with butter herb mixture. Place in air fryer. Cook for 15 minutes.

Baste pork once more with butter mix and cook for an additional 5-10 minutes or until pork is cooked through.

Allow to rest for 5 minutes before slicing.

SERVES 4

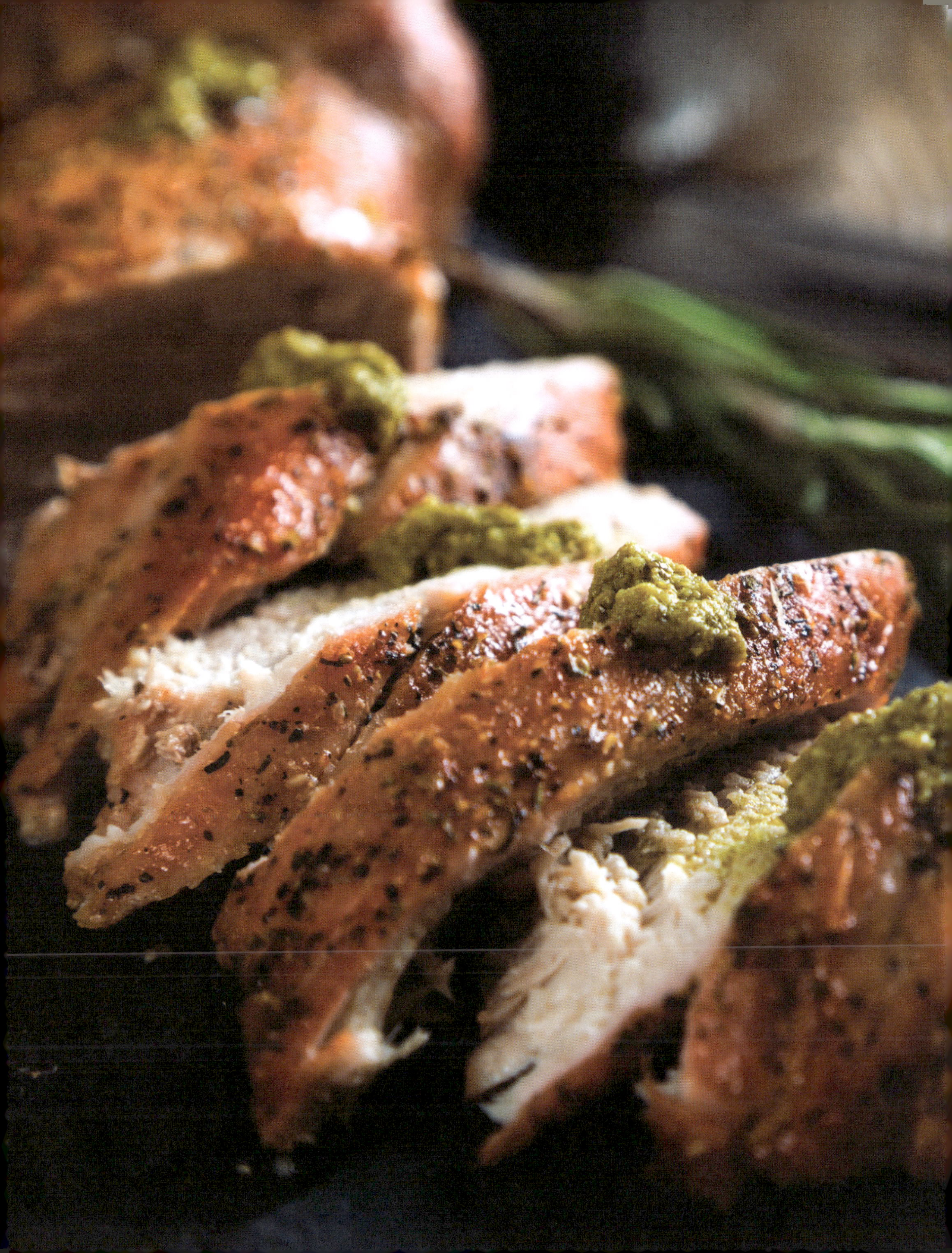

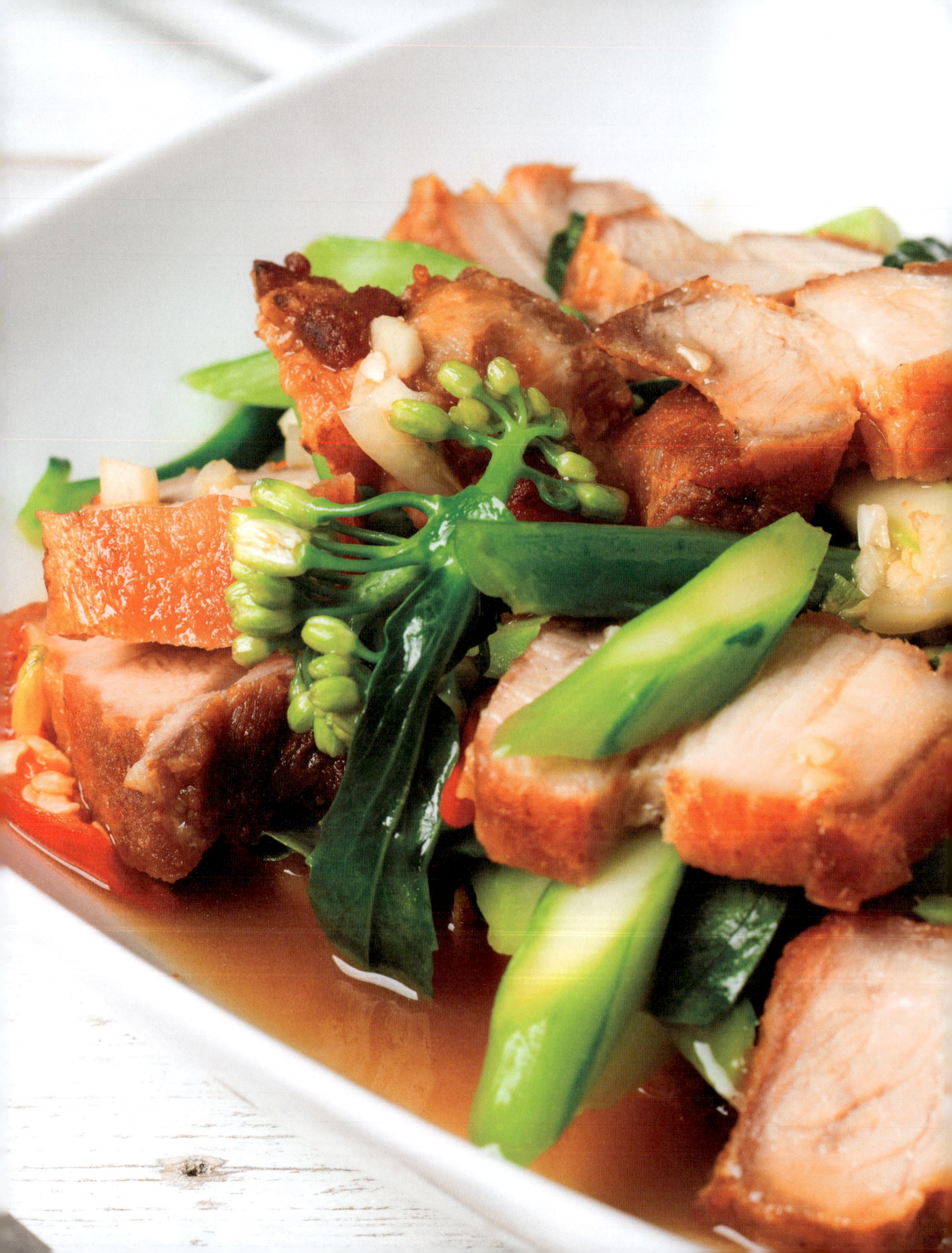

Pork Belly with Stir-Fried Greens

750g pork belly

1½ tsps salt

¼ tsp five-spice powder

2 tsps olive oil

500g Chinese greens, such as gai lan, bok choy or choi sum

1 tbsp peanut oil

2 cloves garlic, finely chopped

Small piece ginger, grated

1 long red chilli, deseeded, finely chopped

3 tbsps tamari

¼ cup (60ml) chicken stock

Place pork belly in a pan of boiling water and simmer for 15 minutes.

Pat dry with a paper towel and place uncovered in fridge for 6-8 hours to dry out.

When ready to cook, remove from fridge and pat dry once again. Score the top of the rind. Mix together ½ teaspoon of the salt and the five-spice powder and rub the base of the pork belly with the spice mix.

Rub the top rind with remaining salt and olive oil, massaging into the creases.

Preheat air fryer to 200°C.

Place pork belly in air fryer basket for 30 minutes.

Reduce temperature to 185°C and bake for another 30 minutes.

Allow to rest for 10 minutes.

Meanwhile cut greens into 5cm lengths. Heat a wok over high heat. Add peanut oil and swirl to coat. Add garlic, ginger and chilli. Stir-fry for 1 minute or until fragrant.

Add stems of the greens. Stir-fry for 2-3 minutes or until bright green and just tender. Add leaves, tamari and chicken stock. Stir-fry for 1-2 minutes or until leaves wilt.

Slice pork belly and serve with cooked greens.

SERVES 4

Herbed Lamb Chops

1 tsp fresh rosemary

1 tsp fresh thyme

1 tsp fresh oregano

1 tsp salt

¼ tsp pepper

1 tsp ground coriander

2 tbsps olive oil

Juice of ½ lemon

500g lamb chops

Finely chop the herbs, then combine with salt, pepper, coriander, olive oil and lemon juice in a large shallow dish.

Add the lamb chops to the dish and coat well with the herb mixture. Cover and refrigerate for 1 hour.

Place the lamb chops into the air fryer. Cook at 200°C for 3 minutes. Flip the lamb chops then cook for a further 4-5 minutes or until cooked to your liking.

SERVES 4

Dry Rub Spare Ribs

¼ tsp cayenne pepper

1 tsp ground cumin

2 tsps paprika

1 tsp dry oregano

1 tsp sugar

1 tsp salt

25 grinds fresh pepper

1.5kg pork ribs

3 tbsps olive oil

Mix herbs, spices, salt and pepper together in a small bowl.

Brush ribs with oil, then rub in herb and spice mix.

Preheat air fryer to 175°C.

Cut ribs into four equal portions and arrange in the air fryer, leaning on edge of basket. Spray with cooking spray.

Cook for 30-35 minutes, turning halfway, until cooked through.

SERVES 4

Lamb Kebabs

350g boneless lamb, (fillet, backstrap, rump, leg or shoulder), cut into 2cm pieces

1 tbsp olive oil

Salt and pepper to taste

2 tsps ground cumin

Chopped parsley, to serve

Skewers

Place the lamb pieces in a large bowl.

Drizzle with olive oil and season with salt and pepper. Add the cumin and toss to coat.

Thread the lamb onto skewers.

Place skewers inside air fryer basket with space between them. Cook in batches or use a double layer accessory if necessary.

Cook at 200°C for 8-10 minutes, turning halfway, until the lamb is cooked to your liking.

Sprinkle with chopped parsley to serve.

SERVES 2

Rare Roast Beef

1kg beef joint

1 tbsp olive oil

Salt and pepper to taste

Preheat air fryer to 200°C.

Pat dry the beef and rub with olive oil. Season well with salt and pepper.

Cook for 15 minutes, then use tongs to carefully turn the beef over.

Reduce temperature to 180°C.

Cook for a further 25 minutes or until internal temperature reaches 52°C for rare beef. For medium rare cook for a further 5 minutes until internal temperature reaches 57°C.

SERVES 4

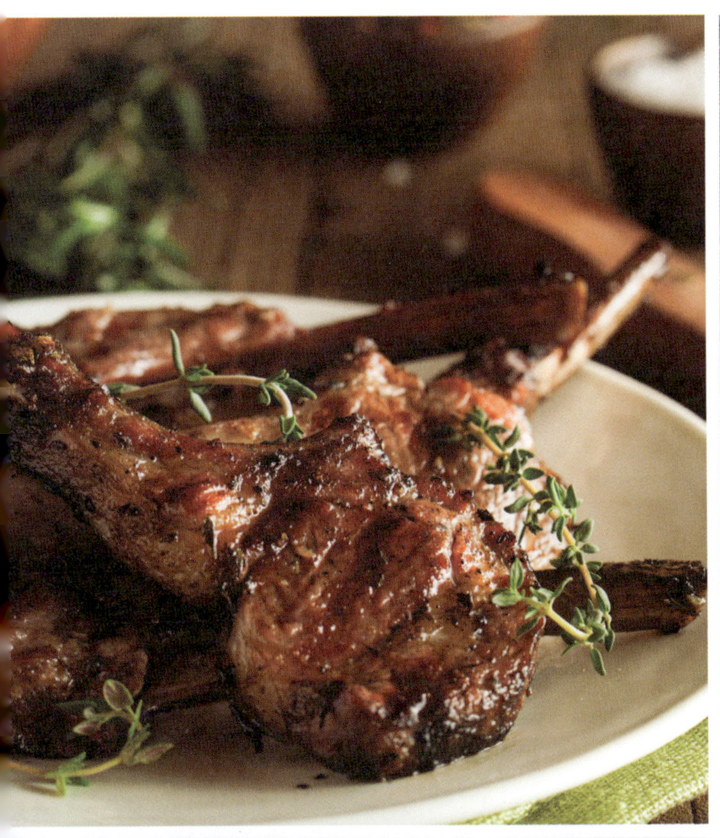
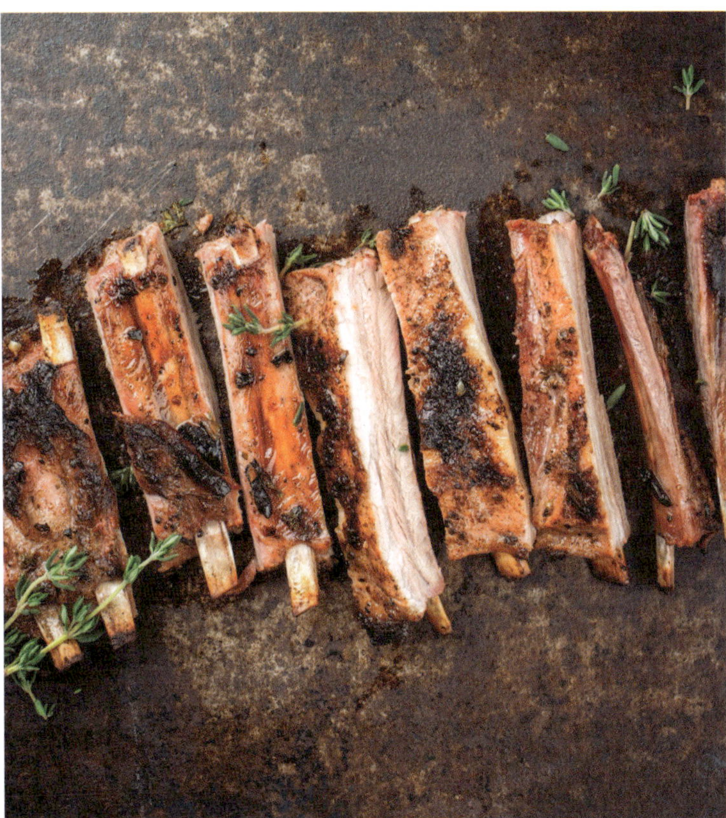
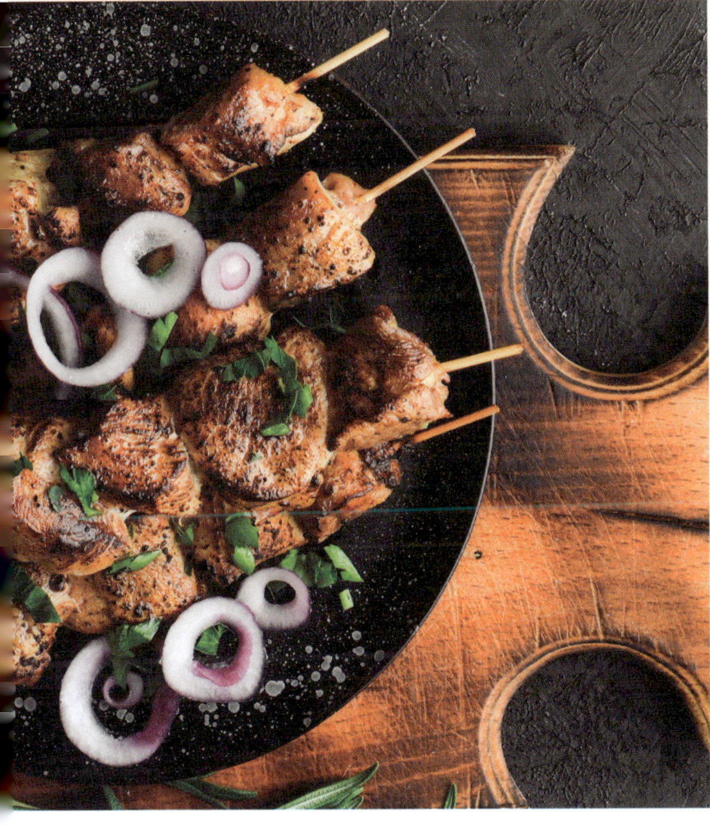
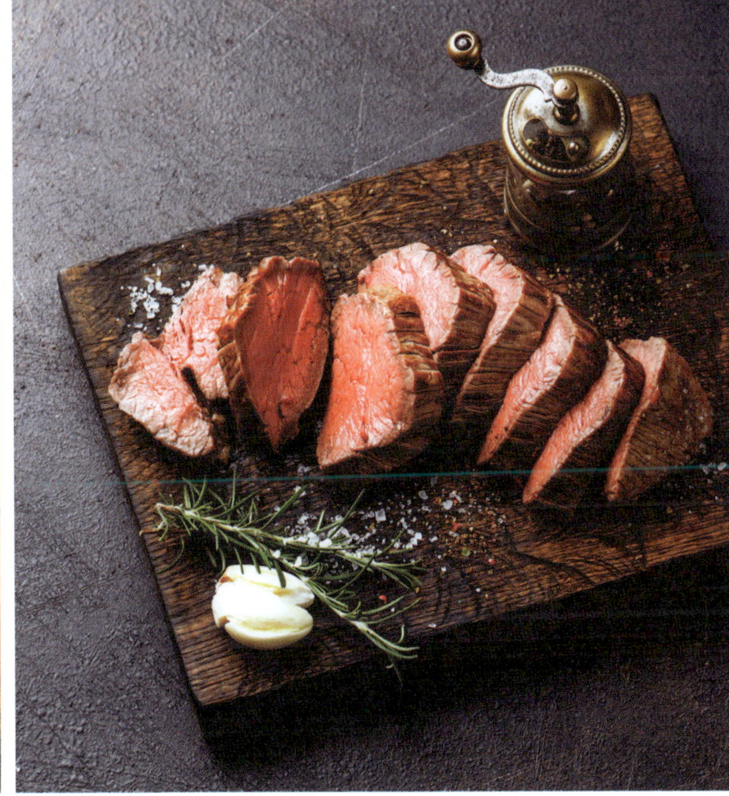

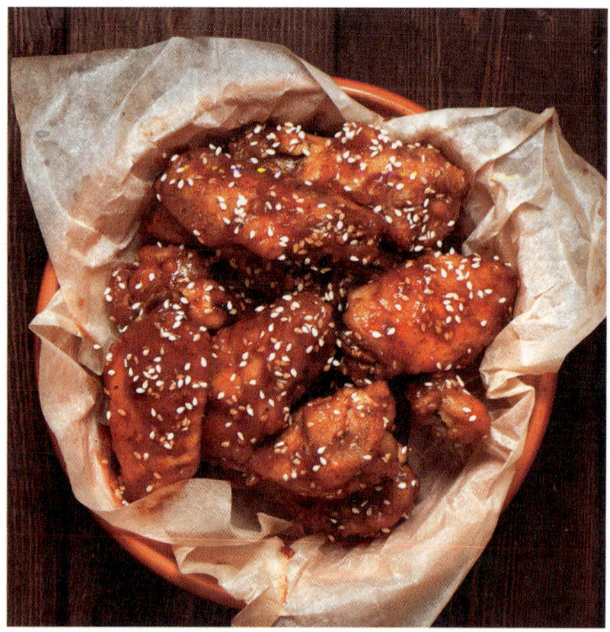

Ginger, Honey and Sesame Chicken Wings

2 cloves garlic, chopped

Small piece ginger, minced

2 tbsps honey

1 tbsp tamari

1 tbsp rice wine vinegar

2 tsps sesame oil

1 tsp Sriracha

6 chicken wings

1 tbsp toasted sesame seeds

Combine the first seven ingredients in a large bowl. Stir to combine. Add the chicken and toss to coat thoroughly. Cover and place in the fridge for at least 30 minutes, preferably overnight.

Place the wings in the air fryer basket. Cook at 190°C for 20 minutes, turning every 5 minutes.

Sprinkle over sesame seeds to serve.

SERVES 2

Maple Duck Breast

2 medium beetroots, peeled and chopped

1 medium sweet potato, peeled and chopped

1 tbsp olive oil

Salt and pepper to taste

2 duck breasts, skin on

2 tbsps maple syrup

¼ tsp cayenne pepper

2 tsps brown sugar

Olive oil cooking spray

Preheat the air fryer to 200°C.

Place beetroot and sweet potato in a bowl with olive oil, salt and pepper. Toss to coat.

Place beetroot in air fryer basket. Cook for 30 minutes, shaking every 10 minutes. After 5 minutes add in sweet potatoes. When tender set aside and keep warm.

Score duck fat several times and rub with salt and pepper.

Combine the maple syrup, cayenne pepper, and sugar in a small pan. Place over medium-low heat and stir until the sugar dissolves.

Place duck in basket skin-side up. Spray with cooking spray. Cook for 10 minutes at 200°C. Flip over and spray once more, and cook for 6-8 minutes.

Flip over once more, brush with the maple glaze and cook for a further 2 minutes. Transfer duck breast to a cutting board and allow to rest for a few minutes.

Slice duck and pour over any remaining sauce. Serve with roast vegetables.

SERVES 2

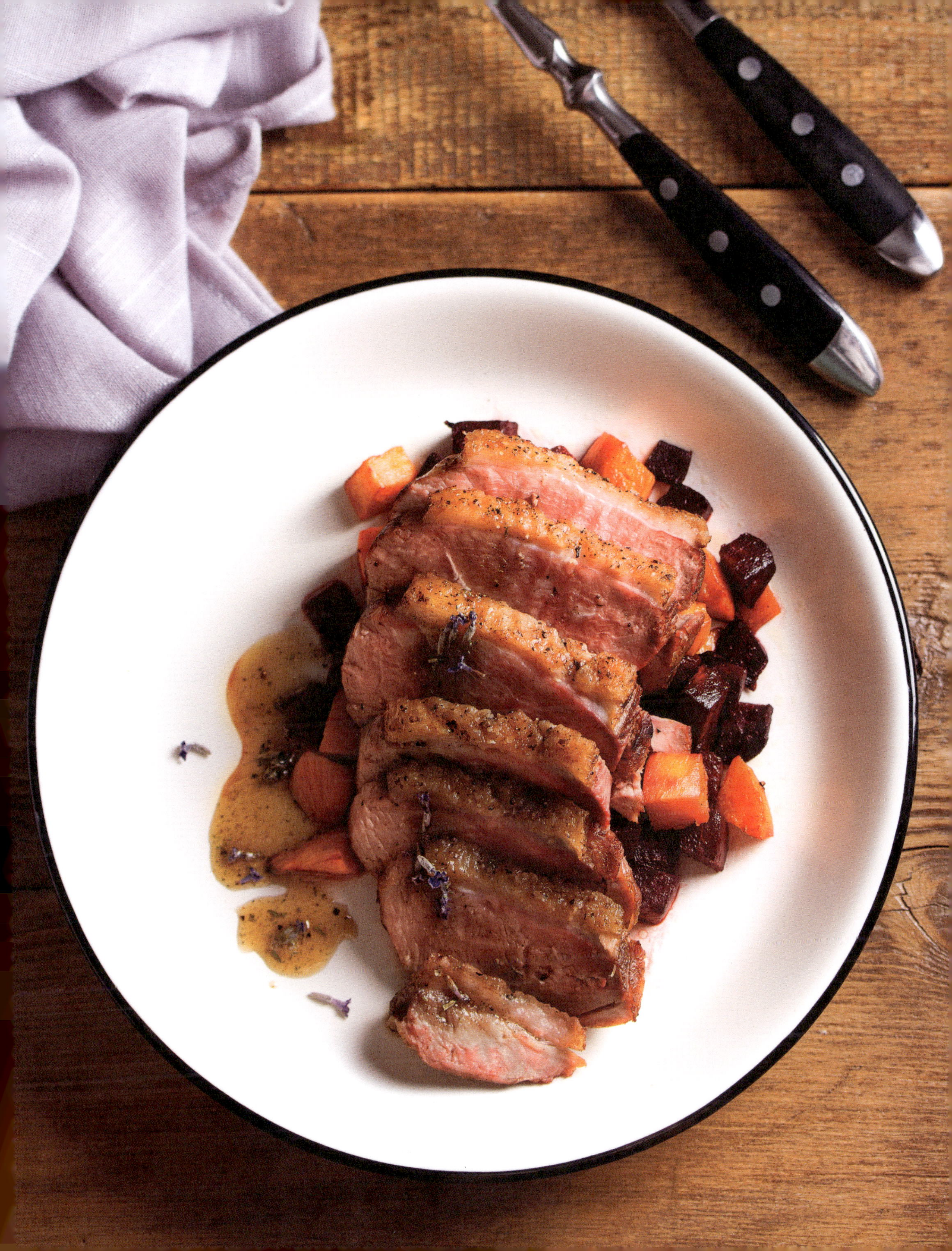

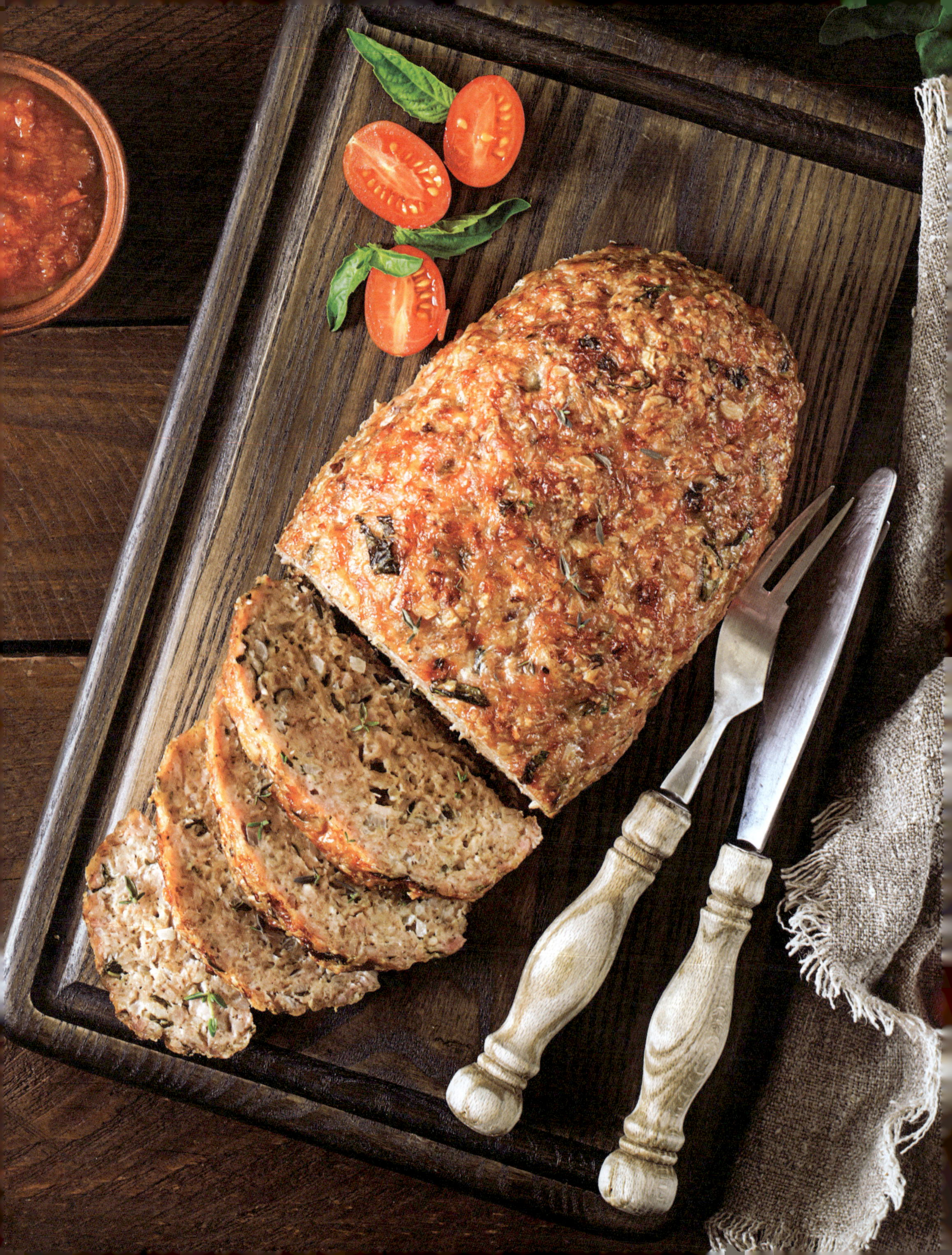

Chicken Meat Loaf

500g chicken mince

½ red onion, grated

¼ cup (10g) basil leaves, chopped

¼ cup (30g) almond meal

¼ cup (55g) canned chopped tomatoes

1 egg

1 tsp salt

¼ tsp ground black pepper

1 tsp garlic powder

Cooking spray

Cake tin or baking pan

Grease a cake tin or baking pan that will fit in your air fryer.

Combine all of the ingredients in a large bowl. Mix together thoroughly.

Use your hands to form mixture into a loaf shape.

Place in cake tin or baking pan. Spay with cooking spray.

Place in air fryer and cook for 20 minutes at 180°C. Cover with foil then cook for a further 10 minutes or until internal temperature is 74°C.

Set aside to rest before slicing.

SERVES 4

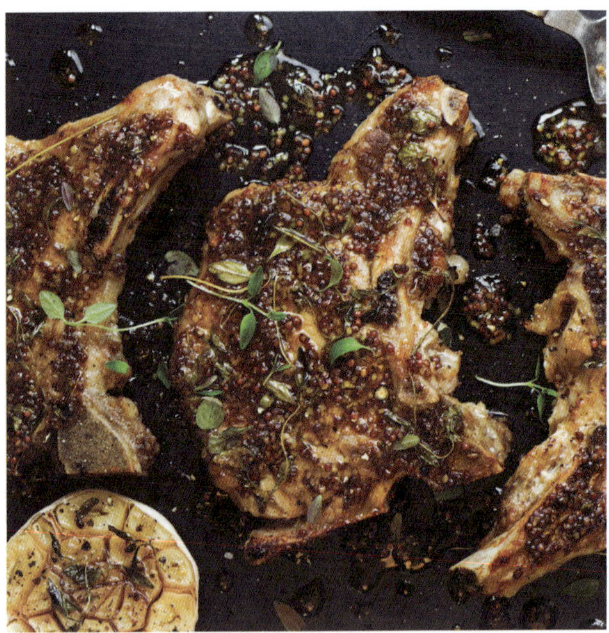

Honey Mustard Pork Chops

4 tbsps wholegrain mustard

2 tbsps honey

2 tbsps garlic, minced

½ tsp salt

¼ tsp pepper

4 pork chops, 1½ cm thick

Olive oil cooking spray

In a large bowl, mix together mustard, honey, garlic, salt and pepper.

Add pork chops and toss to coat.

Spray air fryer basket with cooking spray.

Evenly space pork chops in basket and spray with cooking spray. Cook for 6 minutes at 180°C. Flip chops, spray again and cook for a further 6 minutes until cooked through.

Allow to rest for 5-10 minutes before serving.

SERVES 4

Cajun Spiced Ribs

1 tsp salt

1 tbsp dark brown sugar

1 tbsp sweet paprika

1 tsp garlic powder

1 tsp onion powder

1 tsp rosemary, chopped

1 tsp thyme, chopped

½ tsp mustard powder

½ tsp pepper

1kg individually cut pork ribs

In a large bowl, whisk together salt, brown sugar, paprika, garlic powder, onion powder, rosemary, thyme, mustard powder and pepper. Add ribs and toss. Press gently with hands to coat.

Arrange ribs in air fryer basket standing on end and leaning against wall of basket. Cook at 190°C for 35 minutes until ribs are tender inside and crisp on the outside. Transfer to plates and serve hot.

SERVES 2

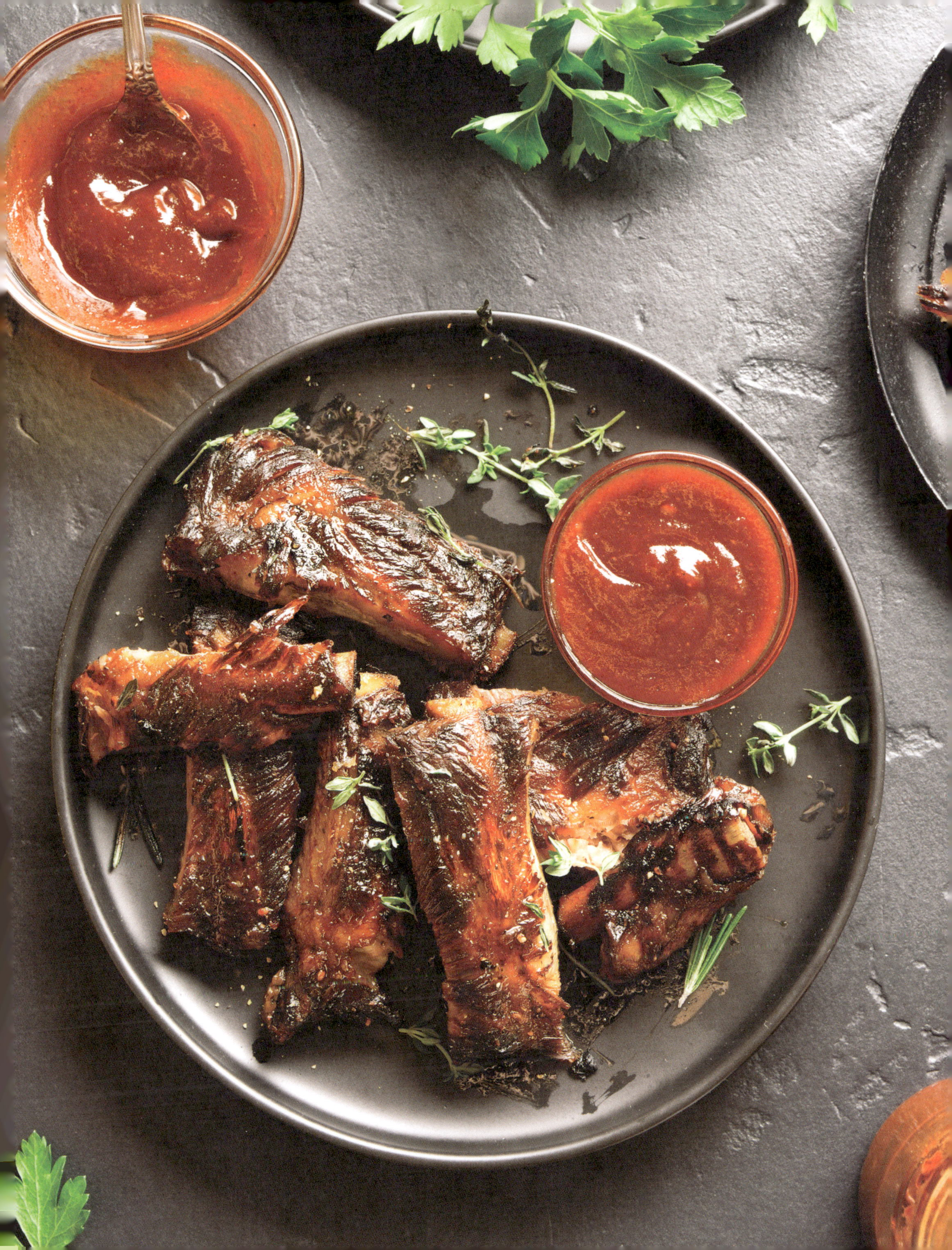

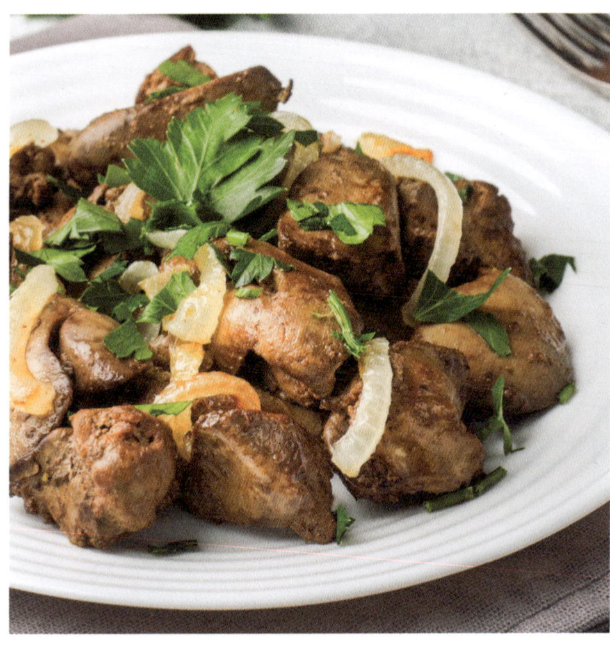

Chicken Livers with Onions

400g chicken livers, washed

1 onion, sliced

25g butter or 2 tbsps olive oil

Salt and pepper

1 tbsp parsley, chopped, to serve

Baking pan

Place chicken livers, onion and butter or olive oil in baking pan.

Cook for 15-20 minutes at 190°C, stirring after 2 minutes then again after 10 minutes.

Season well with salt and pepper, then spoon onto plates and sprinkle with chopped parsley to serve.

SERVES 2

Beef Liver and Apple Salad

400g beef liver, sliced

Olive oil cooking spray

Salt and pepper to taste

3 tbsps olive oil

1 tbsp vinegar

¼ tsp mixed herbs

300g baby spinach leaves

1 green apple, sliced

Baking pan

Place livers in a baking pan that will fit into your air fryer. Spray with olive oil cooking spray and toss to coat.

Place in air fryer and cook for 15-20 minutes at 190°C, stirring every few minutes.

Season well with salt and pepper and set aside.

Combine olive oil, vinegar and mixed herbs in a small bowl or sealable jar with a lid. Season with salt and pepper. Stir or shake to combine.

Arrange spinach leaves, apple and cooked liver on two serving plates. Drizzle with dressing and toss to coat.

SERVES 2

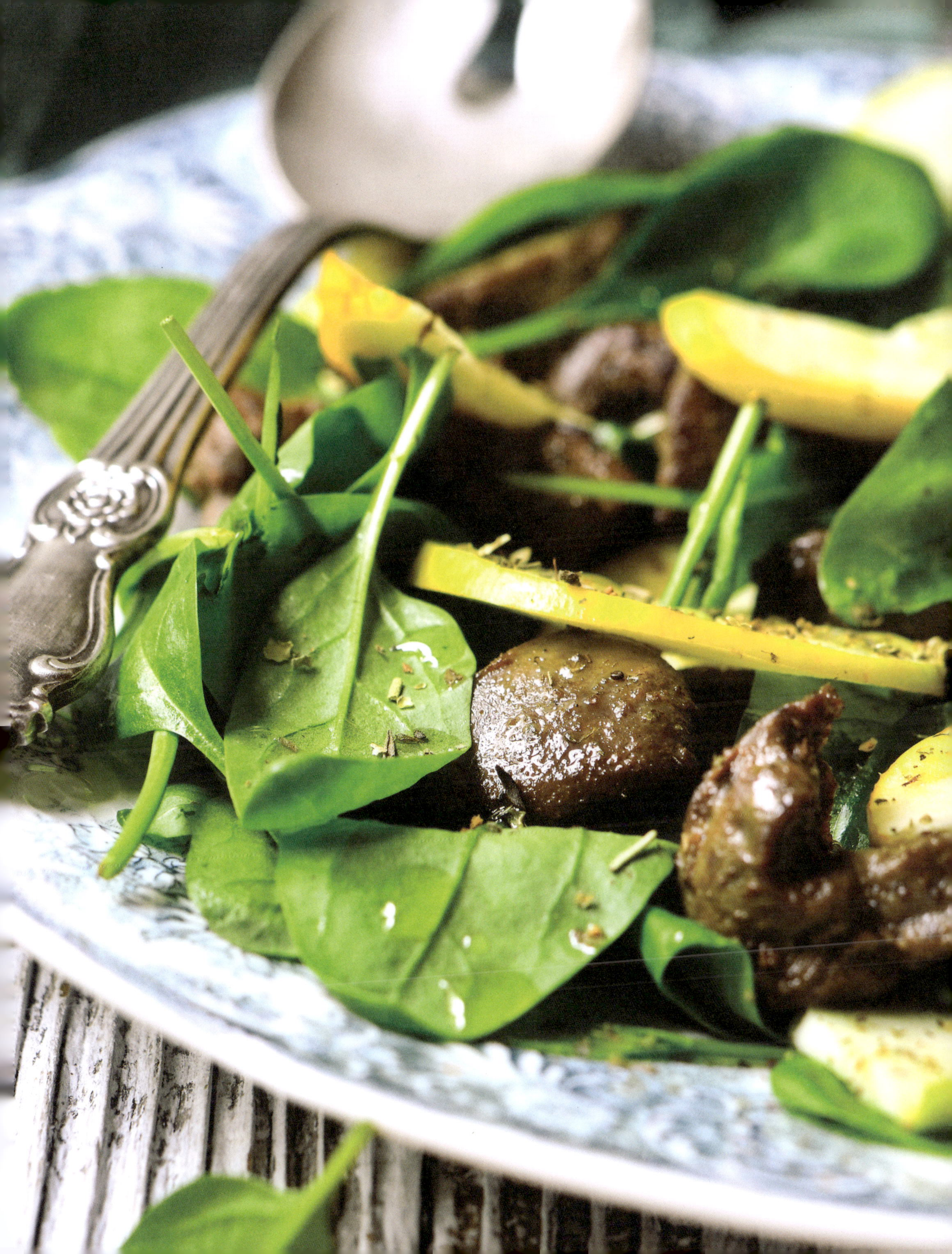

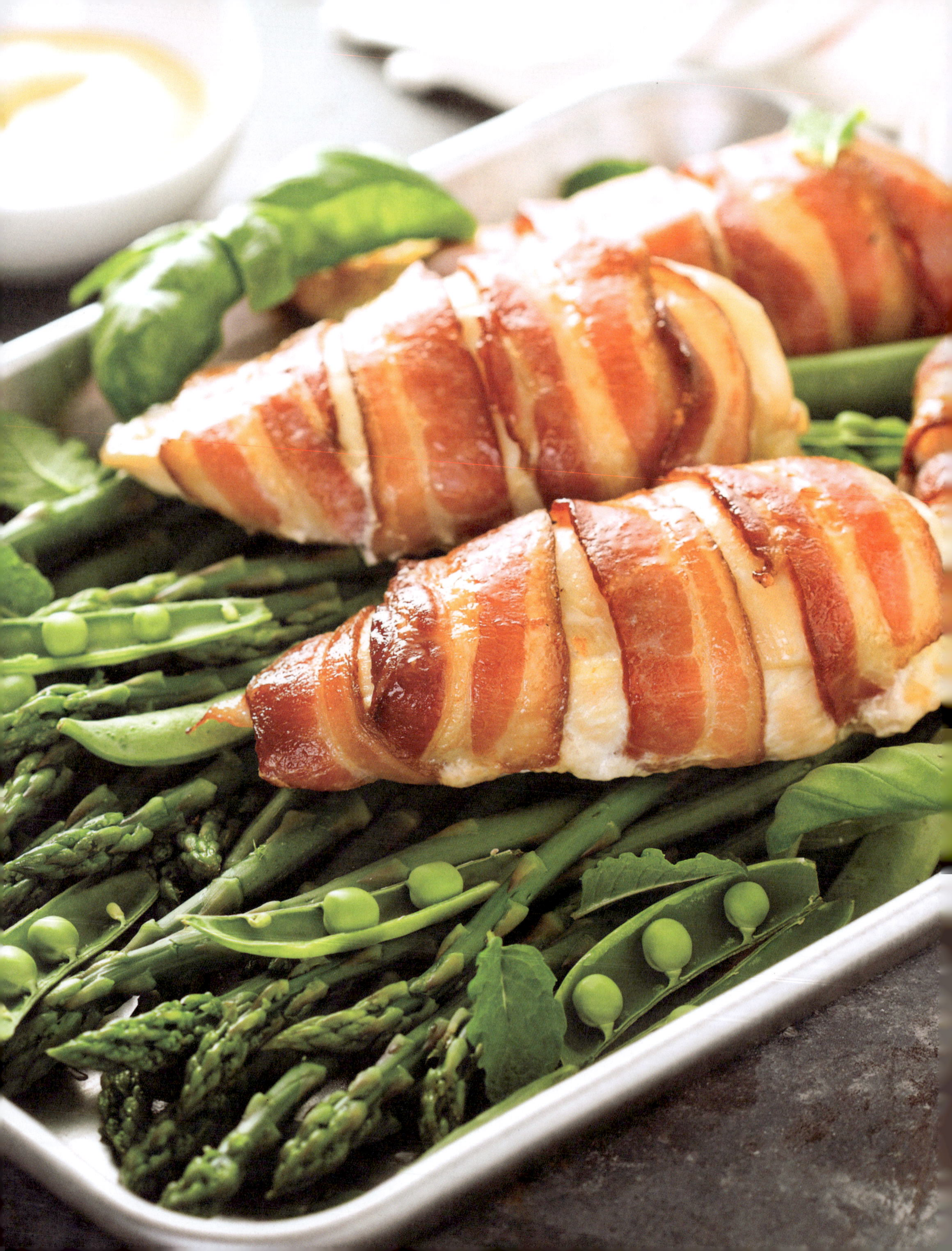

Keto

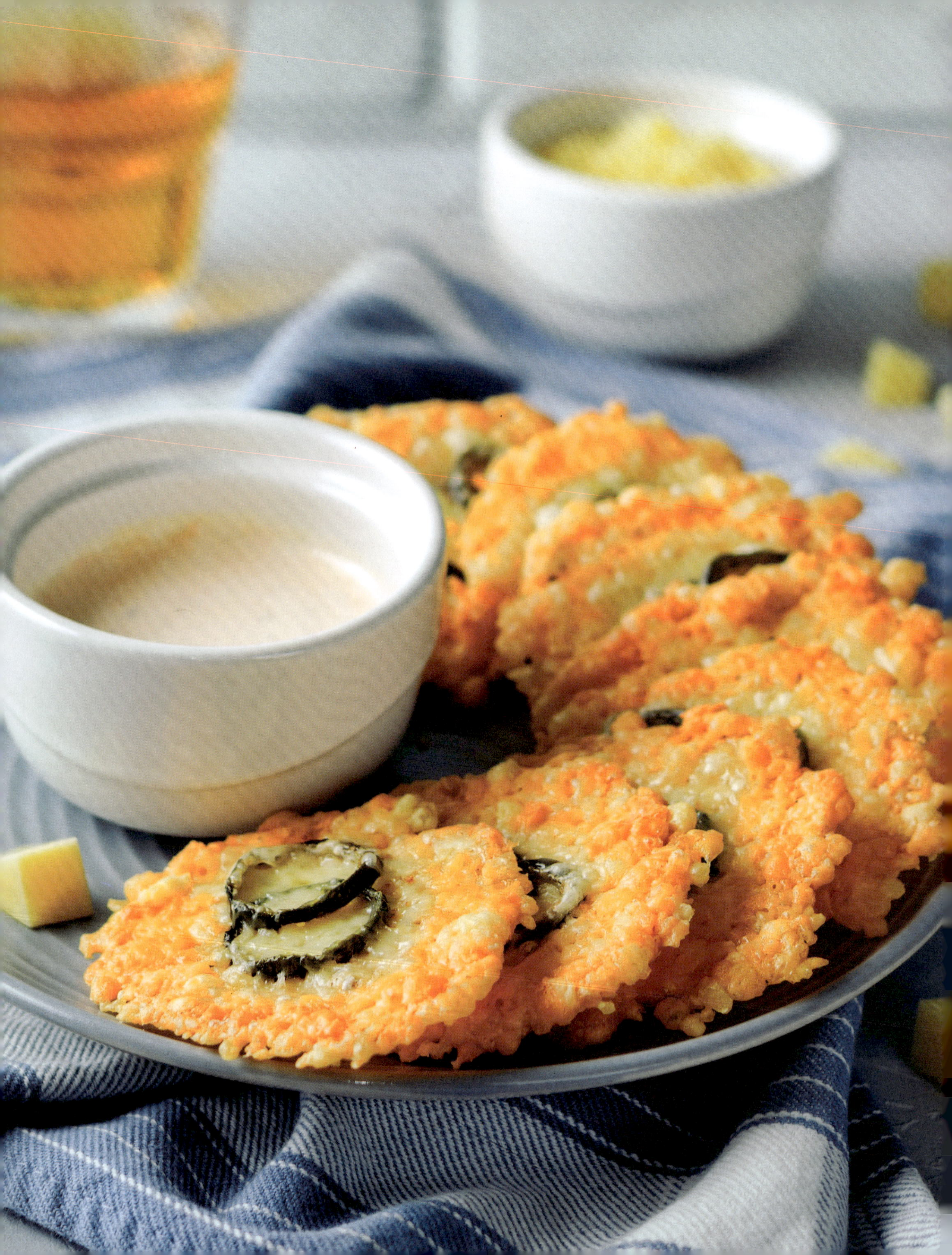

Jalapeno Cheese Crisps with Yoghurt Dip

2 jalapeno chillies, sliced horizontally

Cooking spray

1 cup (100g) Parmesan cheese, grated

½ cup (60g) Cheddar cheese, grated

Salt and pepper to taste

YOGHURT DIPPING SAUCE

⅓ cup (80ml) Greek yoghurt

1 clove garlic, minced

1 tsp lemon juice

1 tsp olive oil

¼ tsp smoked paprika

Pinch of salt

Cake tin or baking pan

Place jalapeno slices into air fryer basket and spray with cooking spray. Cook for 5 minutes at 170°C, turning halfway through cooking.

Remove jalapenos from air fryer basket.

Line a cake tin or baking pan that will fit into your air fryer with greaseproof paper.

In a large bowl combine the two cheeses.

Using 2 tablespoons at a time place small mounds of cheese on the paper about 4cm apart. Cook in batches if necessary. Top each mound with two slices of jalapeno and press down slightly.

Cook for about 10 minutes at 170°C until golden brown.

Allow to cool slightly before peeling off the greaseproof paper.

Repeat with remaining cheese and jalapenos.

Combine all the ingredients for the dipping sauce in a medium bowl. Mix well to combine.

Serve the cooled crisps with the yoghurt dip on the side.

SERVES 4

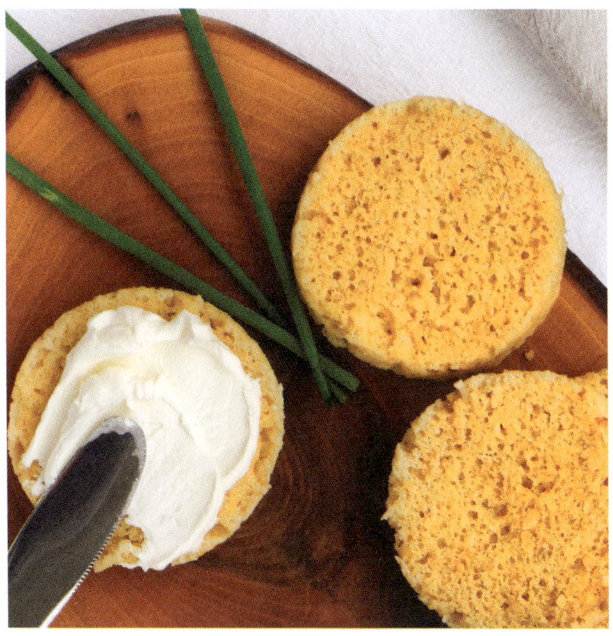

Keto Almond Bread Buns

Avocado oil spray

1½ cups (150g) blanched almond flour

5 tbsps psyllium husk powder

2 tsps baking powder

½ tsp salt

2½ tbsps apple cider vinegar

3 egg whites

1 cup (250ml) boiling water

Cake tin

Spray cake tin with avocado oil spray. Preheat air fryer to 160°C.

In a large bowl, combine almond flour, psyllium husk powder, baking powder and salt. Stir in the vinegar and eggs and mix until a thick dough forms. Add the water and mix well. Set aside for 2 minutes to allow the dough to firm up.

Divide dough into eight equal pieces and shape into buns. Working in batches, place buns into the greased tin, about 3cm apart. Place into air fryer and cook for 20-25 minutes, turning after 15 minutes. Cook until buns are golden brown, puffed and cooked through.

Allow to cool before slicing.

MAKES 8

Chicken Liver and Mushroom Souffle

3 tbsps olive oil

300g mushrooms, finely diced

600g chicken livers, cleaned

¾ cup (200ml) kefir

1 egg

1 onion, diced

1 tbsp fresh rosemary

2 tbsps almond meal

½ tsp garlic powder

Salt and pepper to taste

25g butter

4 ramekins

Heat oil in a large frying pan over medium heat. Add mushrooms and fry for 4-6 minutes until all the liquid evaporates from the pan. Set aside to cool.

Place chicken livers in a large bowl with the kefir, egg, diced onion and rosemary. Use a stick blender to blend until smooth.

Stir in almond meal, garlic powder and salt and pepper. Cover and refrigerate for 1 hour.

Add the cooled mushrooms to the bowl and stir to combine.

Grease four ramekins with butter.

Pour mixture into ramekins and place in air fryer basket.

Cook at 160°C for about 30 minutes or until completely set.

SERVES 4

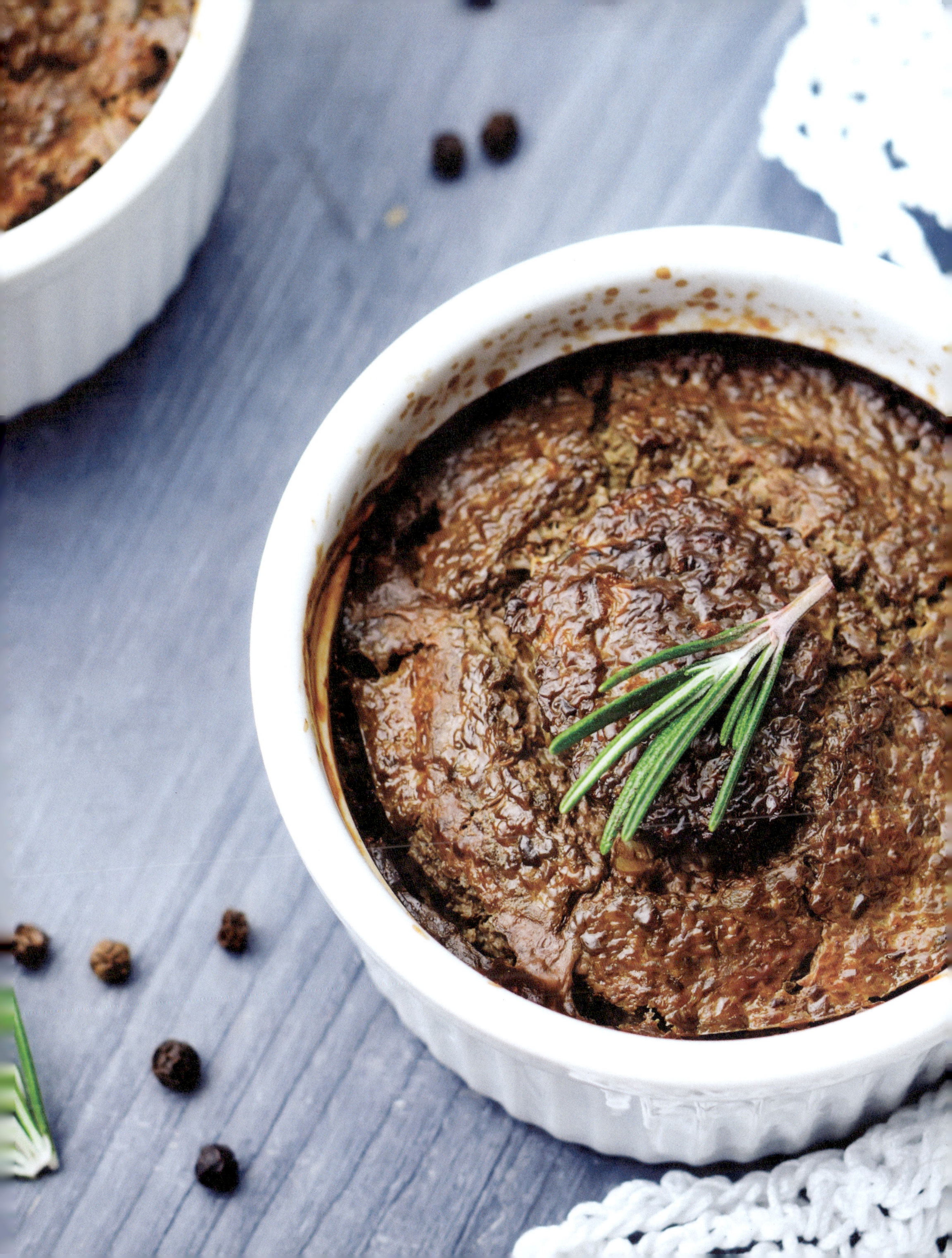

Perfect Crispy Bacon

12 rashers bacon

Arrange the bacon in the air fryer in a single layer. Cook in batches or use a double layer accessory if necessary.

Cook for 5 minutes at 200°C, then use tongs to turn the bacon.

Cook for another 4 minutes until crispy.

Set aside and keep warm.

Repeat with remaining bacon.

SERVES 4

Bacon-Wrapped Scallops

16 large scallops, cleaned and patted dry

8 rashers bacon, cut in half lengthways

Olive oil spray

Pepper to taste

Preheat air fryer to 200°C.

Wrap each scallop in a piece of bacon and secure with a toothpick.

Spray with olive oil and season lightly with pepper.

Arrange scallops in a single layer in the air fryer. Cook in batches or use a double layer accessory if necessary. Cook for 8 minutes, turning halfway through, until scallops are tender and opaque and bacon is cooked through.

Serve hot.

SERVES 4

Avo Eggs with Bacon

2 rashers bacon

2 avocados

4 eggs

Salt and pepper to taste

1 tbsp chives, chopped

Place bacon in air fryer. Cook for 4 minutes at 200°C, then turn with tongs and cook for a further 4 minutes. Set aside to cool.

When bacon is cool enough to handle snip it into small pieces. Set aside.

Cut avocados in half and remove the stone.

Place avocados in air fryer basket then crack an egg into each one, keeping the yolk intact.

Cook at 200°C for 9 minutes or until egg is done to your liking.

Season the eggs with salt and pepper. Sprinkle over bacon pieces and chives to serve.

SERVES 2

Mini Sausages in Bacon

8 rashers of bacon

16 cocktail sausages

Preheat air fryer to 180°C.

Cut each rasher of bacon in half lengthways.

Wrap each sausage in bacon and secure with a toothpick.

Arrange in air fryer basket, making sure there is space between each sausage. Cook in batches or use a double layer accessory if necessary.

Cook for 20 minutes until cooked through, turning sausages halfway through cooking.

Keep warm while you cook the remaining sausages.

SERVES 4

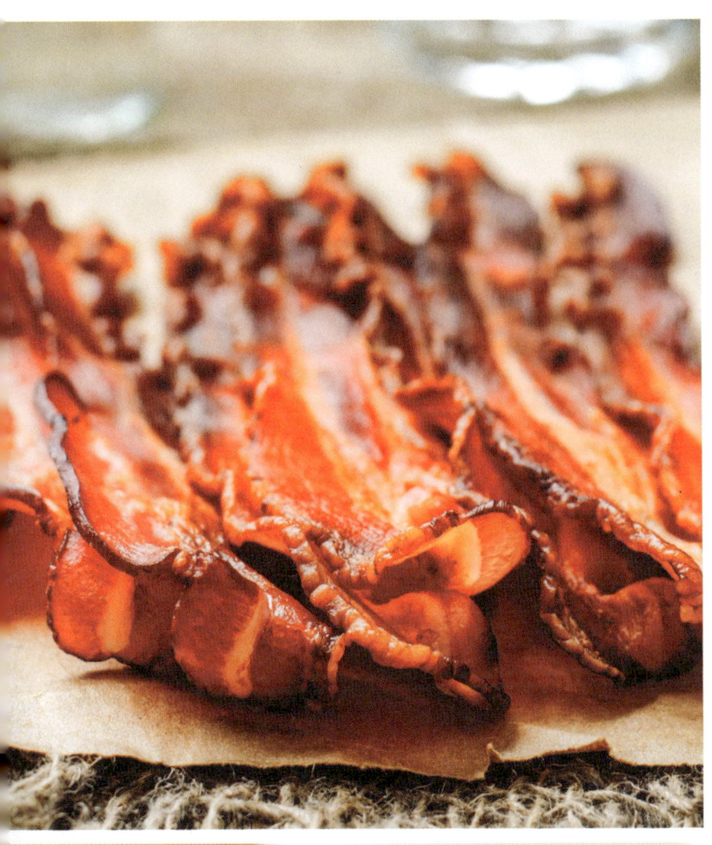
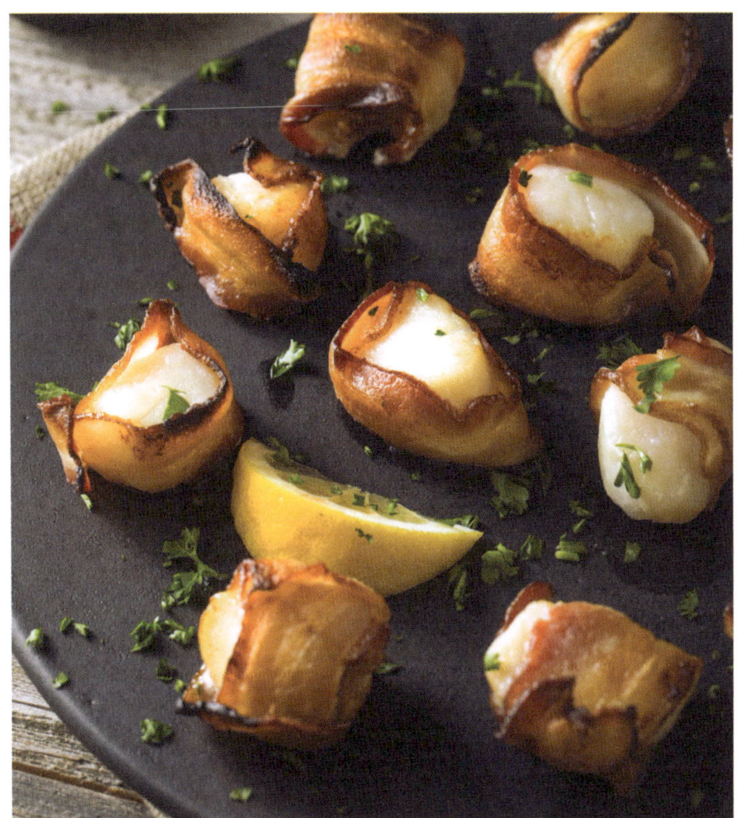
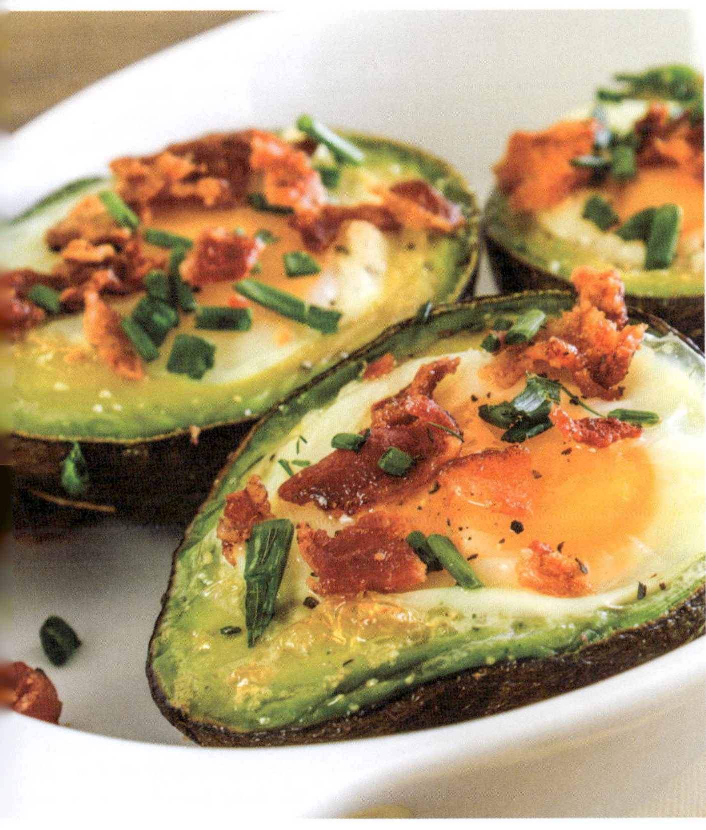
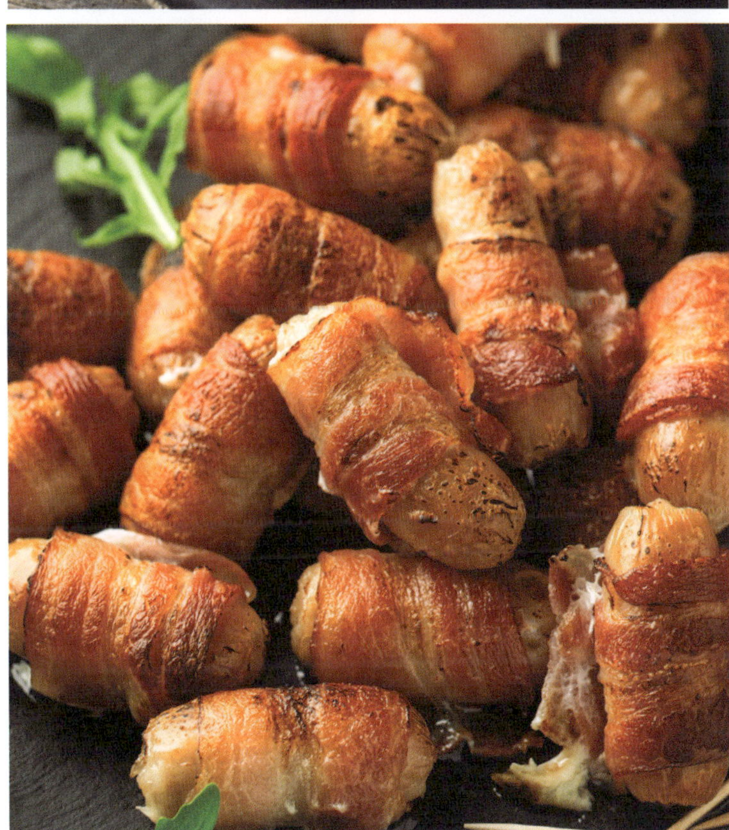

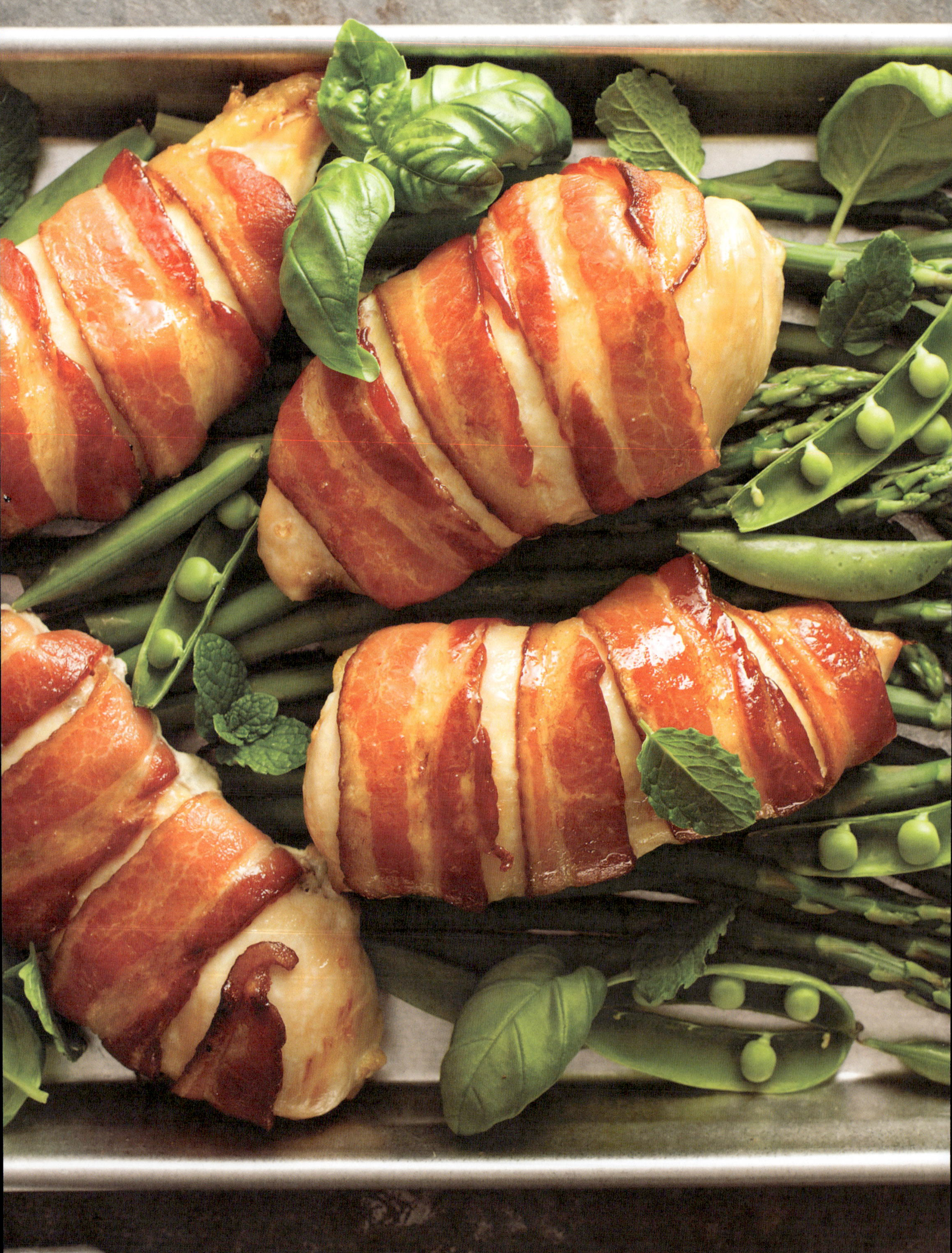

Bacon-Wrapped Chicken Breast

2 skinless chicken breasts

Salt and pepper to taste

½ tsp garlic powder

½ tsp paprika

4-6 rashers bacon

Olive oil or avocado oil cooking spray

Fresh green vegetables to serve (optional)

Pound chicken breasts into an even 2cm thickness.

Rub chicken breasts with salt, pepper, garlic powder and paprika.

Wrap bacon strips around chicken, tuck the ends on the underside of the chicken breasts.

Spray air fryer basket with cooking spray then carefully transfer chicken to basket. Make sure bacon is still tucked under firmly.

Cook at 200°C for 20-25 minutes or until chicken is cooked through and internal temperature reaches 74°C.

Serve with fresh green vegetables.

SERVES 2

Tip: See recipe on page 203 for air fried asparagus.

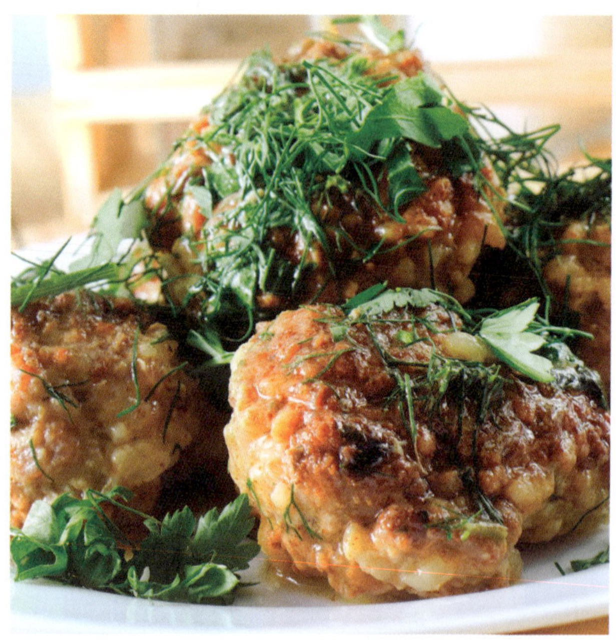

Cheese and Herb Meatballs

½ cup (50g) Parmesan cheese, grated

½ cup (60g) mozzarella cheese, shredded

1 large egg, lightly beaten

2 tbsps thickened cream

1 clove garlic, minced

500g beef mince

2 tbsps fresh parsley, chopped + more to serve

2 tbsps fresh dill, chopped + more to serve

Salt and pepper to taste

Cake tin or baking pan

Preheat air fryer to 175°C. Grease cake tin or baking pan.

In a large bowl, combine cheeses, egg, cream and garlic. Add beef and herbs and season with salt and pepper. Use your hands to mix well.

Shape into golf-ball-sized meatballs.

Place in a single layer in the tin and place in air fryer basket. Cook in batches if necessary. Cook for 8-10 minutes until lightly browned and cooked through.

Keep warm while you cook the remaining meatballs.

Sprinkle with fresh herbs to serve.

SERVES 4

Baked Salmon with Almond and Cheese Crust

2 skin-on salmon fillets

Salt and pepper to taste

25g softened butter

4 tbsps slivered or flaked almonds

100g Gruyère or Emmental cheese, grated

1 tsp dried parsley

Olive oil or avocado oil cooking spray

150g mixed salad leaves, to serve

Preheat air fryer to 160°C.

Season salmon fillets with salt and pepper. Place skin-side down, then smear with softened butter.

Combine almonds, cheese and parsley in a large bowl. Mix gently.

Press cheese mixture onto salmon fillets.

Spray air fryer basket with cooking spray.

Place salmon fillets skin-side down in air fryer basket.

Cook for 12-15 minutes, until the topping is crisp and golden and the salmon cooked.

Allow to rest for 5 minutes before serving with mixed leaf salad.

SERVES 2

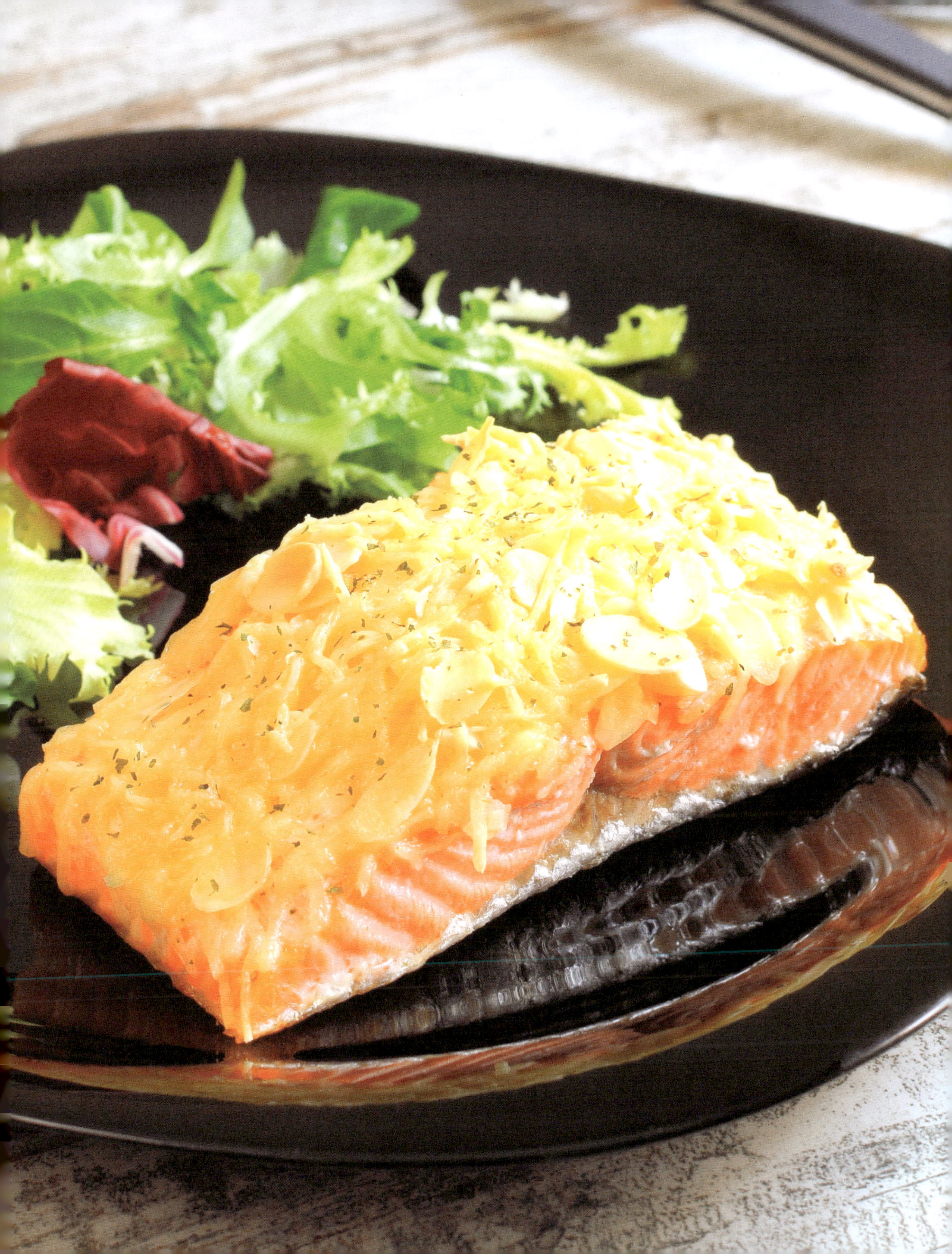

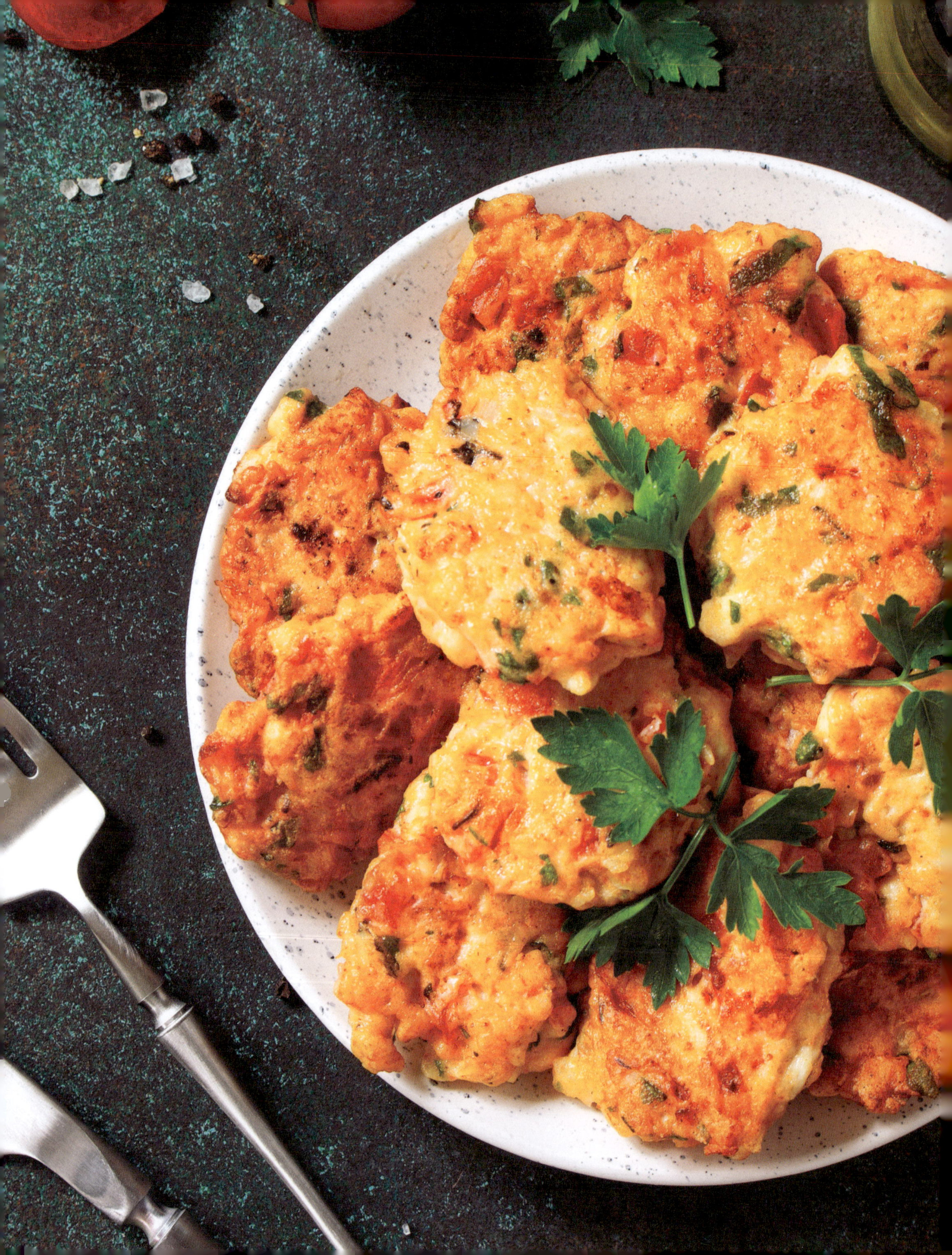

Chicken and Tomato Patties

750g chicken mince

¼ cup (25g) Parmesan cheese

½ tsp salt

¼ tsp pepper

¼ tsp garlic powder

1 tsp dried oregano

½ tsp onion powder

1 tsp paprika

⅔ cup (150g) cherry tomatoes, finely chopped

3 tbsps fresh parsley, chopped

Cooking spray

Place chicken mince in a large bowl with cheese, salt, pepper, garlic powder, oregano, onion powder and paprika. Mix well with your hands.

Add tomatoes and parsley and again use your hands to gently combine.

Form into 12 small patties.

Spray air fryer basket with cooking spray.

Arrange patties in air fryer basket leaving space between each one. Cook in batches or use a double layer accessory if necessary. Spray patties with cooking spray.

Cook for 10 minutes at 175°C until golden brown and cooked through. Turn halfway through cooking.

Repeat with remaining patties.

SERVES 4

Cauliflower Crust Pizza

1 head of cauliflower, broken into florets

½ cup (60g) mozzarella, shredded

¼ cup (25g) Parmesan, grated

½ tsp dried oregano

¼ tsp salt

¼ tsp garlic powder

2 eggs, lightly beaten

100g cream cheese

1 zucchini, thinly sliced

1 tbsp olive oil

1 tbsp chives, chopped

½ red chilli, sliced

Place cauliflower in a food processor and pulse until it resembles rice.

Steam cauliflower in a steamer basket for 5 minutes until tender or microwave for 5 minutes in a covered bowl. Drain well. Pat dry with a clean tea towel or paper towels.

In a large bowl, combine mozzarella, Parmesan, oregano, salt, garlic powder and eggs. Add the cauliflower and use a rubber spatula to mix.

Transfer mixture to a piece of greaseproof paper and shape into a pizza crust that will fit into your air fryer. If you have a regular-sized air fryer you will need to make two crusts and cook one at a time.

Use the greaseproof paper to lift the pizza crust into the air fryer.

Cook for 14 minutes at 175°C.

Using the greaseproof paper, gently lift the crust out of the air fryer. Place an upturned plate on top of the crust. With one hand under the greaseproof paper and one hand on the plate, flip the crust over onto the plate, then carefully slide back onto the greaseproof paper, so now the bottom side is up.

Spread the crust with cream cheese. Arrange zucchini slices on the cream cheese and drizzle with oil.

Return crust to air fryer and cook for 3-4 minutes at 175°C.

Remove from air fryer and scatter with chives and chillies to serve.

SERVES 2

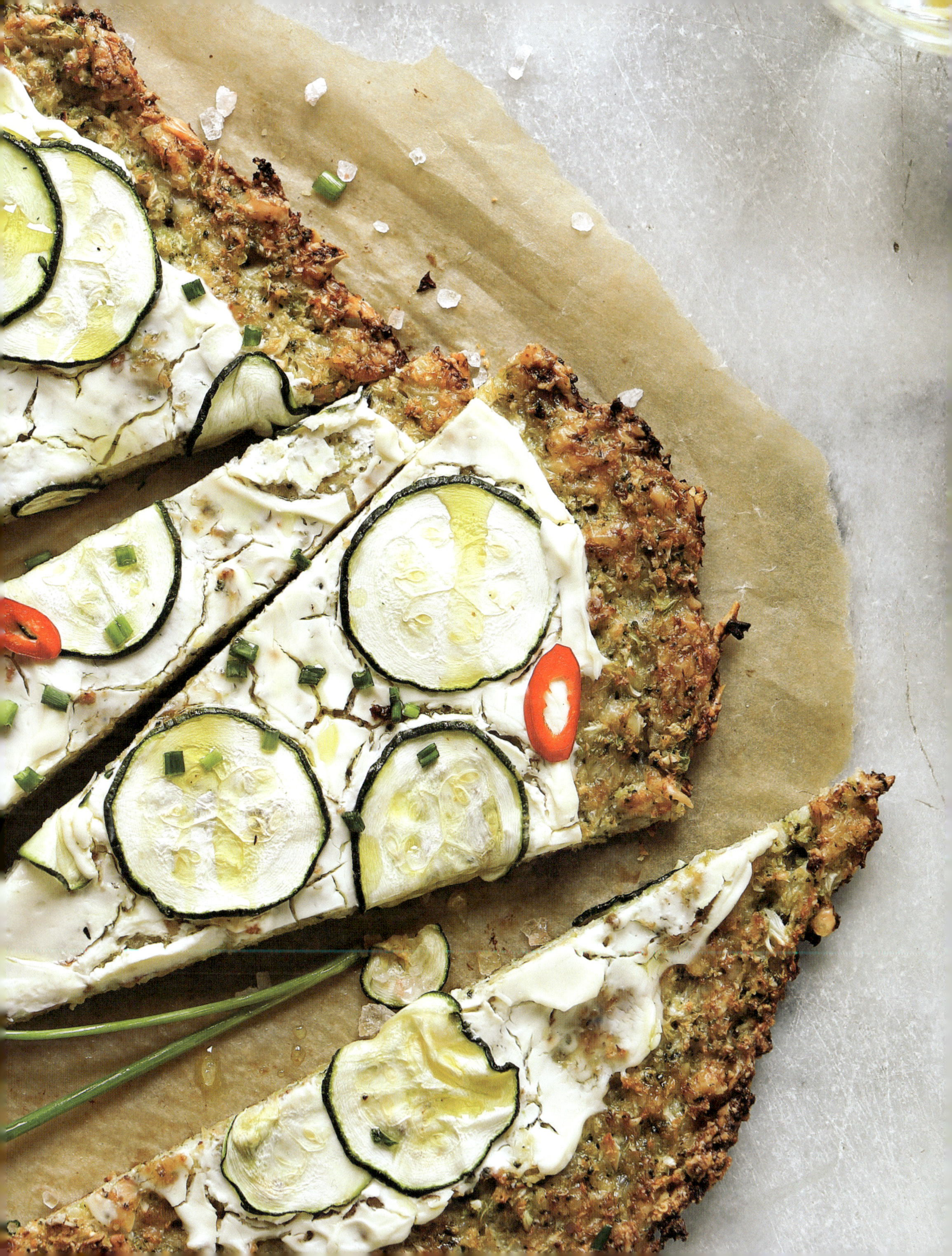

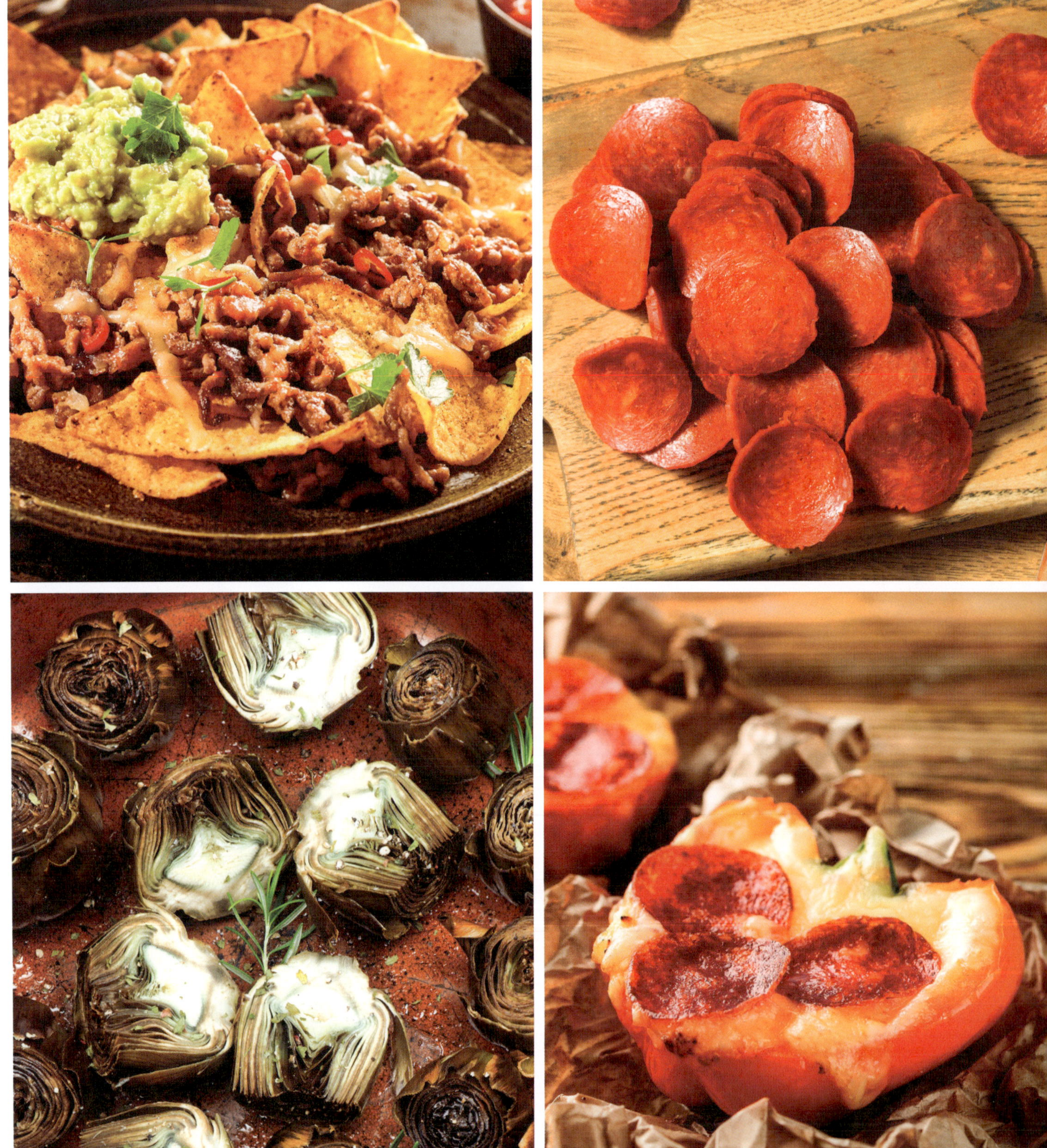

Nachos

1 ripe avocado

½ clove garlic, crushed

Pinch of salt

Juice of ½ lime

2 cups (55g) corn chips

1 cup (245g) warm chilli con carne (see recipe page 159)

1 cup (125g) Cheddar cheese, grated

½ red chilli, sliced

2 tbsps fresh coriander leaves

Use a fork to mash avocado in a small bowl with garlic, salt and lime juice. Mix well and set aside.

Line base and two sides of air fryer basket with aluminium foil. Preheat air fryer to 190°C.

Place corn chips in basket, spoon over chilli con carne and sprinkle with cheese. Cook for 1-2 minutes, until cheese is just melted.

Remove nachos from the air fryer and top with avocado, chilli slices and fresh coriander. Serve immediately.

SERVES 4

Pepperoni Chips

200g Pepperoni Salami (whole or sliced)

Baking tray (optional)

Preheat air fryer to 200°C and the line the air fryer basket (or ovenproof baking tray) with baking paper.

Cut the Pepperoni into slices, if required, and place on the prepared tray, being careful not to overcrowd the tray.

Cook at 190°C for about 5 minutes until cooked and slightly crispy.

Drain well on paper towels before serving.

SERVES 2

Roasted Artichokes

500g artichokes

Juice of 2 lemons

2 tbsps olive oil

2 sprigs fresh rosemary

2 tsps salt

Freshly ground mixed peppercorns

Preheat the air fryer to 170° C.

Remove outer leaves of artichokes, cut 3cm off the tips and remove stems. Cut larger artichokes in half, lengthways, keep smaller artichokes whole.

Place artichokes in a large bowl and drizzle with lemon juice and olive oil. Add rosemary sprigs to bowl and season with salt and pepper. Toss well to coat.

Place artichokes in air fryer basket. Place the halves cut-side down. Cook in batches or use a double layer accessory if necessary.

Cook for 12-15 minutes or until tender.

Serve with a dip of your choice.

SERVES 2

Cheese and Salami Stuffed Capsicums

2 red capsicums

Olive oil cooking spray

Salt and pepper to taste

2 cups (250g) Cheddar cheese, grated

150g salami sausage, thinly sliced

Cut the capsicums in half lengthways and scoop out the seeds and membranes.

Spray inside and out with olive oil cooking spray and season with salt and pepper.

Place capsicums in air fryer basket cut-side up and cook for 6 minutes at 175°C.

Remove from air fryer and when cool enough to handle fill each half with equal amounts of cheese. Top with sausage slices.

Return to the air fryer and cook for a further 4-5 minutes at 175°C until the cheese is melted.

SERVES 2

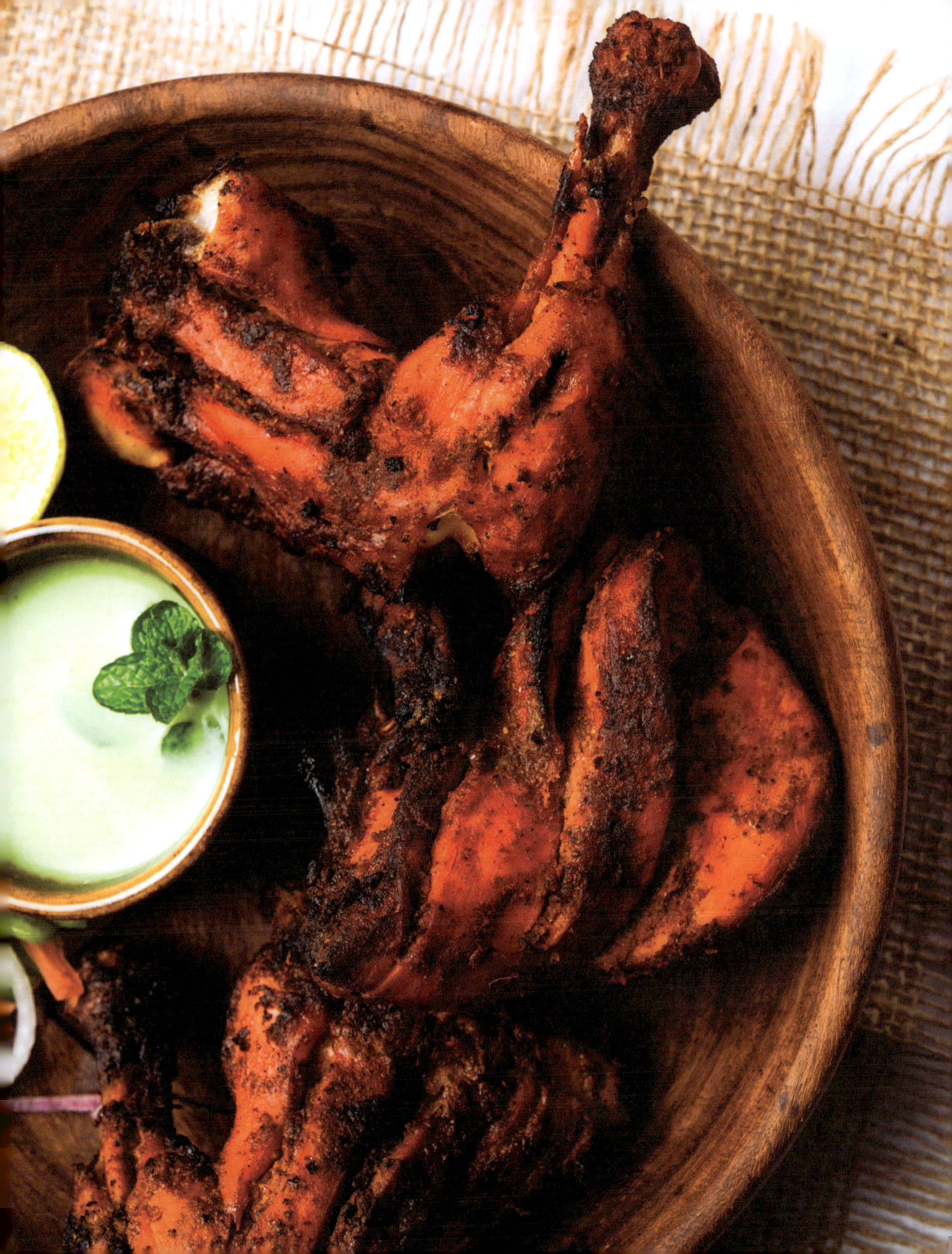

Tandoori Roasted Chicken Legs

2 chicken Marylands

MARINADE

1 cup (250ml) Greek yoghurt

1 tbsp peanut oil

1 tbsp lemon juice

Small piece of ginger, grated

3 cloves garlic, minced

2 tsps garam masala

1 tbsp smoked paprika

½ tsp ground turmeric

2 tsps ground cumin

2 tsps ground coriander

½ tsp chilli powder

½ tsp salt

MINT YOGHURT

⅔ cup (160ml) Greek yoghurt

⅓ cup (5g) mint leaves

Salt and pepper

1 tsp olive oil

Place all the marinade ingredients in a large bowl. Mix well then add the chicken. Coat the chicken in the marinade, then cover and refrigerate for 12-24 hours.

Preheat air fryer to 200°C.

Remove chicken from marinade (retaining marinade for later). Place chicken in air fryer basket, in a single layer, skin-side down. Cook for 10 minutes.

Baste with marinade and cook for a further 15 minutes.

Flip over and baste once more. Cook for a further 10-12 minutes or until cooked through.

Allow the chicken to rest for 5 minutes before serving.

To make the mint yoghurt, place all of the ingredients into a food processor and blitz until smooth. Serve with the chicken.

SERVES 2

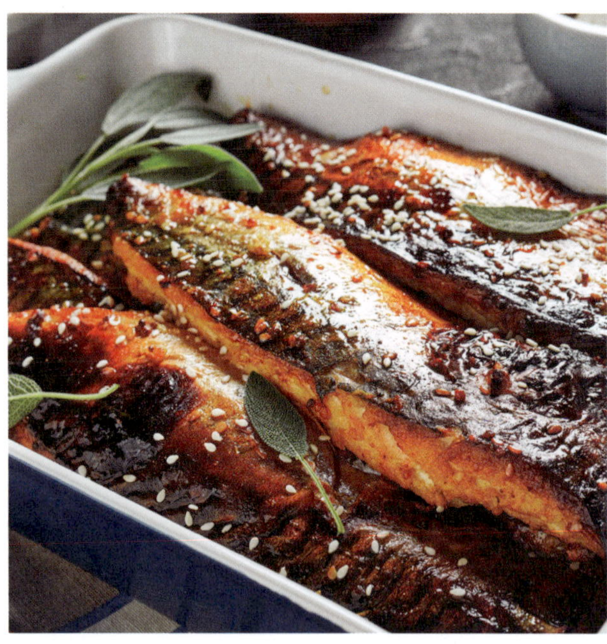

Roasted Mackerel Fillets

1 fresh chilli, finely chopped

2 cloves garlic, finely minced

2 tbsps soy sauce

Juice and zest of 1 lime

1 tsp honey

4 tbsps olive oil

1 tbsp sesame oil

500g mackerel fillets

Avocado or olive oil cooking spray

In a small bowl whisk together chilli, garlic, soy sauce, lime juice, lime zest, honey, olive oil and sesame oil.

Place fish in a shallow dish. Pour marinade over fish. Coat well then cover and refrigerate. Marinate the fish for 30 minutes.

Preheat air fryer to 180°C.

Spray air fryer basket with cooking spray. Arrange mackerel fillets in basket.

Cook for 15-20 minutes until just cooked through.

SERVES 2

Cajun Salmon

2 skin-on salmon fillets

Olive oil cooking spray

½ tsp salt

¼ tsp pepper

½ tsp garlic powder

1 tsp paprika

½ tsp onion powder

⅛ tsp cayenne pepper

¼ tsp dried oregano

1 tsp brown sugar

Preheat air fryer to 200°C.

Dry salmon fillets with paper towel. Spray with olive oil.

Combine seasonings, spices, herbs and brown sugar in a shallow dish. Press flesh sides of fillets into seasoning.

Spray air fryer basket with cooking spray and place salmon fillets skin-side down. Spray salmon once again.

Cook for 8 minutes. Rest for 2 minutes before serving.

SERVES 2

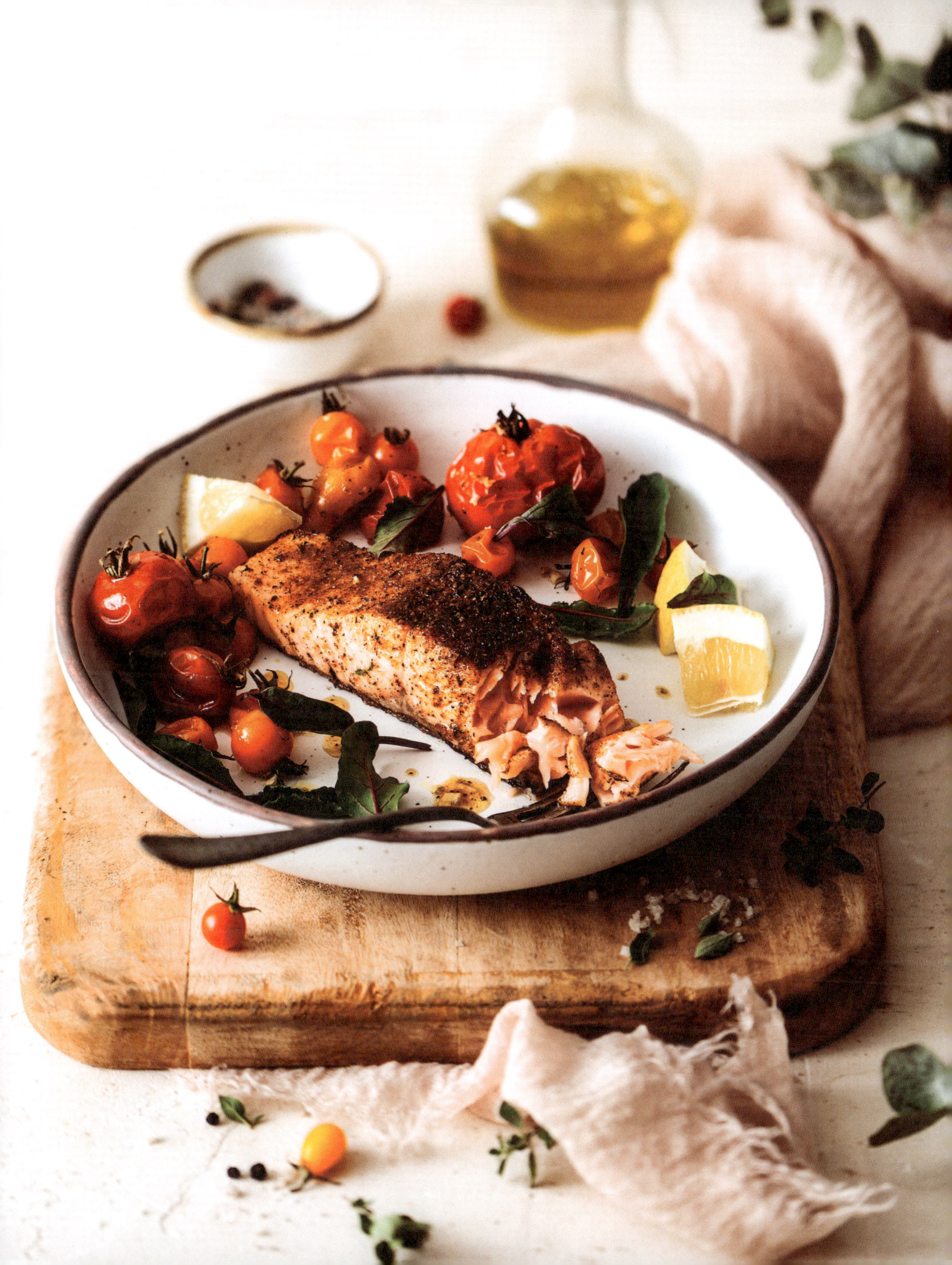

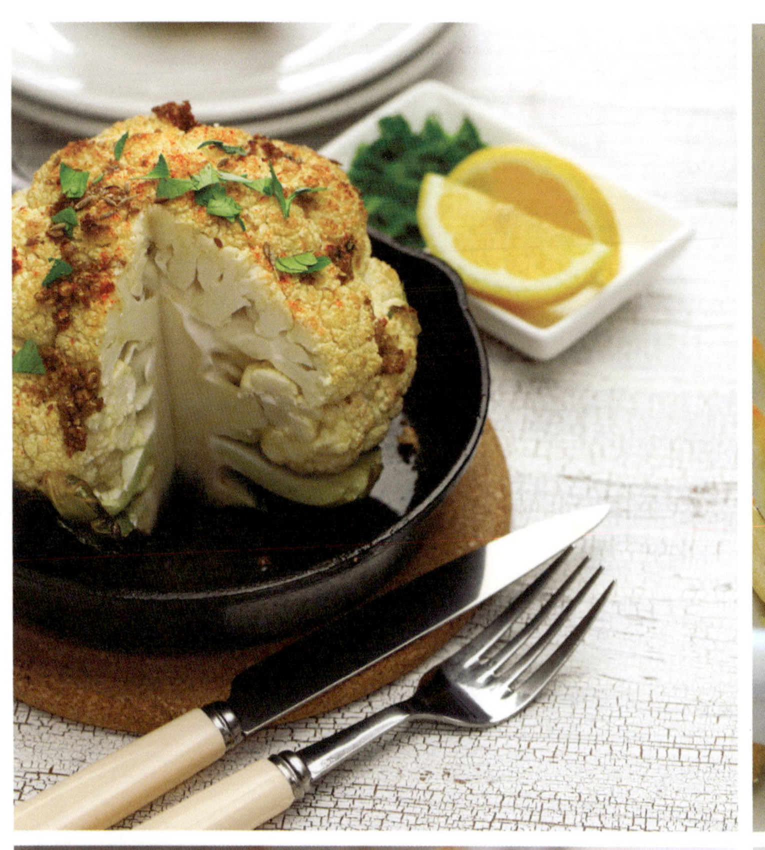
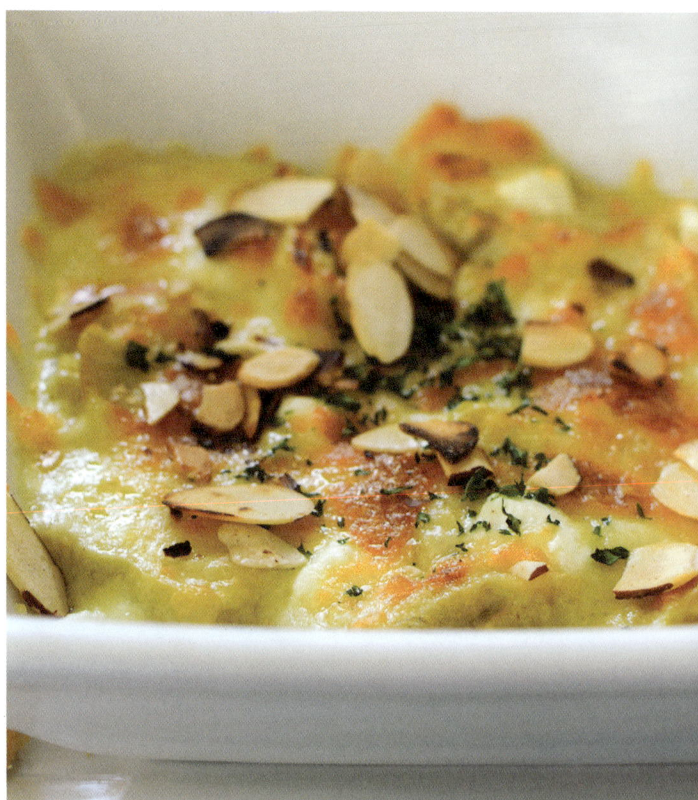
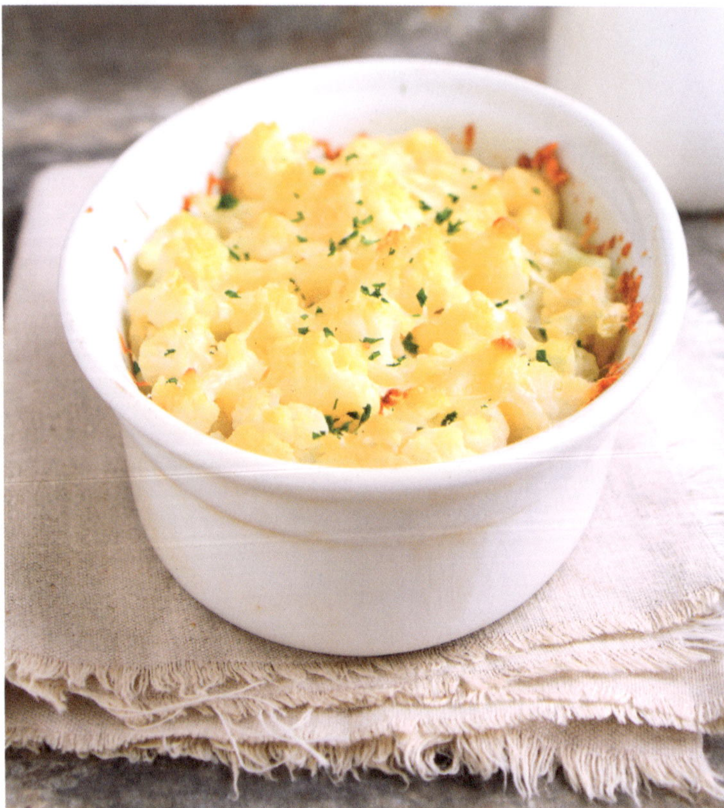
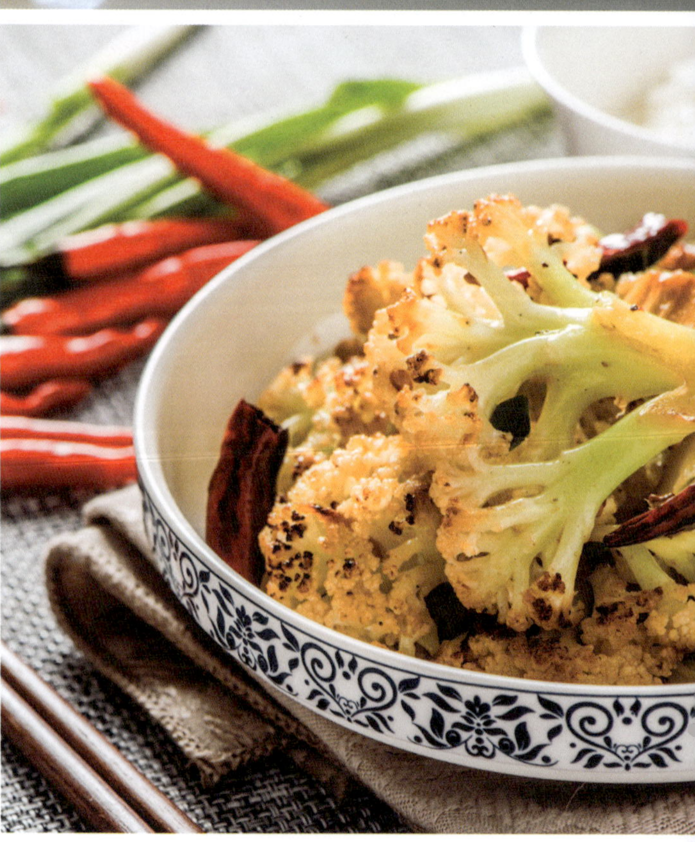

Whole Roasted Cauliflower

⅓ cup (80ml) Greek yoghurt

1 tbsp honey

2 tsps cumin

½ tsp ground coriander

½ tsp paprika

Salt and pepper to taste

1 small head cauliflower

In a large bowl mix together the yoghurt with the honey and spices. Season with salt and pepper.

Place cauliflower into bowl and use your hands to coat cauliflower with this mixture. Set aside for 30 minutes at room temp to marinate.

Preheat air fryer to 180°C.

Place the cauliflower into air fryer basket and cook for 10-12 minutes until it is starting to soften.

Increase heat to 200°C and cook for 3 minutes until browned and tender.

SERVES 4

Artichokes Gratin

1 x 280g jar artichoke hearts, drained

2 tsps lemon juice

1 clove garlic, minced

Salt and pepper to taste

¼ cup (30g) Cheddar cheese, grated

25g goat's cheese, crumbled

¼ cup (25g) Parmesan cheese, grated

¼ cup (60g) mayonnaise

2 tbsps flaked almonds

1 tsp fresh parsley, finely chopped

Baking pan

Place artichokes in a large bowl with lemon juice, garlic, salt and pepper. Toss gently to coat.

In another bowl combine cheeses and mayonnaise.

Arrange artichokes in baking pan. Spoon over cheese mixture. Place dish in air fryer.

Cook for 10 minutes at 170°C. Sprinkle with almonds and cook 2 minutes more. Sprinkle with parsley to serve.

SERVES 2

Cauliflower Gratin

1 head cauliflower, cut into florets

1 tbsp olive oil

Salt and pepper to taste

¾ cup (185ml) thickened cream

½ cup (60g) Cheddar cheese, grated

½ cup (60g) mozzarella, grated

¼ cup (25g) Parmesan, grated

½ tsp garlic powder

Baking pan

Toss the cauliflower florets in olive oil, salt and pepper. Place in air fryer basket and cook for 16-17 minutes at 190°C until just tender.

Meanwhile in a small saucepan over medium-low heat combine cream, cheeses and garlic powder. Cook, stirring until the sauce thickens.

Arrange the cooked cauliflower in baking pan. Pour cheese sauce over cauliflower.

Place pan in air fryer and cook for a 12 minutes at 190°C until sauce is bubbling.

SERVES 4

Cauliflower Stir-Fry

1 head cauliflower, cut into florets

5 cloves garlic, finely sliced

5-7 whole dried chillies

1 tbsp tamari

1 tbsp rice wine vinegar

½ tsp coconut sugar

1 tbsp Sriracha

Salt and pepper to taste

Baking pan

Place cauliflower in baking pan in the air fryer.

Cook for 20 minutes at 175°C, shaking halfway through.

Add garlic and chillies, stir and cook for 5 more minutes.

Mix tamari, vinegar, coconut sugar, Sriracha, salt and pepper together in a small bowl.

Add the mixture to cauliflower and stir. Cook for 5 more minutes until cauliflower is tender.

SERVES 4

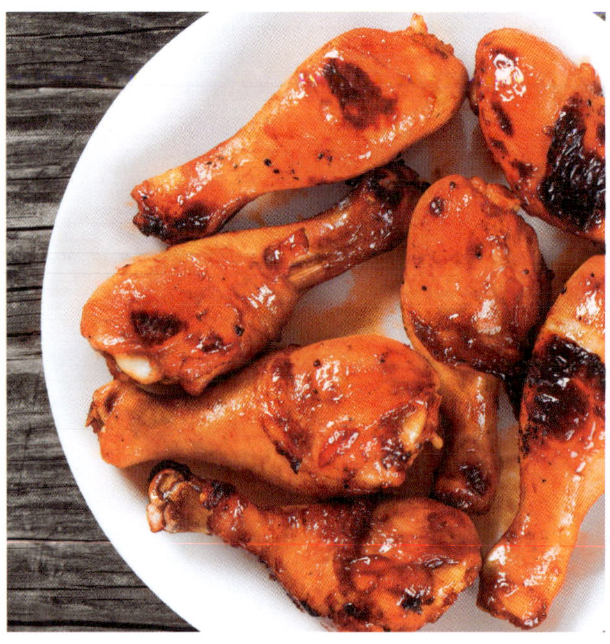

Marinated Chicken Drumsticks

2 tbsps sweet chilli sauce

1 tbsp lime juice

1 tbsp tamari

4 chicken drumsticks

Olive oil cooking spray

Whisk together the sweet chilli sauce, lime juice and tamari in a large bowl.

Add chicken drumsticks and mix to coat thoroughly.

Cover and place in fridge for at least 1 hour or overnight.

Spray air fryer basket with cooking spray. Place chicken drumsticks spaced out in a single layer in air fryer basket. Spray chicken with cooking spray.

Cook for 20-25 minutes at 200°C, turning halfway through, until chicken is cooked through or internal temperature reaches 74°C.

Allow to rest for 5 minutes before serving.

SERVES 2

Chilli Sesame Salmon

2 tbsps Sriracha

2 tbsps soy sauce

1 tbsp sesame oil

1 tbsp rice wine

1 garlic clove, minced

Small piece of ginger, grated

2 salmon fillets

Avocado or olive oil cooking spray

1 tbsp sesame seeds

1 spring onion, chopped

Boiled rice, to serve

1 avocado sliced, to serve

Wilted greens, to serve

In a shallow dish, mix together Sriracha, soy sauce, sesame oil, rice wine, garlic and ginger. Lay the pieces of salmon in the marinade, skin-side up, and set aside for 15 minutes.

Preheat air fryer to 200°C.

Spray air fryer basket with cooking spray.

Place salmon fillets in air fryer, skin-side down. Cook for 6-8 minutes until flesh flakes away easily with a fork.

Sprinkle salmon with sesame seeds and chopped spring onion.

Serve with boiled rice, avocado and wilted greens.

SERVES 2

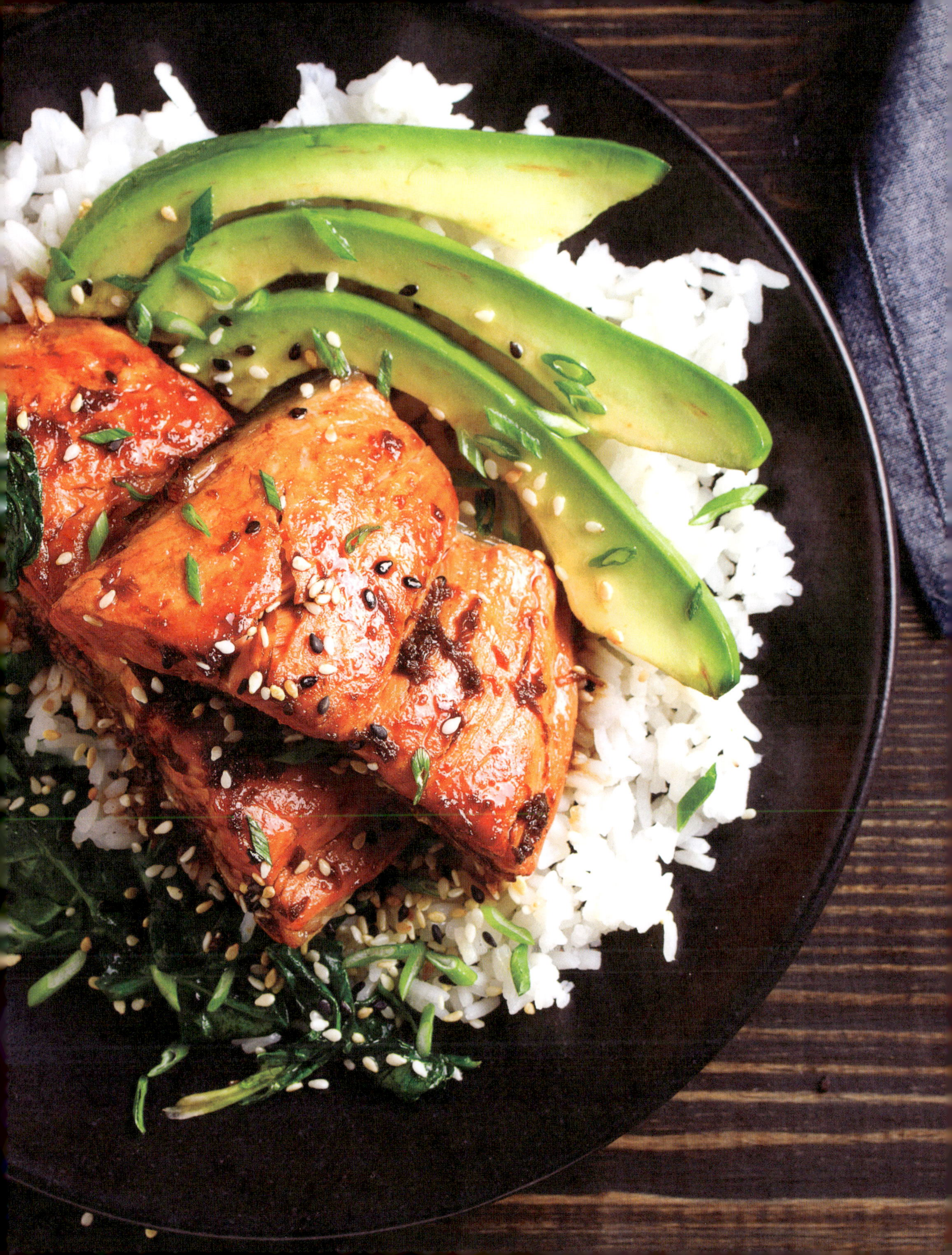

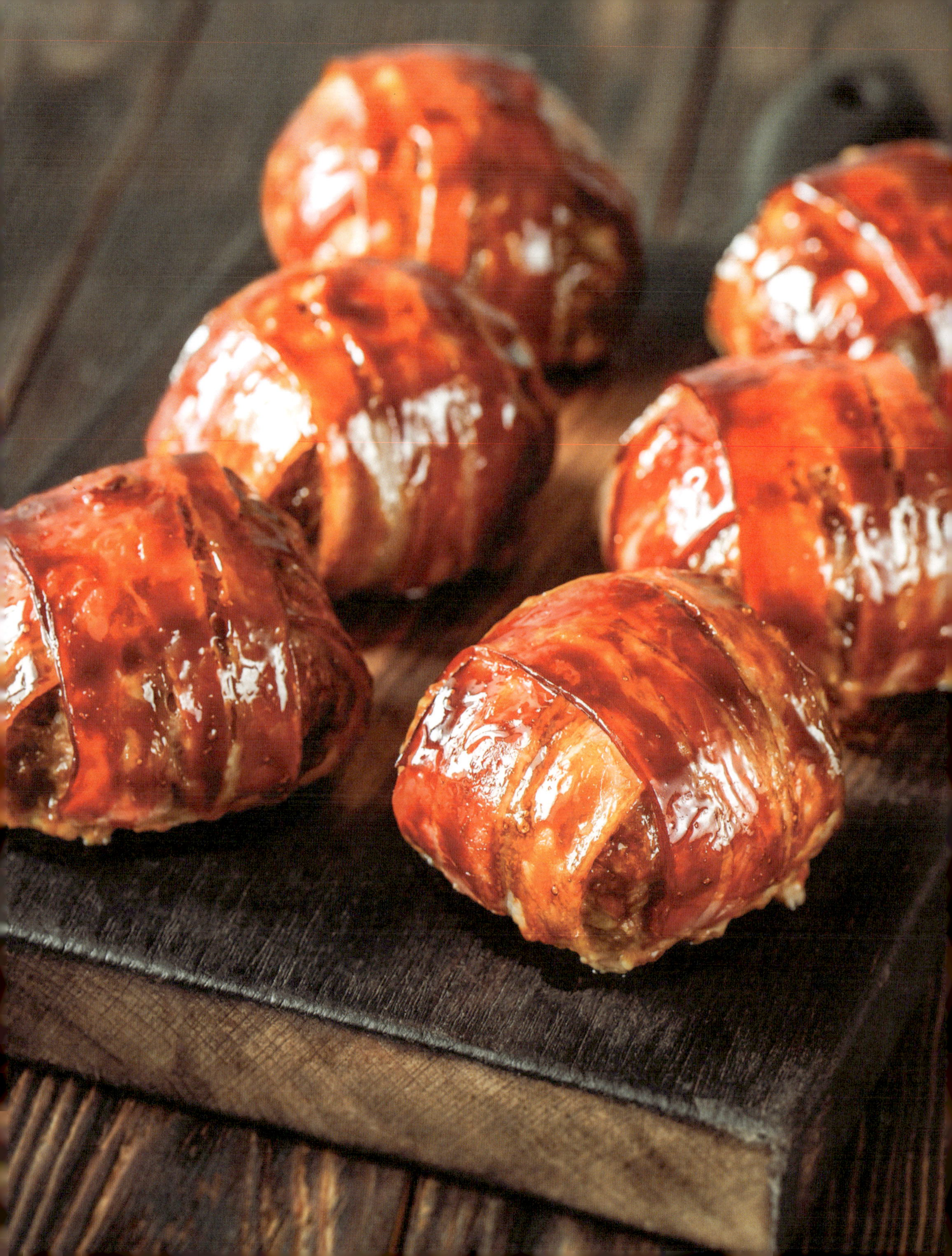

Bacon-Wrapped Cheese Meatballs

500g beef mince

2 cloves garlic, minced

1 tsp onion powder

½ tsp salt

½ tsp cracked pepper

125g Cheddar cheese

8 rashers bacon, cut in half lengthways

Place beef mince in a large bowl with garlic, onion powder, salt and pepper. Use your hands to combine.

Divide the mixture into eight equal portions, then form into balls.

Cut the cheese into eight small cubes. Flatten each meatball and place a cube of cheese in the centre. Form the meat into a ball around the cheese, sealing the cheese in the centre.

Wrap each meatball with a half rasher of bacon. Take another half rasher and make cross with the bacon on top of the meatball and wrap in the other direction.

Preheat air fryer to 175°C.

Arrange meatballs in one layer in the air fryer basket and cook for 28-32 minutes or until the beef is cooked through.

SERVES 2

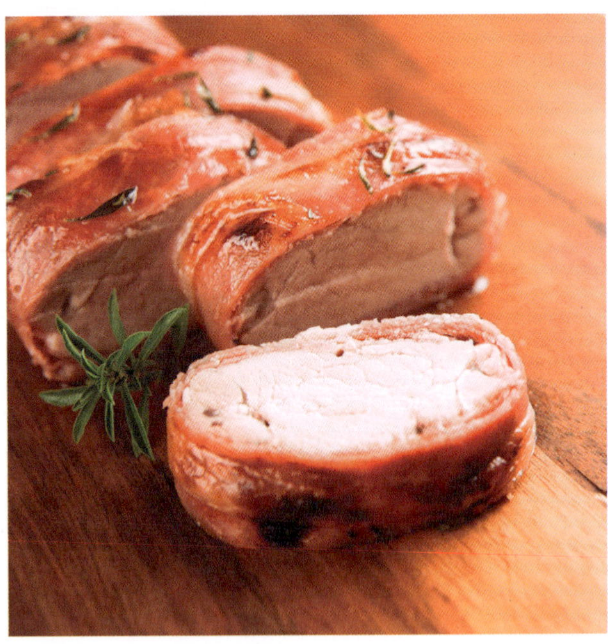

Prosciutto-Wrapped Pork Tenderloin

1kg pork tenderloin

50g prosciutto

¼ cup (65g) Dijon mustard

Salt and pepper to taste

1 sprig of rosemary, leaves picked

Preheat air fryer to 180°C.

Lay out prosciutto slices on a piece of greaseproof paper, overlapping slightly.

Place pork on prosciutto.

Brush pork with Dijon mustard and season with salt and pepper.

Wrap pork tightly in the prosciutto and sprinkle with rosemary leaves.

Place pork into air fryer and cook for 20-30 minutes or until meat is cooked through.

Rest meat for 10 minutes before slicing.

SERVES 4

Piccata

1 tbsp olive oil

1 onion, diced

1 clove garlic, chopped

1 x 400g can tomatoes

Salt and pepper to taste

2 x 200g boneless pork chops

¼ cup (25g) powdered Parmesan

1 tsp garlic powder

2 eggs

½ cup (60g) Cheddar cheese, grated

Steamed broccoli, to serve

Baking pan or cake tin

Heat olive oil in a pan over medium-high heat. Add onion and cook, stirring, for 3-5 minutes until soft and translucent. Add garlic and cook for 1 minute more until fragrant. Add tomatoes, season with salt and pepper, then simmer for 10 minutes stirring occasionally. Set aside and keep warm.

Preheat air fryer to 200°C.

Pound the pork chops with a meat mallet to an even 1cm thickness. Season with salt and pepper.

Place powdered Parmesan and garlic powder in one bowl. Mix together egg and grated cheese in another.

Dip pork chops into powdered Parmesan and coat evenly, then dip into cheese and egg mix.

Place pork chops into baking pan or cake tin and place in air fryer. Spoon over any remaining cheese from egg mix.

Cook for 10-12 minutes, turning halfway through cooking.

Serve with tomato sauce and steamed broccoli.

SERVES 2

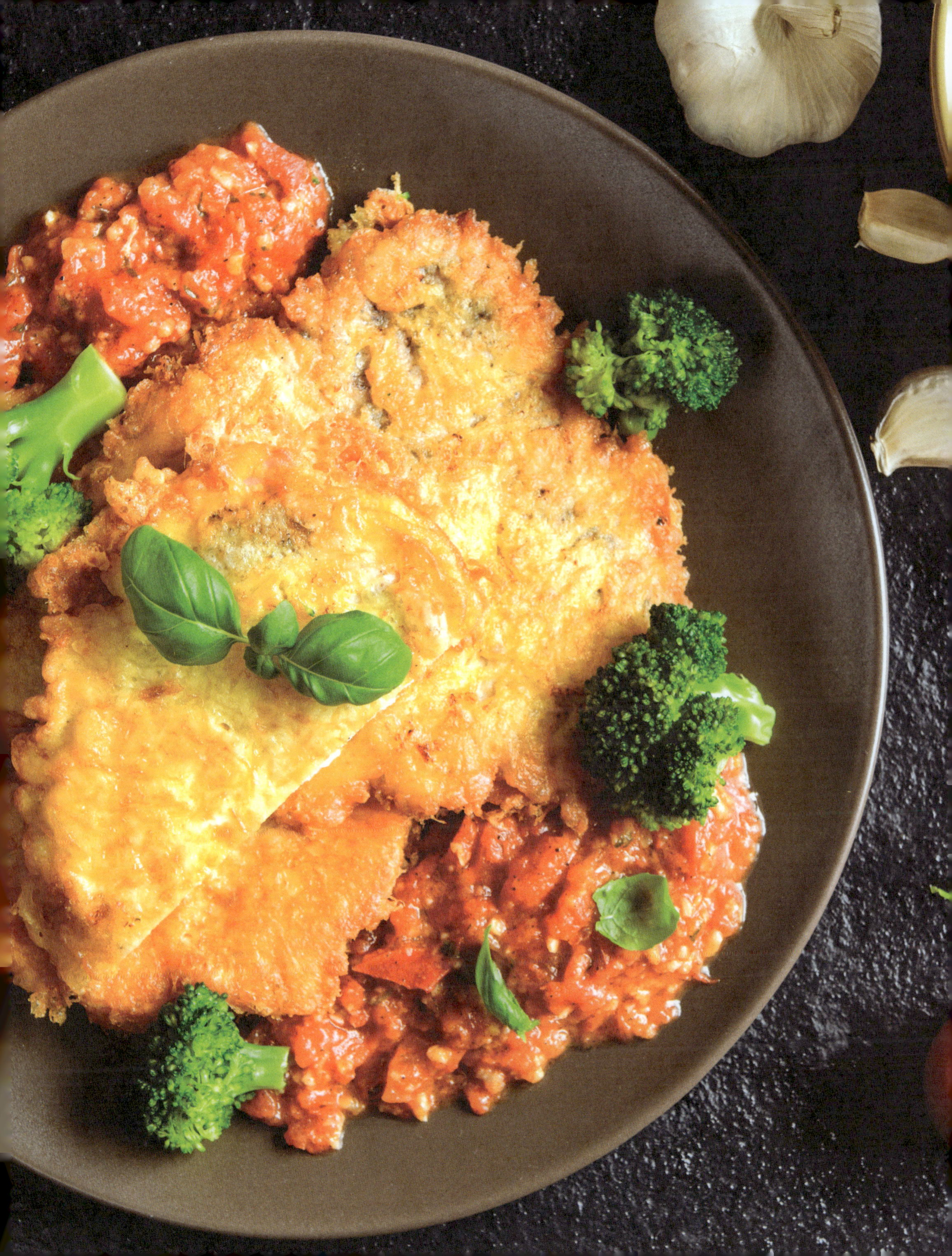

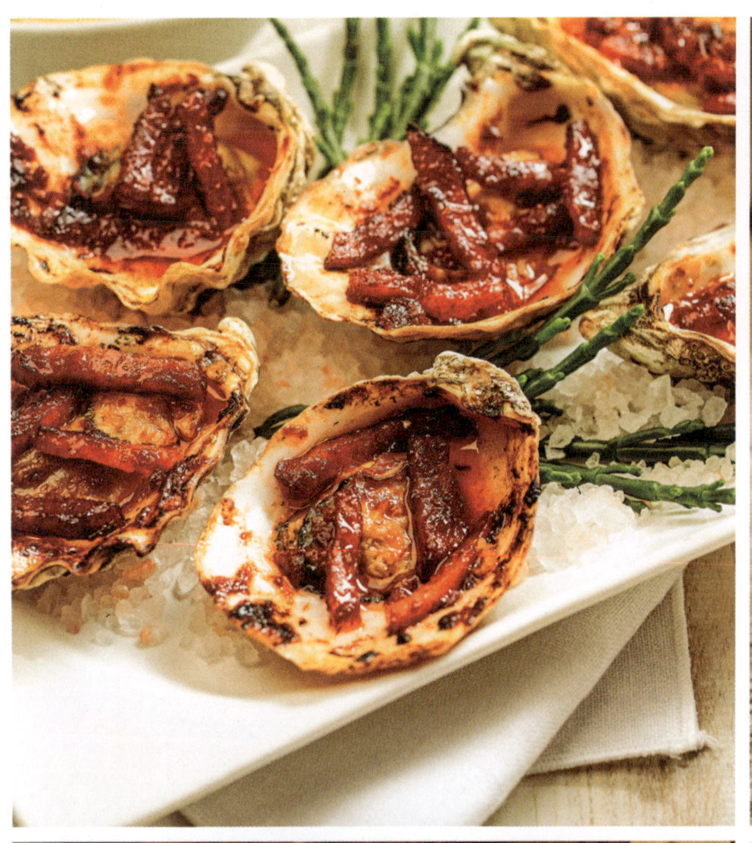
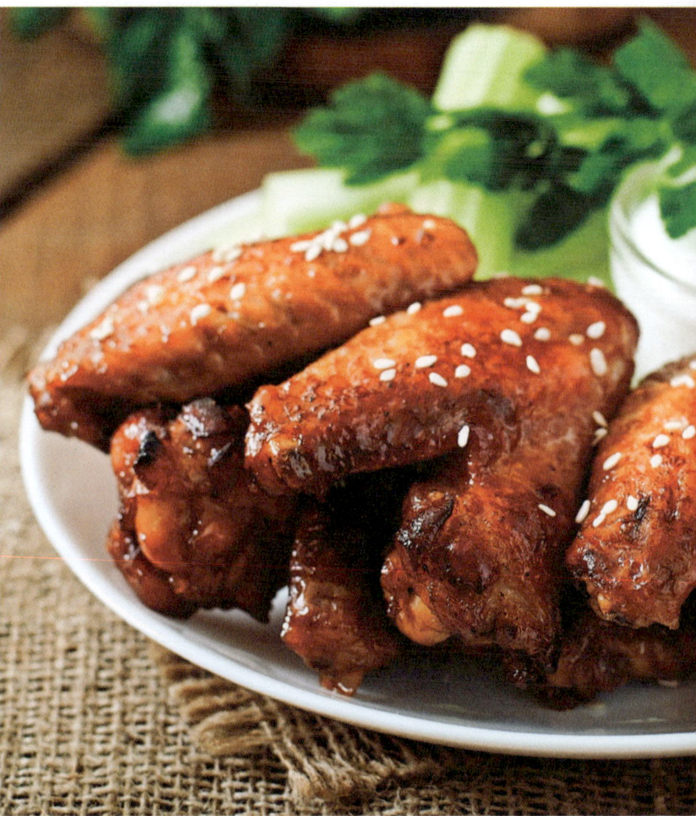
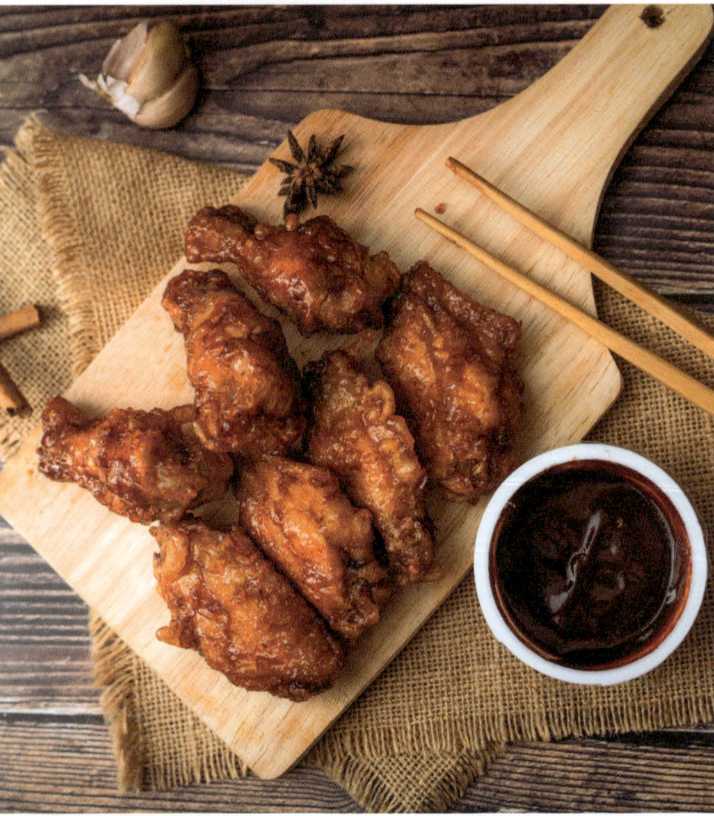
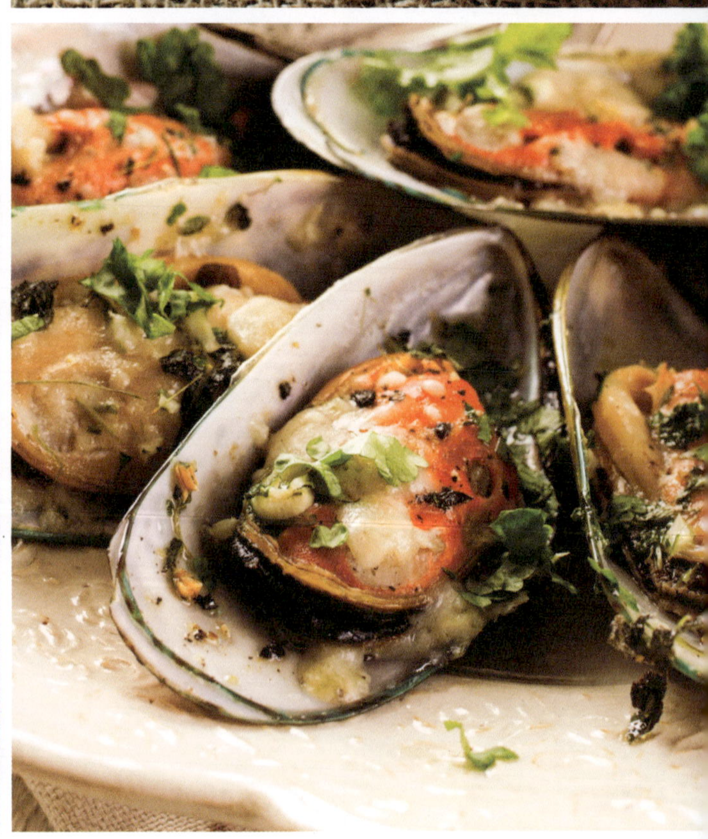

Oysters Kilpatrick

2 rashers thick-cut bacon

2 tbsps butter, melted

4 tbsps balsamic vinegar

2 tbsps Worcestershire sauce

Dash of Tabasco sauce

16 oysters, shucked

Place bacon in air fryer and cook for 6 minutes at 200°C.

Slice into small strips.

Combine butter, vinegar, Worcestershire sauce and Tabasco sauce in a small bowl.

Pour ½ tablespoon of sauce over each oyster and top with bacon strips. Pour over any remaining sauce.

Place oysters in air fryer basket and cook for 10 minutes at 180°C.

SERVES 4

Barbecue Chicken Wings

1kg chicken wings

1 tsp garlic powder

1 tsp smoked paprika

1 tsp olive oil

Salt and pepper to taste

2 tbsps tomato ketchup

1 tsp brown sugar

½ tsp white wine vinegar

½ tsp Worcestershire sauce

2 tsps sweet paprika

In a large bowl combine chicken wings with garlic powder, smoked paprika, oil, salt and pepper. Mix well.

Preheat air fryer to 180°C. Working in batches, arrange chicken wings in a single layer in air fryer basket. Cook for 12 min. Flip wings and cook further for 5 min.

Mix together remaining ingredients. Brush over chicken wings and cook for an additional 2 min.

SERVES 4

Korean Chicken Drumsticks

8 chicken drumsticks or thighs

¼ cup (75g) gochujang (Korean chilli paste)

2 tbsps tamari

2 tbsps mirin

2 tbsps brown sugar

2 tbsps sesame oil

2 cloves garlic, minced

Combine the gochujang, tamari, mirin, brown sugar, sesame oil and garlic in a large bowl.

Add the chicken and toss to coat. Cover and refrigerate for at least 1 hour.

Preheat air fryer to 200°C.

Arrange chicken in one layer in air fryer basket. Cook in batches or use a double layer accessory if necessary.

Cook for 15 minutes, then flip over and baste with remaining marinade. Cook for a further 10-12 minutes until cooked through. Allow to rest for 5 minutes before serving.

SERVES 4

Baked Mussels with Parmesan and Parsley

25g butter, softened

2 tsps lemon juice

1 clove garlic, minced

2 tbsps fresh parsley, chopped

10 mussels on the half shell

½ cup (50g) Parmesan cheese, grated

Preheat air fryer to 180°C.

Combine the butter, lemon juice, garlic and parsley in a small bowl. Mix thoroughly.

Top each mussel with some butter-garlic mixture.

Place in a single layer in the air fryer basket. Cook for 7 minutes. Sprinkle with cheese and cook for a further 3 minutes or until cheese is melted.

SERVES 2

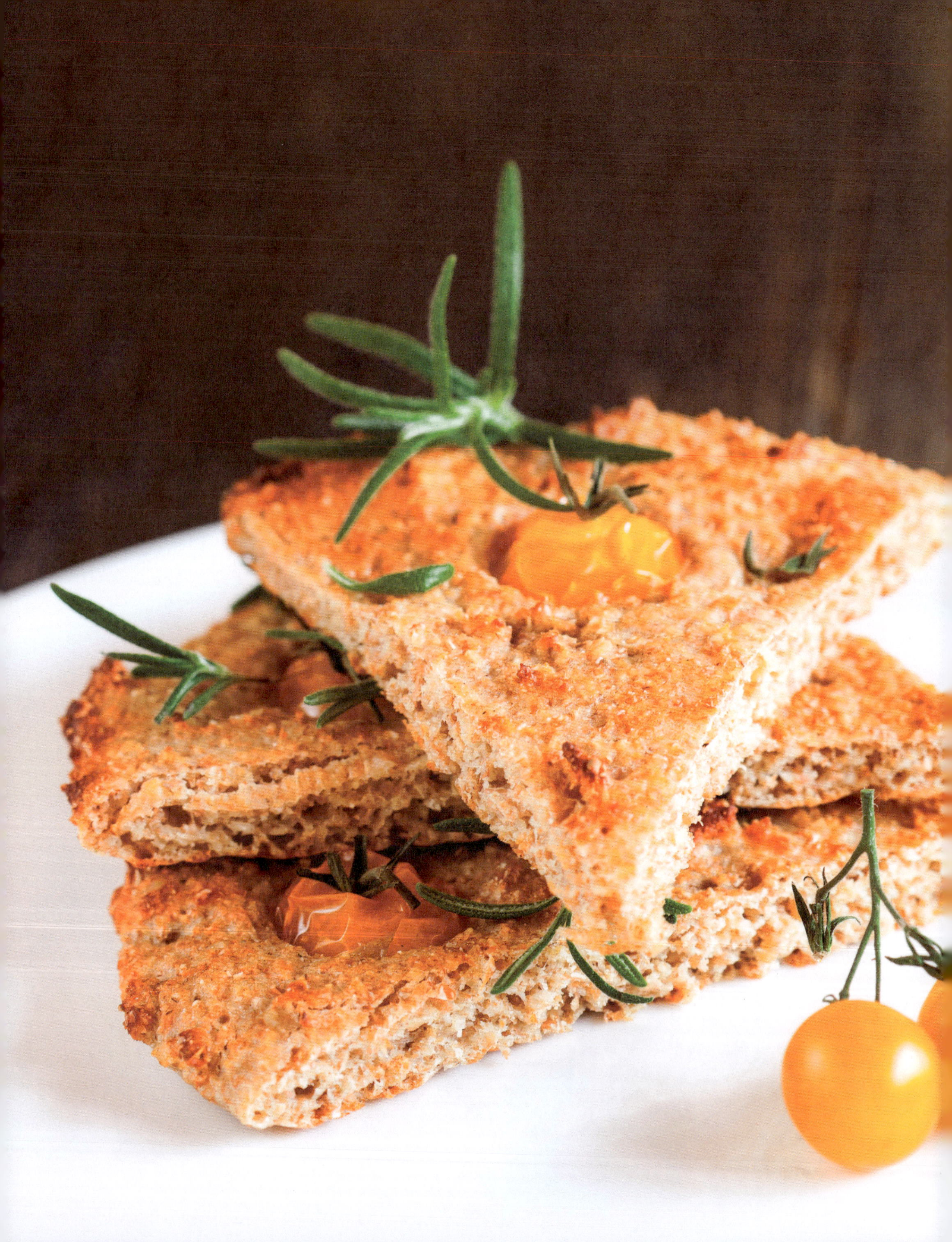

Keto Rosemary Focaccia

1½ tsps active dry yeast

1½ tsps maple syrup or honey (this is to feed the yeast, no sugar will remain post cooking)

¼ cup (55ml) lukewarm water

¾ cup (100g) almond meal

¼ cup (20g) finely ground psyllium husk powder

2 tsps ground flaxseed

1 tsp baking powder

⅛ tsp salt

1 egg

1 egg white

1 tbsp olive oil + more for greasing

1½ tsps apple cider vinegar

8 yellow cherry tomatoes

8 rosemary sprigs

½ tsp salt flakes

Cake tin

Mix together yeast and maple syrup in a large bowl. Pour lukewarm water over yeast mixture. Cover bowl with a tea towel and rest for 7 minutes until mixture is bubbly.

Place almond meal, psyllium husk, flaxseed, baking powder and salt a medium bowl. Whisk together, then set aside.

Add egg, egg white, olive oil and vinegar to the yeast mixture and whisk until light and frothy. Add in flour mixture and stir to incorporate.

Line cake tin with greaseproof paper and grease with olive oil. Place the dough in the tin and spread out evenly.

With wet fingers make indentations in the dough. In some place cherry tomatoes, in others rosemary sprigs, and in others some salt flakes.

Cover with a tea bowl and place in a warm draught-free place for 40 minutes.

Preheat air fryer to 160°C.

Place cake tin in air fryer and cook for 8 minutes. Cover with a dome of foil then continue to cook for a further 12-15 minutes until golden brown.

Allow the focaccia to cool before cutting.

SERVES 4

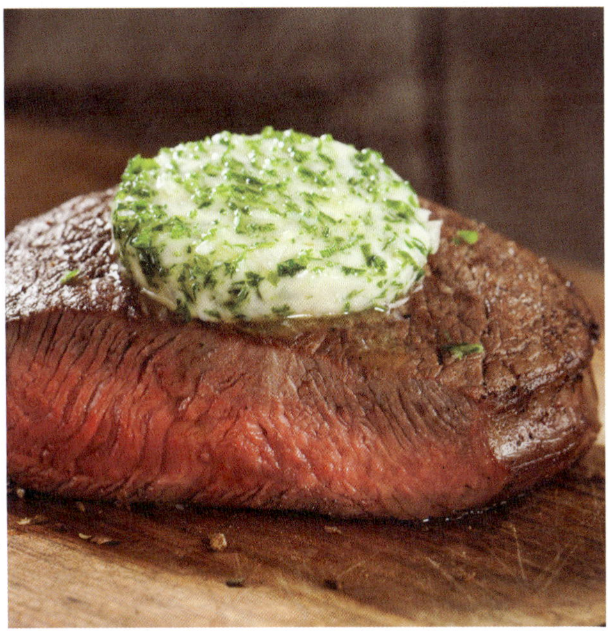

Steak with Herb Butter

1 x 500g sirloin steak, about 3cm thick

Salt and pepper to taste

4 tbsps unsalted butter, room temperature

2 tbsps fresh parsley, finely chopped

1 small clove garlic, minced

Allow the steak to sit at room temperature for 30 minutes before cooking.

Preheat air fryer to 200°C. Generously season steak on both sides with salt and pepper.

Place steak in the centre of air fryer basket. Cook for 10 minutes for medium-rare, 12 minutes for medium and 14 minutes for medium-well. Transfer the steak to a cutting board and allow to rest for about 10 minutes.

Meanwhile, mash together the butter, parsley and garlic in a small bowl until combined. Slice the steak against the grain. Top with the garlic-herb butter.

SERVES 2

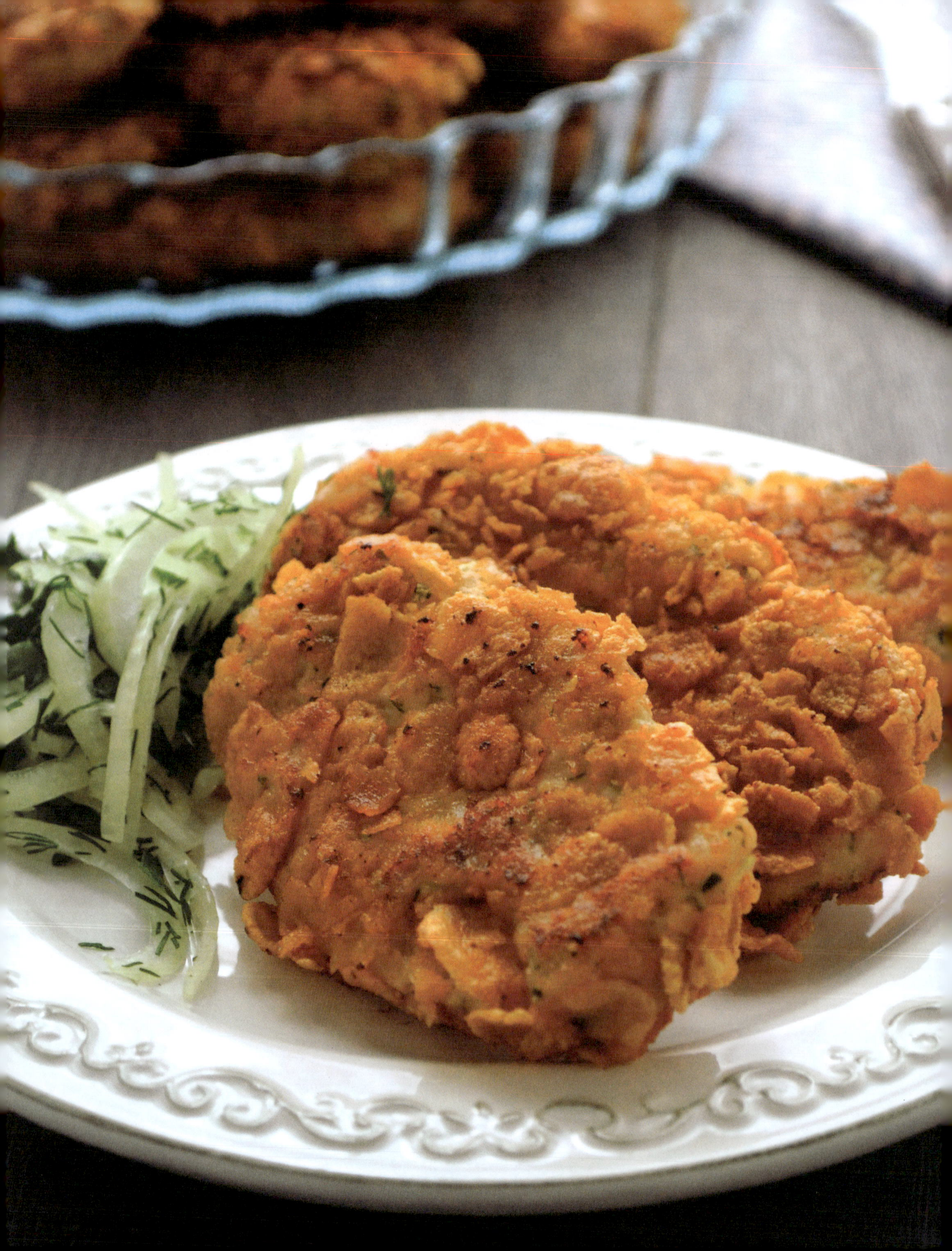

Gluten-Free

Sesame-Crusted Chicken

500g chicken breasts

2 tsps sesame oil

3 tsps tamari

½ cup (80g) toasted sesame seeds

½ tsp salt

¼ tsp pepper

Olive oil cooking spray

Cut the chicken breasts into pieces approximately 10cm long x 5cm wide.

Combine the sesame oil and tamari in one bowl and place the sesame seeds and salt and pepper in another.

Place each chicken piece into the bowl with the oil and tamari, flip over to coat both sides. Next place chicken into the bowl with the sesame seed mixture and gently press with your fingers to coat well.

Preheat the air fryer to 200°C.

Spray air fryer basket with cooking spray. Place chicken in the basket ensuring there is space between each piece (cook in batches or use a double layer accessory if necessary). Spray with cooking spray.

Cook for 5 minutes then flip and spray once more. Cook for a further 5-6 minutes until cooked through, crispy and golden.

SERVES 4

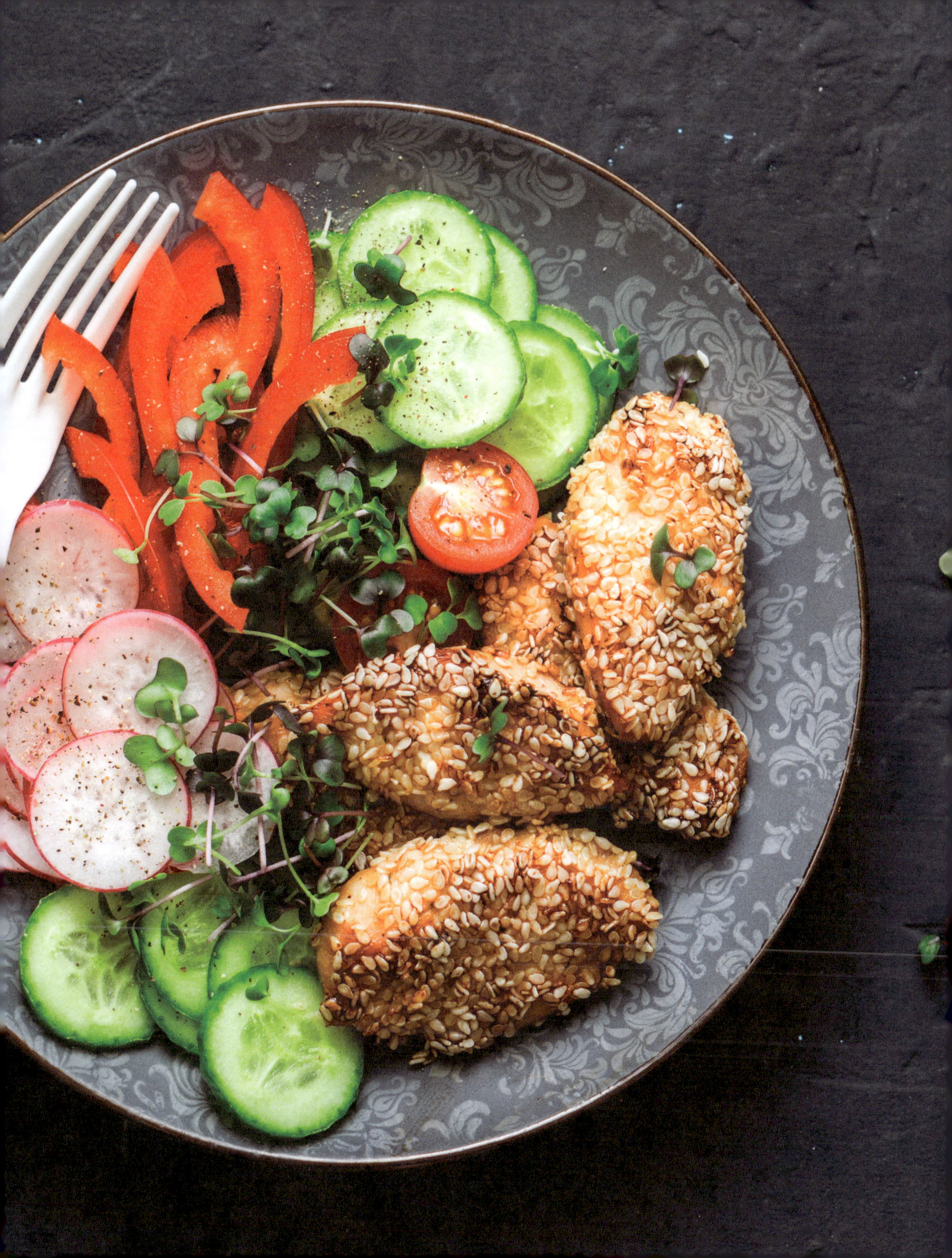

Jerk Chicken Wings

750g chicken wings

1 tsp brown sugar

½ tsp dried thyme

½ tsp garlic powder

½ tsp ground allspice

⅛ tsp cinnamon

Pinch of cayenne pepper (optional)

1 tbsp gluten-free cornflour

2 tbsps olive oil

Salt and pepper to taste

Ranch dressing, to serve

Place chicken wings in a large bowl with sugar, herbs, spices, cornflour, oil, salt and pepper. Rub well to coat.

Arrange in air fryer basket, overlapping slightly.

Cook for 20 minutes at 190°C, turning halfway through.

Serve with Ranch Dressing.

SERVES 2

Sun-Dried Tomato Stuffed Chicken

2 chicken breasts

Salt and pepper to taste

2 tsps dried oregano

1½ cups (80g) sun-dried tomatoes in oil

100g fresh mozzarella, diced

Season chicken breasts with salt, pepper and dried oregano.

Cut a deep slit lengthways into each breast. Place a layer of sun-dried tomato inside the chicken, top with mozzarella then finish with more sun-dried tomato.

Use toothpicks to hold the chicken together.

Drizzle oil from sun-dried tomatoes over chicken.

Place chicken in air fryer basket.

Cook at 180°C for 20-22 minutes, turning halfway through cooking.

Allow to rest for 5 minutes before removing toothpicks and slicing.

SERVES 2

Mac and Cheese

350g gluten-free macaroni

4 tbsps olive oil

4 cloves garlic, minced

4½ tbsps arrowroot powder

2 cups (500ml) milk

Salt and pepper to taste

5 tbsps nutritional yeast + more to taste

½ cup (50g) Parmesan cheese, grated + more to serve

Baking pan

Cook pasta in a large pan of boiling water until al dente.

Heat oil in a pan over medium heat. Add garlic and cook for 1 minute until fragrant. Immediately add arrowroot and whisk for 1 minute.

Slowly pour in milk while whisking, then cook for 2 minutes, stirring constantly. Add nutritional yeast and cheese. Cook for a further 2 minutes, stirring.

Transfer pasta and sauce to baking pan. Place in air fryer and cook for 10 minutes at 170°C. Sprinkle with Parmesan and thyme leaves to serve.

SERVES 4

Gluten-Free Meatballs

500g beef mince

1 cup (100g) Parmesan cheese, grated

¼ cup (60ml) milk

2 cloves garlic, minced

2 tsps Italian seasoning

Salt and pepper to taste

Homemade or store-bought pasta sauce, to serve

Combine mince, cheese, milk, garlic and herbs in a bowl. Season with salt and pepper and mix well. Roll into golf-ball-sized meatballs.

Place meatballs into air fryer basket in a single layer, making sure they are spaced apart.

Air fry the meatballs at 190°C for 15 minutes.

Serve meatballs with pasta sauce.

SERVES 4

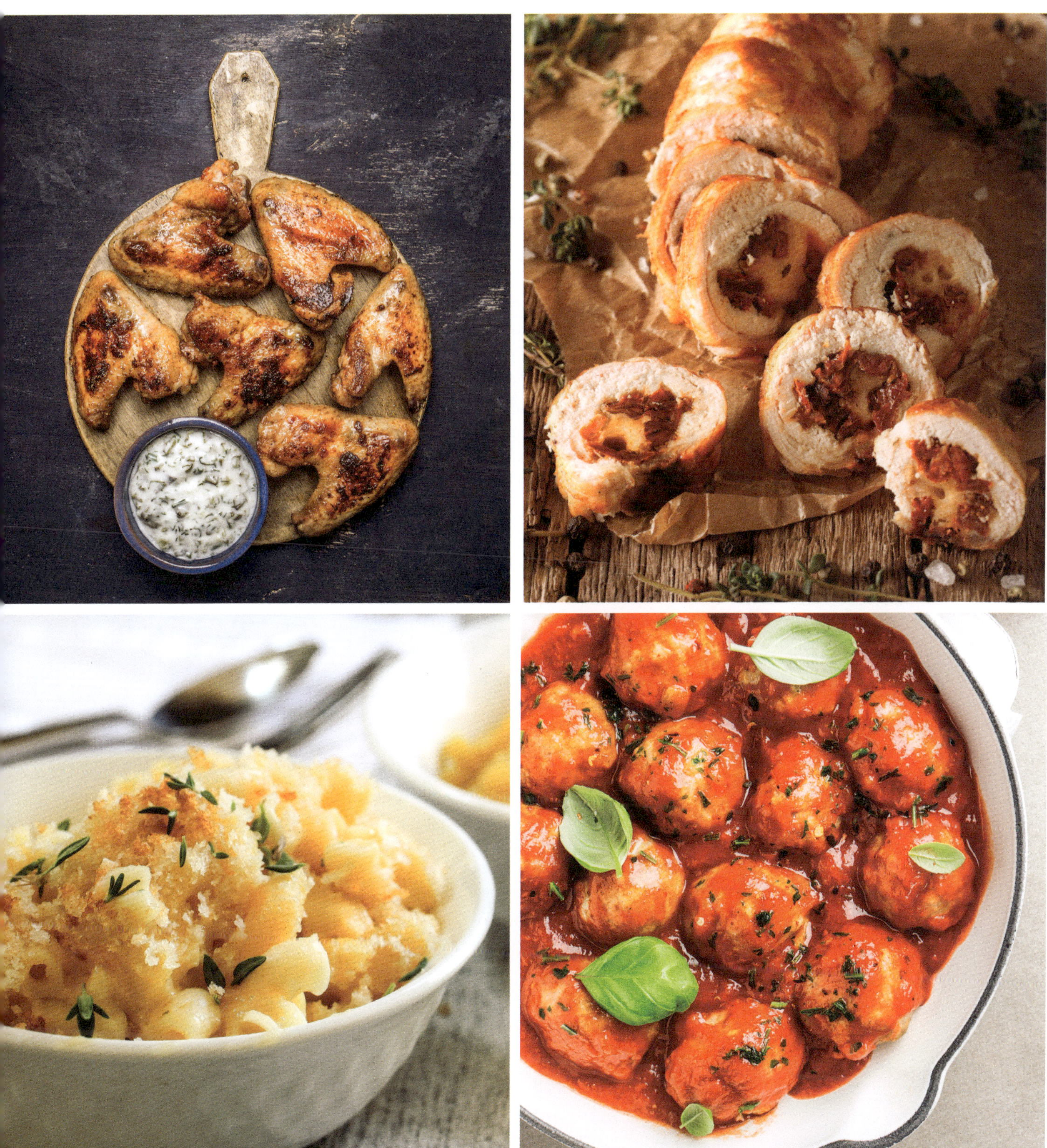

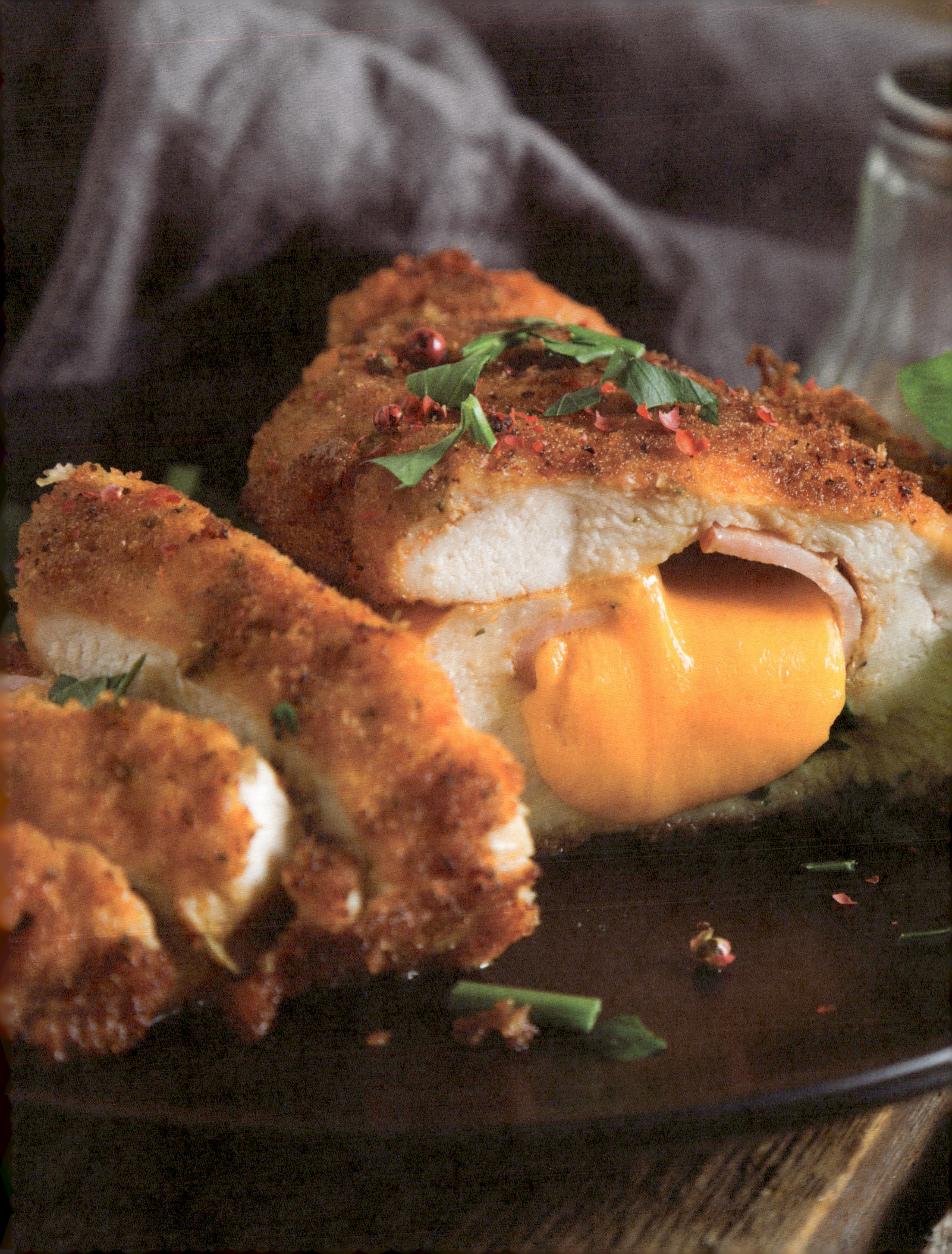

Gluten-Free Chicken Cordon Bleu

500g chicken breast, cut into 4 even pieces

4 slices ham

4 slices Jarlsberg cheese

1 egg, beaten

¼ cup (30g) gluten-free breadcrumbs

¼ cup (25g) Parmesan cheese, grated

½ tsp garlic powder

½ tsp onion powder

½ tsp ground paprika

Salt and pepper to taste

Cooking spray

Preheat air fryer to 200°C.

Use a meat mallet to pound each piece of chicken to 1cm thick.

Place a slice of ham then a slice of cheese on top of each piece of chicken.

Carefully roll up chicken and place seam side down.

Place the egg in one bowl and combine the breadcrumbs, Parmesan and seasonings in another bowl. Dip the chicken first into the beaten egg and then into the breadcrumb mixture and gently press to coat evenly.

Spray air fryer basket with cooking spray. Place chicken seam side down into air fryer basket. Spray with cooking spray. Cook for 12 -15 minutes until crisp and golden brown.

SERVES 4

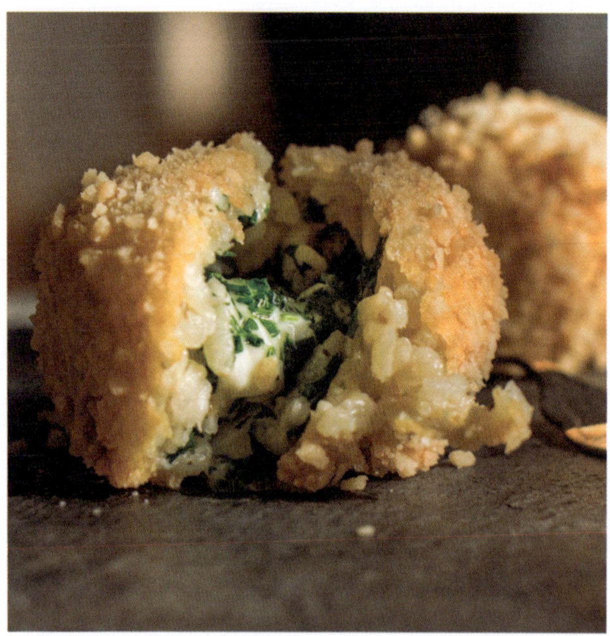

Gluten-Free Stuffed Arancini

1 tbsp olive oil

1 onion, finely diced

1 cup (155g) Arborio rice

4 cups (1L) vegetable stock

Salt and pepper to taste

1 cup (100g) Parmesan cheese

1½ cups (185g) gluten-free breadcrumbs

2 eggs, beaten

75g mozzarella, cut into 1cm cubes

¼ cup (60g) pesto

Heat oil in a large pan over medium heat. Add onions and saute until soft. Add rice and fry for 1 minute.

Add stock, ½ cup at a time, stirring until liquid is absorbed. Continue until all liquid is absorbed and rice is soft. Season with salt and pepper. Stir in Parmesan.

Pour risotto into a large dish. Refrigerate for 2 hours.

In a small bowl, place the breadcrumbs. In another bowl, place the beaten eggs.

Remove chilled rice from the fridge. Shape into 3cm balls with a piece of mozzarella and a dollop of pesto in the centre encased by the rice. Dip each ball into eggs then into breadcrumbs. Refrigerate for 45 minutes.

Place into air fryer in small batches. Cook at 200°C for 10 minutes shaking halfway through.

SERVES 4

Stuffed Capsicums

1 tsp olive oil

1 onion, diced

250g beef mince

½ tsp salt

¼ tsp pepper

¼ tsp garlic powder

1 cup (165g) cooked rice

1 cup (225g) passata

2 large or 3 small capsicums, halved lengthways

¾ cup (90g) mozzarella cheese, grated

Heat the olive oil in a large pan over medium heat.

Add the onion and cook, stirring, for 3-5 minutes until soft and translucent. Add beef mince, salt, pepper and garlic powder. Cook, stirring occasionally, for about 10 minutes until beef is browned. Stir in rice and passata until well combined. Remove from the heat.

Place capsicum halves into the air fryer basket. Fill each with the beef and rice mixture.

Cook for 15 minutes at 180°C.

Sprinkle over cheese and cook for a further 2 minutes.

SERVES 2

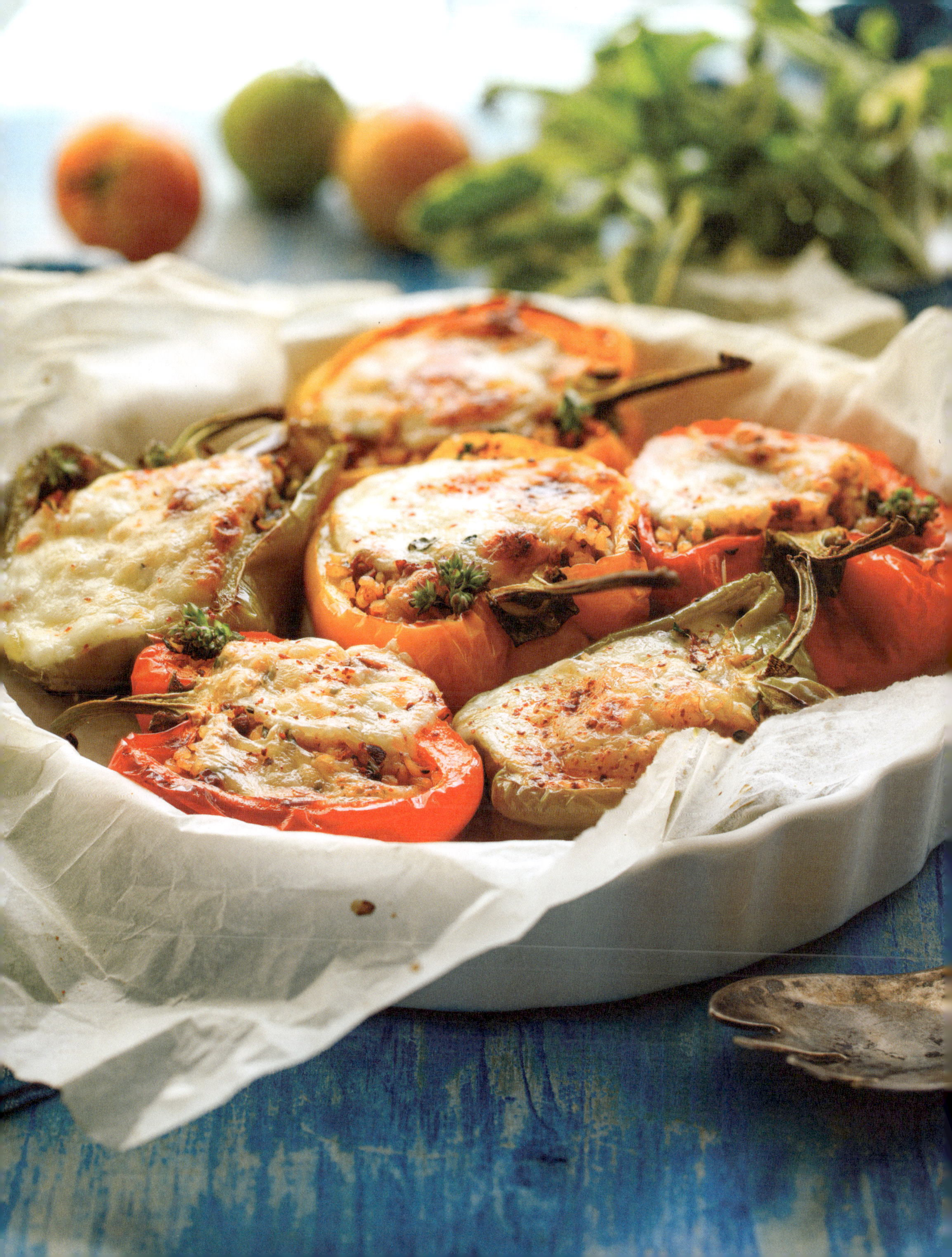

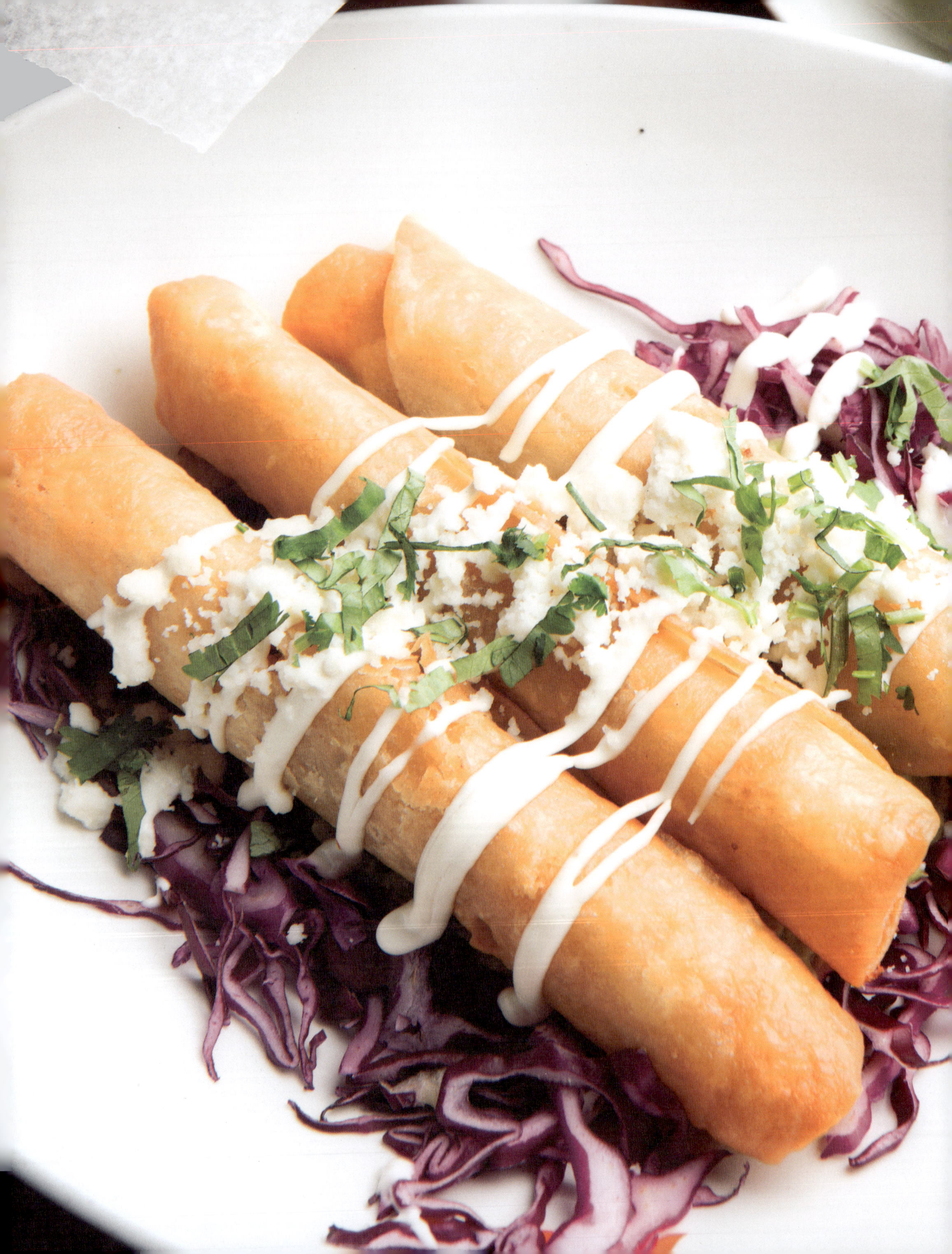

Chicken Taquitos

1 tbsp olive oil

½ onion, diced

2 cloves garlic, minced

1 tbsp dried oregano

1 tsp ground cumin

½ tsp smoked paprika

600g cooked chicken, shredded

¼ cup (60g) passata

Salt and pepper to taste

12 corn tortillas

½ cup (60g) Cheddar cheese, grated

Olive oil cooking spray

½ cup (25g) red cabbage, finely sliced, to serve

2 tbsps sour cream, to serve

1 tbsp fresh coriander, chopped, to serve

Heat the oil in a large frying pan over medium-high heat. Add the onion and fry for 3-5 minutes until soft and translucent. Add the garlic, oregano, cumin and paprika. Fry for 1 minute until fragrant. Add the chicken and passata. Season with salt and pepper and cook for 2-3 minutes until chicken is heated through.

Spoon small amounts of chicken mix along the centre of the tortillas. Top with cheese and roll into taquitos. Secure with a toothpick. Repeat with the remaining tortillas.

Preheat air fryer to 200°C. Spray the basket with cooking spray.

Place four taquitos at a time into the air fryer basket. Spray with cooking spray. Cook for 5-6 minutes until golden brown and crispy. Repeat with the remaining taquitos.

Remove toothpicks and place cooked taquitos on a bed of shredded cabbage, drizzle with sour cream and sprinkle with chopped coriander to serve.

SERVES 4

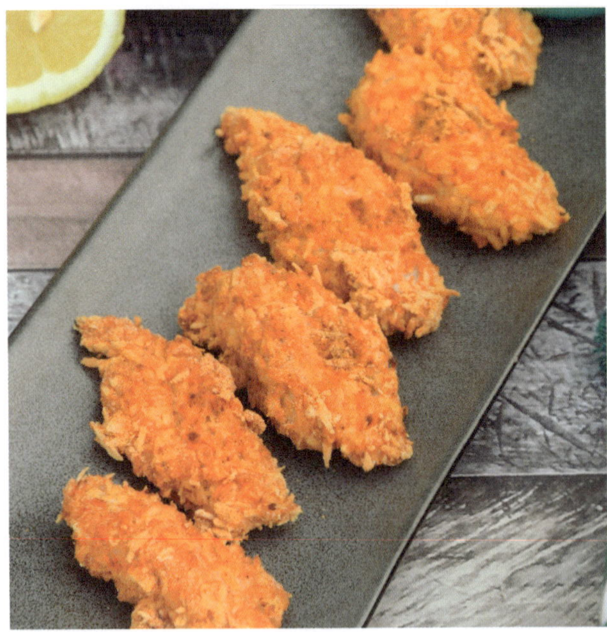

Coconut-Crusted Chicken Tenders

½ cup (75g) gluten-free cornflour

¼ tsp salt

⅛ tsp pepper

1 tsp cayenne pepper {optional}

3 large eggs, beaten

3 cups (270g) shredded coconut

750g chicken tenders

Avocado oil cooking spray

Preheat air fryer to 180°C.

In one bowl mix together cornflour, salt, pepper and cayenne pepper.

In another bowl, pour the beaten eggs.

In a third bowl add shredded coconut.

Take each piece of chicken and coat first in cornflour mixture, then dip in egg and finally dip in coconut. Use your fingers to press gently to coat well.

Spray air fryer basket with cooking spray. Place chicken in basket and spray top with cooking spray.

Cook for 12-14 minutes, flipping halfway through, until cooked through, golden brown and crunchy.

SERVES 4

Salmon and Quinoa Patties

2 cups (370g) cooked quinoa

350g cooked salmon, flaked apart

1 spring onion, sliced

2 tbsps fresh parsley, chopped

¼ cup (60g) mayonnaise

2 tsps Dijon mustard

1 egg, beaten

2 tsps fresh lime juice + extra for serving

Salt and pepper to taste

Olive oil or avocado oil cooking spray

Combine quinoa, salmon, spring onions, parsley, mayonnaise, mustard, egg and lime juice. Season to taste with salt and pepper. Form into eight patties.

Preheat air fryer to 180°C.

Spray basket and patties with cooking spray.

Cook patties for 6-8 minutes, flipping halfway through, until crisp and golden brown.

SERVES 4

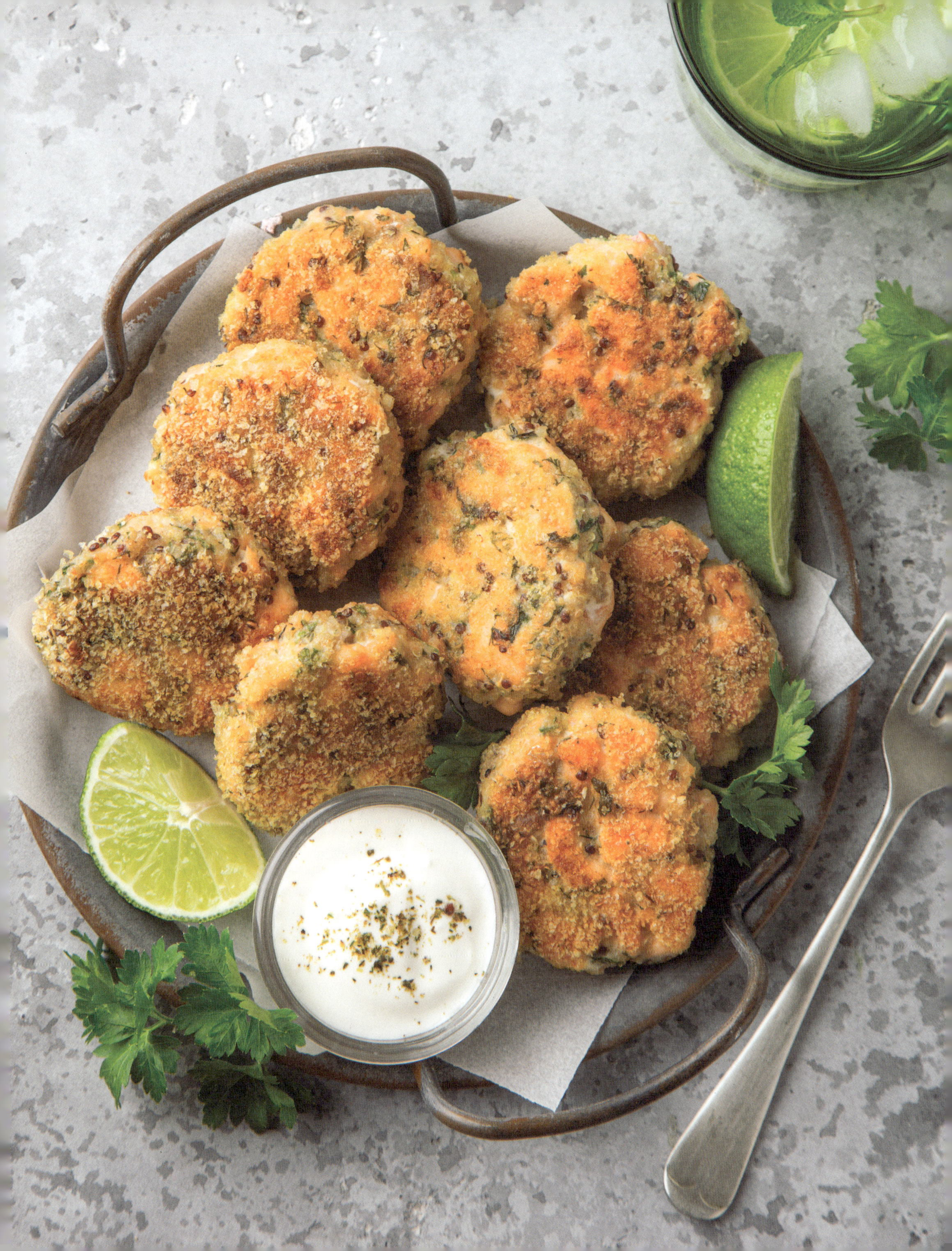

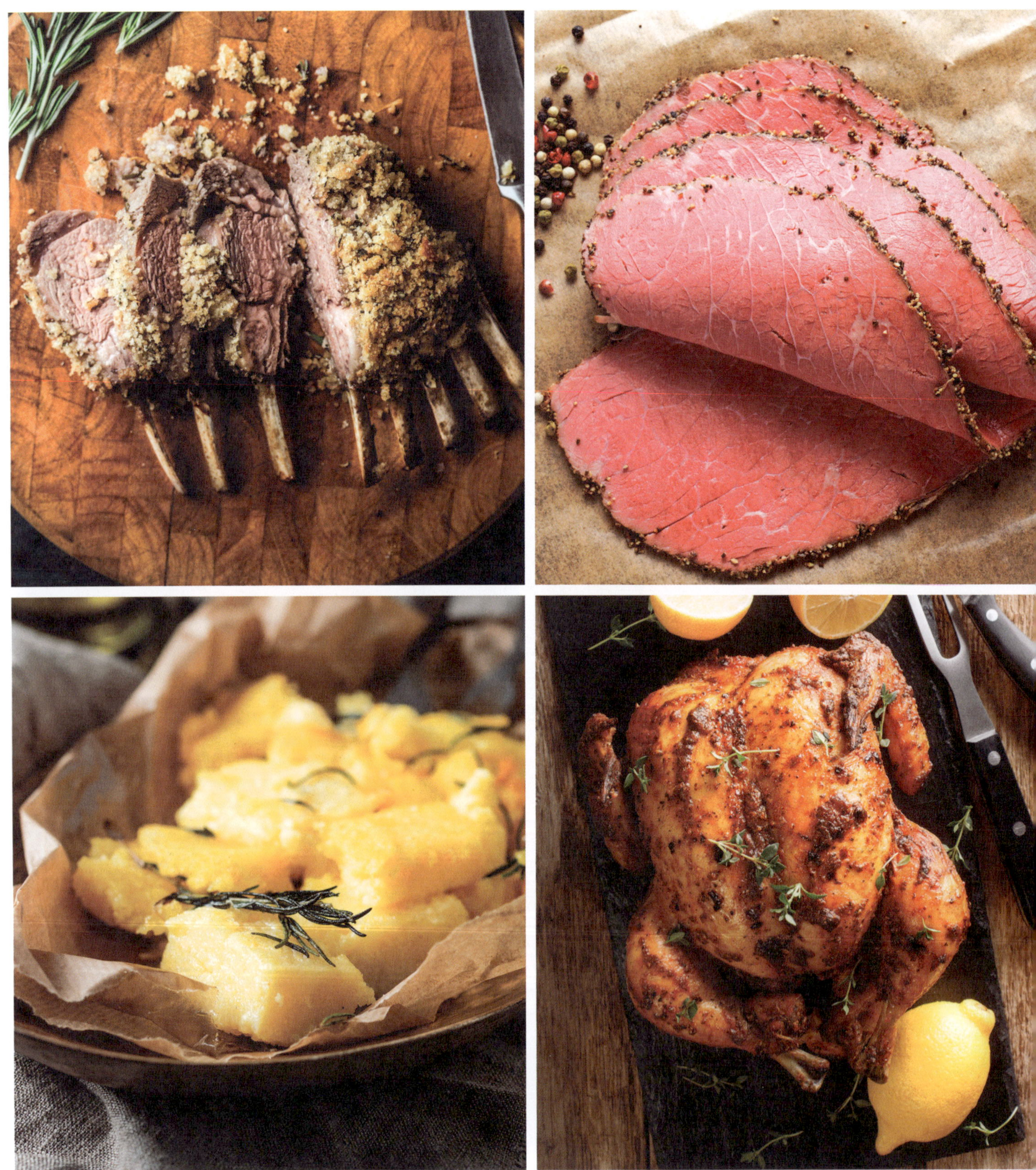

Rack of Lamb with Herb Crust

1 rack of lamb (4 lamb cutlets per person)

Salt and pepper to taste

½ cup (60g) macadamia nuts

¼ cup (10g) parsley, chopped

1 tbsp rosemary, chopped

1 large clove of garlic, peeled

2 tbsps olive oil

½ tsp salt

Season lamb with salt and pepper.

Place nuts, parsley, rosemary, garlic, olive oil and salt into a food processor. Process into a thick, sticky paste.

Press paste with your fingers onto meatier side of rack.

Preheat air fryer to 100°C.

Place lamb in air fryer basket. Cook for 25 minutes. Increase temp to 200°C and cook for a further 25 minutes.

Rest for 10 minutes before slicing and serving.

SERVES 2

Corned Beef

½ cup (80g) brown sugar

¼ cup (65g) Dijon mustard

1 tbsp apple cider vinegar

1 tbsp crushed mixed peppercorns

1.2kg beef silverside

Mix together brown sugar, Dijon mustard, apple cider vinegar and crushed peppercorns.

Rub the mixture all over the beef.

Place beef in air fryer basket.

Cook for 30 minutes at 170°C. Carefully turn the beef over and cook for another 30 minutes. Turn over once more and cook at 160°C for 10 minutes.

Allow to rest for 5-10 minutes before slicing.

SERVES 6

Polenta Fries

3 cups (750ml) water

1 cup (160g) polenta

3 tbsps olive oil

Salt and pepper to taste

Line a baking tray with greaseproof paper.

Bring water to a boil. Reduce to a simmer. Pour in polenta steadily, stirring constantly. Continue to stir for 20-30 minutes until polenta is thickened. It should come away from sides of the pan, and be able to support a spoon.

Spoon polenta onto baking tray and spread out evenly with a spatula. Chill for at least 2 hours or overnight to set.

Cut polenta into 5cm-long wedges. Brush with olive oil and sprinkle with salt. Place in air fryer basket, overlapping slightly if needed.

Cook for 10 minutes at 180°C. Use a spatula to flip polenta then cook for a further 10-15 minutes, shaking occasionally, until crispy. Season to taste before serving.

SERVES 4

Harissa Spiced Chicken

1 x 1.3kg whole chicken

Salt and pepper to taste

2 tbsps harissa paste

2 tbsps olive oil

1 tsp ground cumin

Olive oil cooking spray

Preheat air fryer to 180°C.

Season the chicken with salt and pepper.

In a small bowl whisk together the harissa paste, olive oil and cumin. Rub all over the chicken skin.

Spray the air fryer basket with cooking spray. Place the chicken in the basket, breast side down. Cook for 30 minutes.

Using tongs carefully flip the chicken and continue to cook for 20-25 minutes until the juices run clear and the internal temperature reaches 74°C.

Allow the chicken to rest for a few minutes before serving.

SERVES 4

Shepherd's Pie

500g potatoes, peeled and quartered

½ cup (125ml) milk

2 tbsps butter

1 onion, diced

2 carrots, diced

1 tsp melted ghee or olive oil

500g lamb mince

250g mushrooms, diced

2 cloves garlic, minced

2 tbsps tomato paste

1 tbsp Worcestershire sauce

1⅔ cups (400ml) lamb or chicken stock

½ cup (60g) Cheddar cheese, grated

Baking pan

6 ramekins

Preheat air fryer to 180°C.

Bring potatoes to boil in a pan of salted water over medium-high heat. Cook for 15-20 minutes or until soft.

Drain the cooked potatoes and add milk and butter. Mash until smooth. Set aside.

Place onion and carrot in baking pan. Drizzle with ghee or oil and toss to coat. Place pan in air fryer and cook for 5 minutes, stirring halfway through cooking.

Add mince, mushrooms and garlic to the pan. Break up mince with a fork. Cook for 5 minutes to brown the meat.

In a medium bowl or jug, mix together tomato paste, Worcestershire sauce and stock. Add stock mixture to the air fryer pan. Stir well. Cook for 30-35 minutes, stirring about every 5 minutes.

Spoon meat and veggie mix into six ramekins. Divide mashed potato between each dish and top each with a little grated cheese.

Place each dish into the air fryer basket and cook for 8 minutes, or until cheese is melted and golden.

SERVES 6

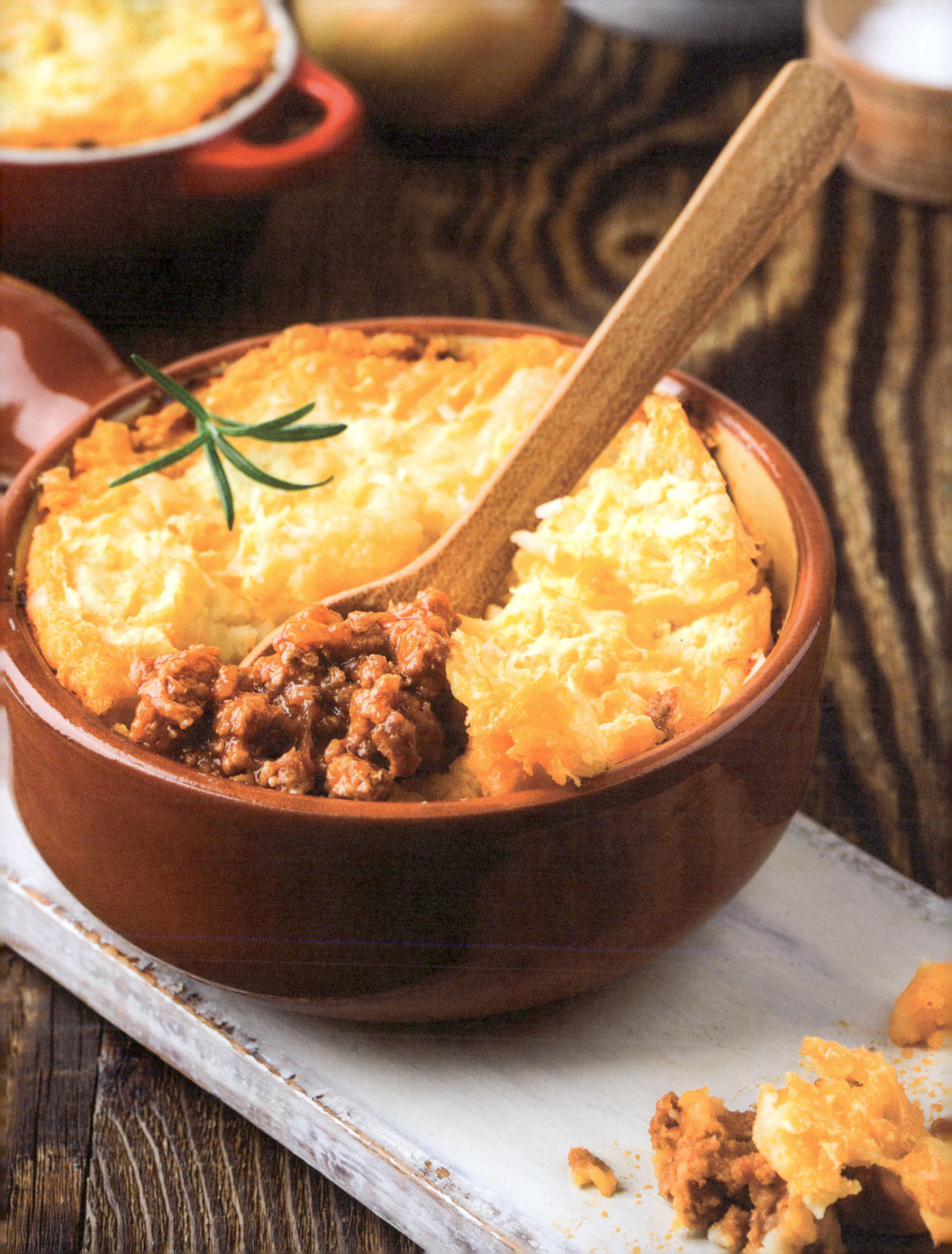

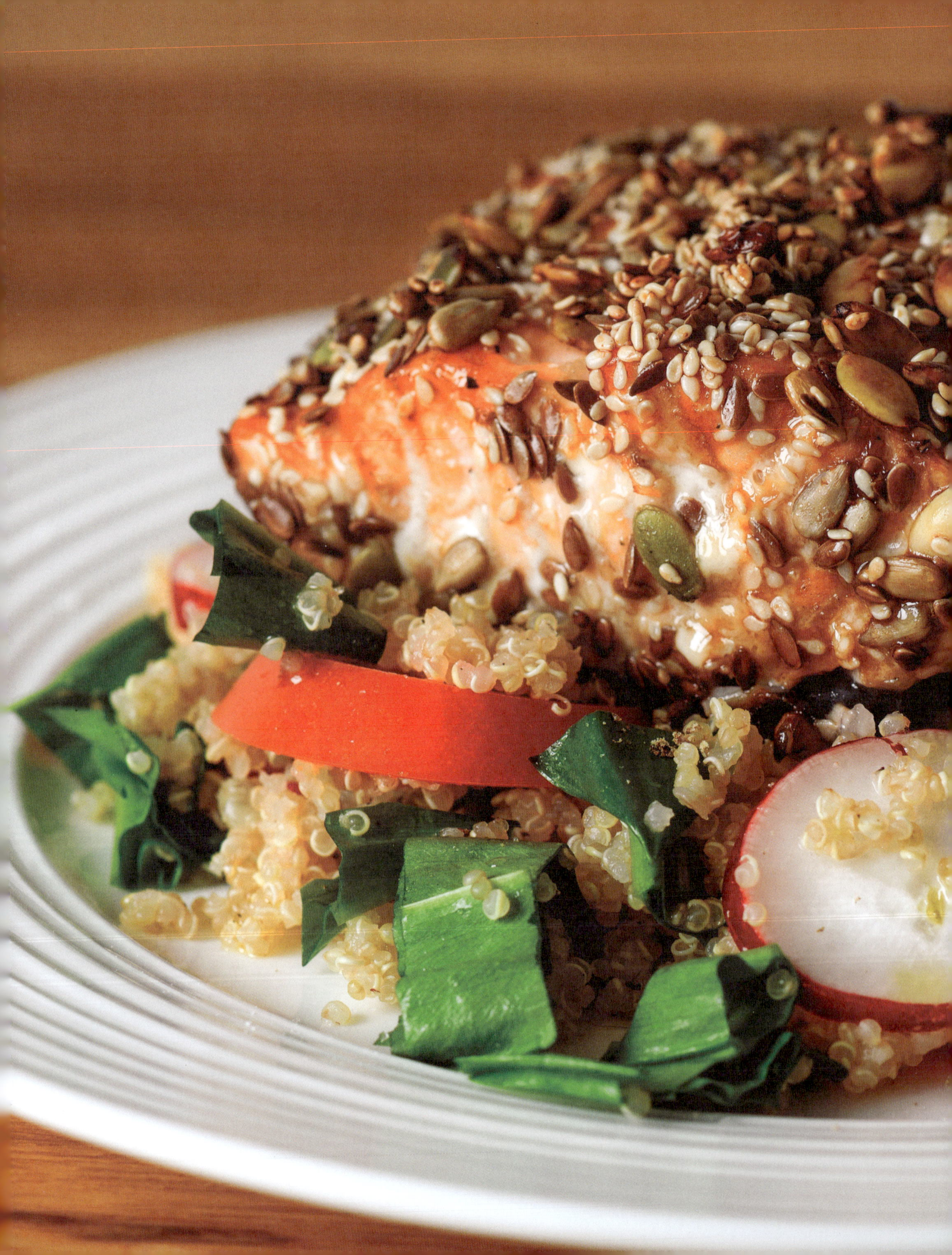

Seed-Coated Salmon with Quinoa Salad

¾ cup (120g) quinoa, rinsed

2 cups (500ml) vegetable stock

Avocado oil cooking spray

2 salmon fillets

2 tbsps sesame oil

2 tbsps coconut aminos

2 tsps pepitas

1 tsp sesame seeds

1 tsp flaxseed

1 tsp sunflower seeds

2 radishes, sliced

1 tomato, sliced

½ lettuce, shredded

Salt and pepper to taste

DRESSING

1 tbsp tamari

1 tsp rice wine vinegar

1 tsp sesame oil

Place quinoa and stock in a saucepan over medium heat. Bring to a boil. Reduce heat and simmer, covered, for 15 minutes. Drain and set aside.

Spray air fryer basket with avocado oil cooking spray.

Place salmon fillets skin-side down in the basket. Brush salmon with sesame oil and coconut aminos.

Scatter seeds over the salmon and press gently to coat.

Cook at 190°C for 12-13 minutes or until salmon flakes easily with a fork. Set aside to rest.

Place quinoa in a large bowl with radish, tomato and lettuce. Season with salt and pepper.

Combine dressing ingredients in a small bowl. Pour over quinoa and toss to coat.

Spoon quinoa salad onto plates and serve with salmon fillets.

SERVES 2

Cornflake Chicken Cutlets

750g chicken tenders or quartered chicken breasts

Salt and pepper to taste

½ cup (125ml) milk

2 eggs

4 cups (120g) gluten-free cornflakes

1 tsp smoked paprika

¼ tsp onion powder

Olive oil cooking spray

Season the chicken pieces with salt and pepper.

Place the milk and eggs in a bowl and whisk to combine.

Place cornflakes, paprika, onion powder, salt and pepper in another bowl and mix.

Dip each chicken piece into the milk mixture, then roll in the cornflakes.

Spray air fryer basket and chicken with cooking spray.

Arrange chicken in one layer and cook for 15 minutes at 200°C, turning halfway, until chicken is cooked.

SERVES 4

Spinach Fish Cakes

300g skinless white fish fillets

150g spinach leaves

Salt and pepper to taste

1 egg

450g potatoes, boiled and mashed

2 spring onions, finely chopped

½ cup (60g) almond meal

Avocado or olive oil cooking spray

In a food processor combine fish, spinach, salt, pepper, and egg. Pulse until smooth.

Place the fish mixture, mashed potatoes and spring onion in a large bowl. Mix well then form into 16 patties.

Place the almond meal in a shallow dish. Coat each patty on all sides with almond meal.

Cover and refrigerate for at least 30 minutes to chill.

Preheat air fryer to 220°C. Working in batches, spray patties with oil and arrange in basket. Cook for 10-15 minutes until golden brown, turning halfway through cooking.

SERVES 4

Coconut Crust Fish

¾ cup (65g) shredded coconut

½ cup (50g) coconut flour

1 tsp salt

3 eggs, beaten

4 x 120g firm white fish fillets (such as whiting)

Avocado or olive oil spray

In one bowl mix together shredded coconut, coconut flour and salt.

In another bowl place beaten eggs.

Dip fish fillets into beaten eggs and then into coconut mixture.

Spray air fryer basket with avocado or olive oil spray.

Place fish into air fryer basket and spray with oil spray.

Cook for 4 minutes at 200°C. Flip the fish and cook for another 4 minutes until fish is cooked and crust is golden brown.

SERVES 4

Gluten-Free Pork Schnitzel

4 x boneless pork chops, pounded to 1cm thin pieces

100g corn chips

¼ cup (25g) Parmesan cheese, grated

1 cup (120g) almond meal

1 tsp dried sage

Salt and pepper to taste

2 eggs, beaten

Olive oil cooking spray

Place corn chips in a food processor and blitz to a fine crumb. Combine crumbs with Parmesan, almond meal, sage, salt and pepper in a shallow dish.

Place the beaten egg in another shallow dish.

Dip each piece of pork first into egg then into the crumb mixture and press gently to coat.

Preheat air fryer to 200°C.

Spray pork with cooking spray and place in air fryer. Cook for 12-14 minutes until cooked through, turning and spraying at 6 minutes.

SERVES 4

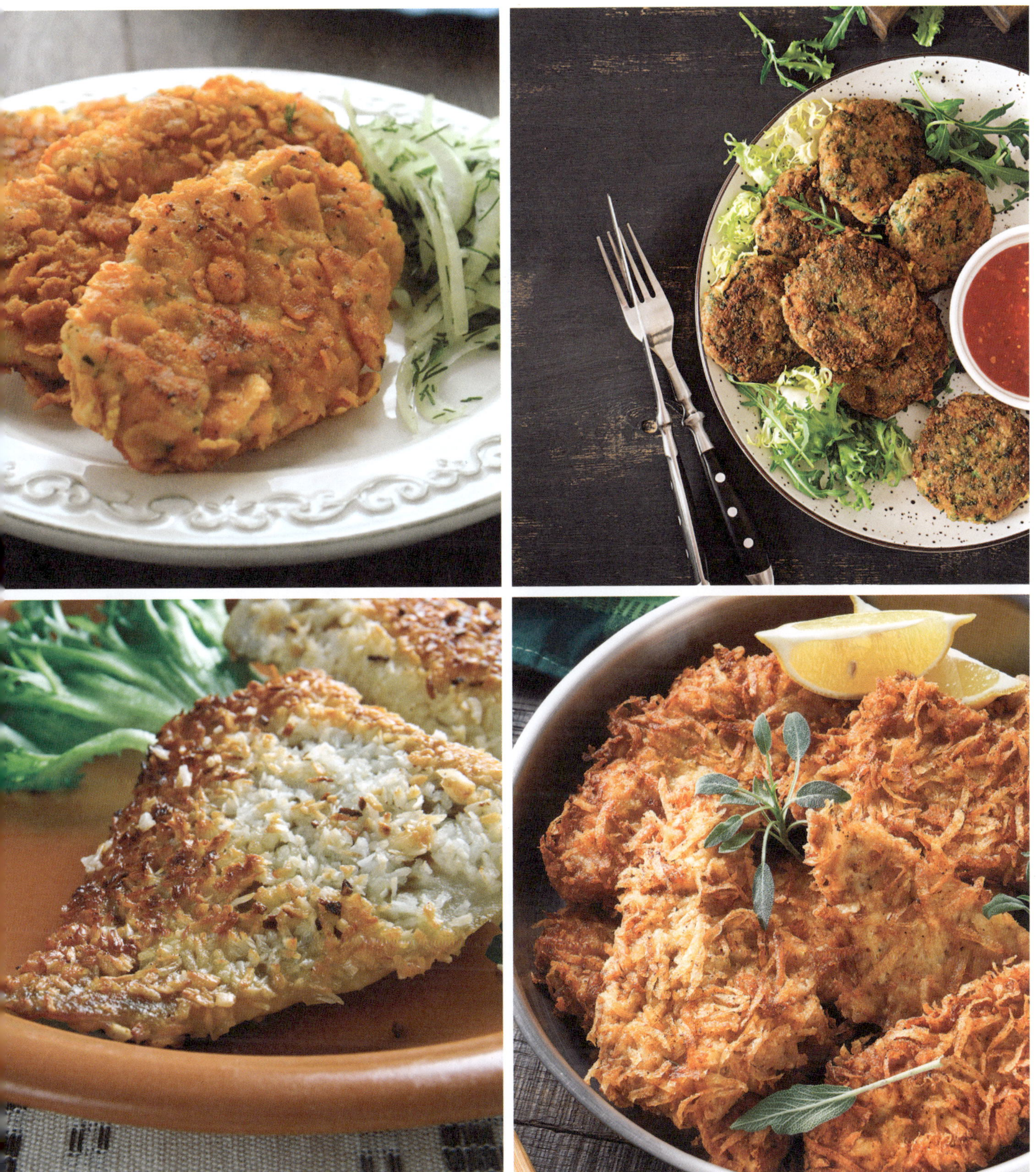

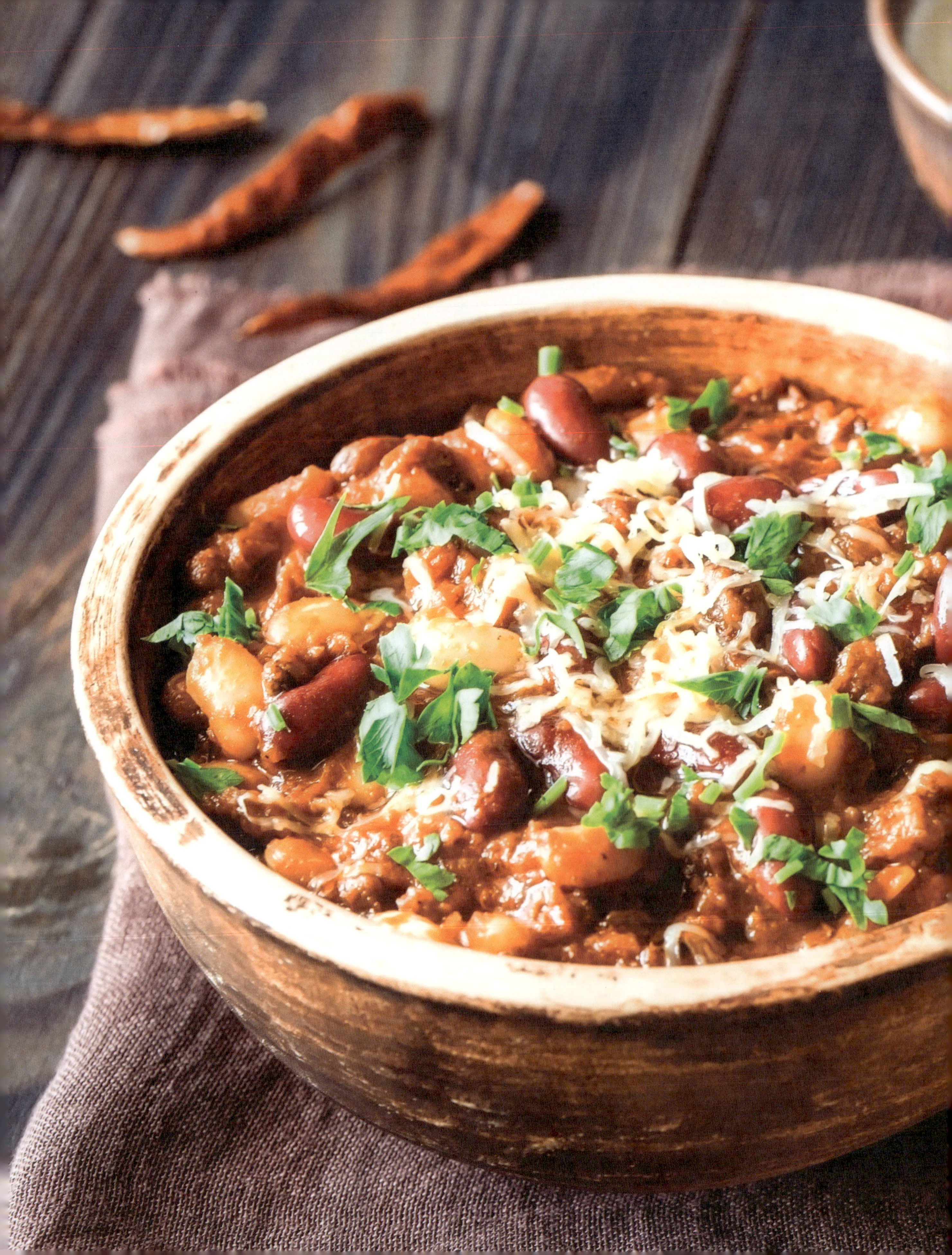

Chilli Con Carne

1 onion, thinly sliced

1 red capsicum, seeded and finely diced

1 red chilli, deseeded and finely chopped

1 tbsp olive oil

500g beef mince

2 cloves garlic, minced

2 tsps chilli powder, or to taste

1 tsp ground coriander

1 tsp ground cumin

2 tbsps tomato paste

1⅔ cups (400ml) hot beef stock

1 x 400g can chopped tomatoes

Salt and pepper, to taste

1 x 400g can kidney beans, drained and rinsed

1 x 400g can cannellini beans, drained and rinsed

2 tsps cacao powder (optional)

Chopped coriander and grated cheese, to serve

Baking pan

Preheat air fryer to 180°C.

Place the onion, capsicum and chilli in baking pan, drizzle evenly with oil and place in air fryer. Cook for 5 minutes.

Add the mince and garlic to the pan. Break up the mince with a fork. Cook for 5 minutes to brown the meat.

In a medium bowl or jug, mix together the spices with the tomato paste. Pour in half of the stock and stir to combine. Add the stock mixture and canned tomatoes to the air fryer pan. Stir well and season to taste. Cook for 25 minutes, stirring about every 5 minutes.

Add the canned beans, the remaining stock and cacao if using. Cook for a further 5-10 minutes, stirring halfway through.

Spoon into bowls and top with chopped coriander and grated cheese to serve.

SERVES 4

Zucchini Tater Tots

2½ cups (560g) zucchini, grated

1 tsp salt

1 clove garlic, minced

1 small onion, finely diced

1 egg

½ tsp pepper

3 tbsps coconut flour

1 tbsp nutritional yeast (optional)

⅓ cup (40g) Parmesan cheese, grated

Avocado or olive oil cooking spray

Place the zucchini in a large bowl. Sprinkle with salt and allow to sit for 20 minutes, then transfer to a clean tea towel and squeeze out the water.

Put the squeezed zucchini in a large clean bowl. Add the garlic, onion, egg, pepper, coconut flour, nutritional yeast and Parmesan and stir well to combine.

Preheat the air fryer to 200°C.

Scoop out tablespoons of the mixture and squeeze gently in the palm of your hand to form small, thick sausage shapes.

Set aside on a plate.

Spray the air fryer basket with cooking spray. Evenly space the zucchini tots in one layer in the air fryer basket. Cook in batches or use a double layer accessory if necessary. Lightly spray the tots with cooking spray.

Cook for 10 minutes, turning halfway through cooking, until nicely golden brown.

SERVES 4

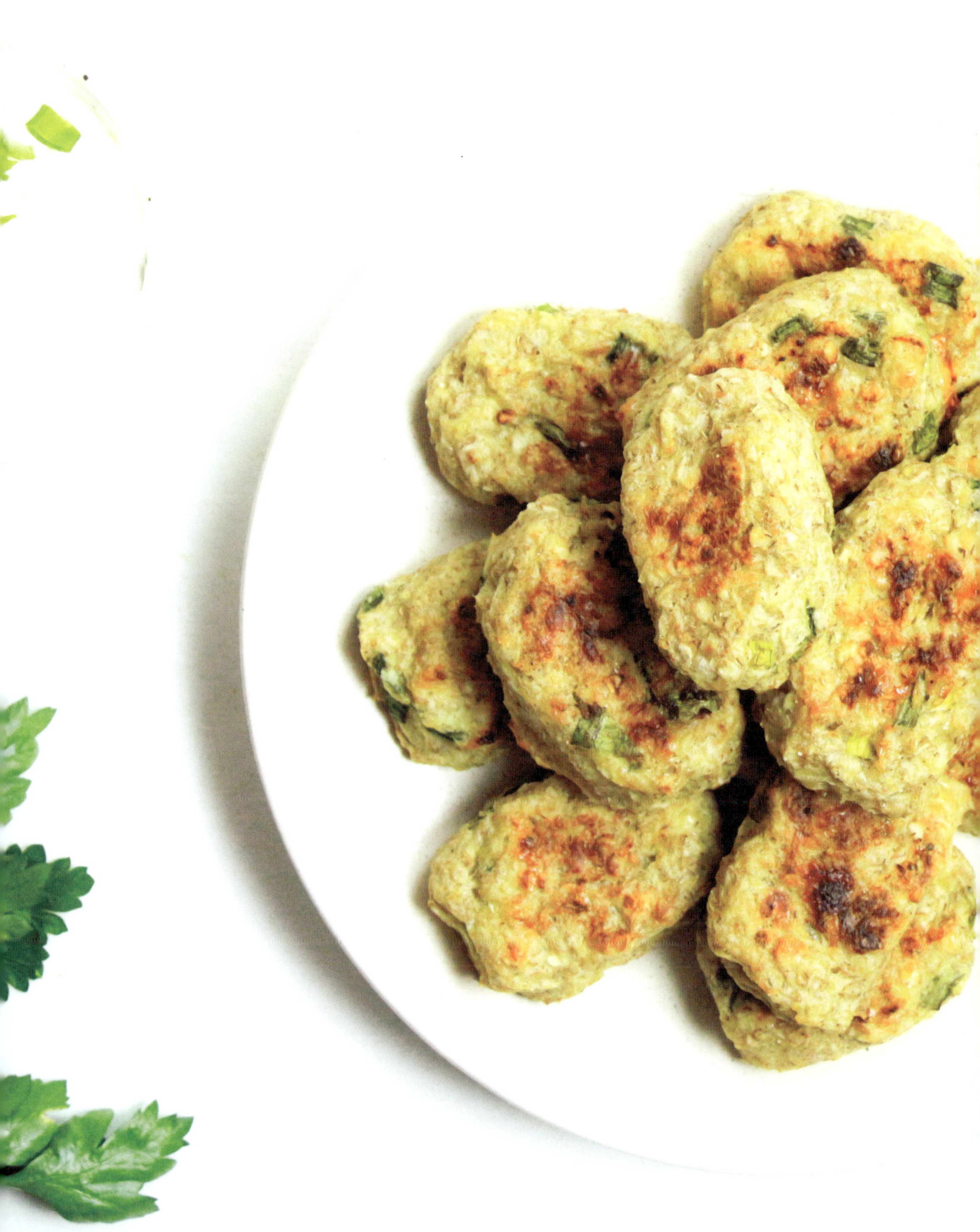

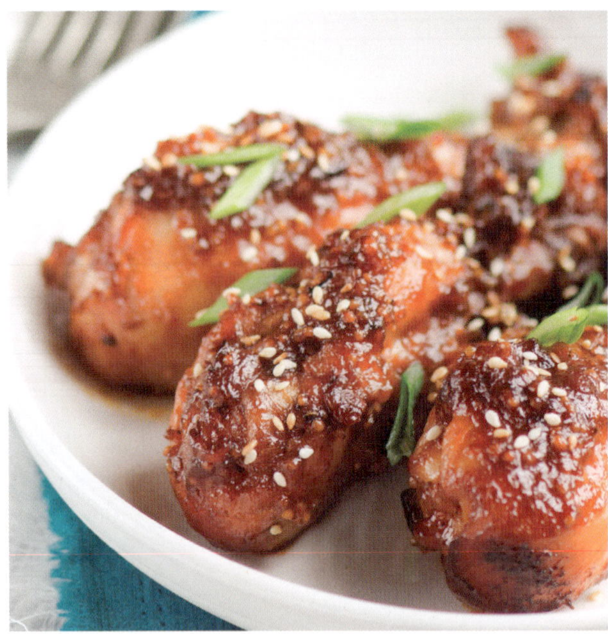

Sticky Chicken Drumsticks

8 chicken drumsticks

½ tsp salt

2 tbsps olive oil

1 tbsp sesame oil

4 tbsps tamari

1 tbsp Worcestershire sauce

2 tbsps lime juice

2 tbsps honey

1 tsp garlic powder

¼ tsp cayenne pepper

In a large bowl mix together all of the ingredients except for the chicken. Mix well then add chicken and toss to coat well. Cover and refrigerate for at least 30 minutes.

Preheat air fryer to 200°C.

Arrange chicken in air fryer basket, cook in batches or use a double layer accessory if necessary to prevent overcrowding. Cook for 15 minutes, then flip and cook for 15 minutes more or until cooked through.

SERVES 4

Pork Tacos

2 tbsps smoked paprika

2 tbsps ground cumin

¼ cup (40g) brown sugar

1 cup (250ml) pineapple juice

1½ cups (375ml) smoky barbecue sauce

1.5kg boned pork shoulder, cut into 4cm-thick slices

Juice of 1 orange

12 corn tortillas, warmed

1 cup (100g) red cabbage, shredded

½ red onion, thinly sliced

¼ cup (10g) fresh coriander leaves

Combine paprika, cumin, sugar, pineapple juice and barbecue sauce in a large bowl. Mix well. Add the pork and toss to combine.

Place in fridge for at least 30 minutes or overnight.

Preheat air fryer to 190°C. Spray air fryer basket with cooking spray. Arrange pork in basket and cook for 45 minutes, flipping every 15 minutes.

Remove pork from air fryer and wrap in foil with the orange juice. Seal the foil to keep in steam and place in air fryer. Cook for 30 minutes. Remove pork and shred with forks.

Divide shredded pork between warm tortillas. Top with shredded cabbage, red onion and coriander to serve.

SERVES 4

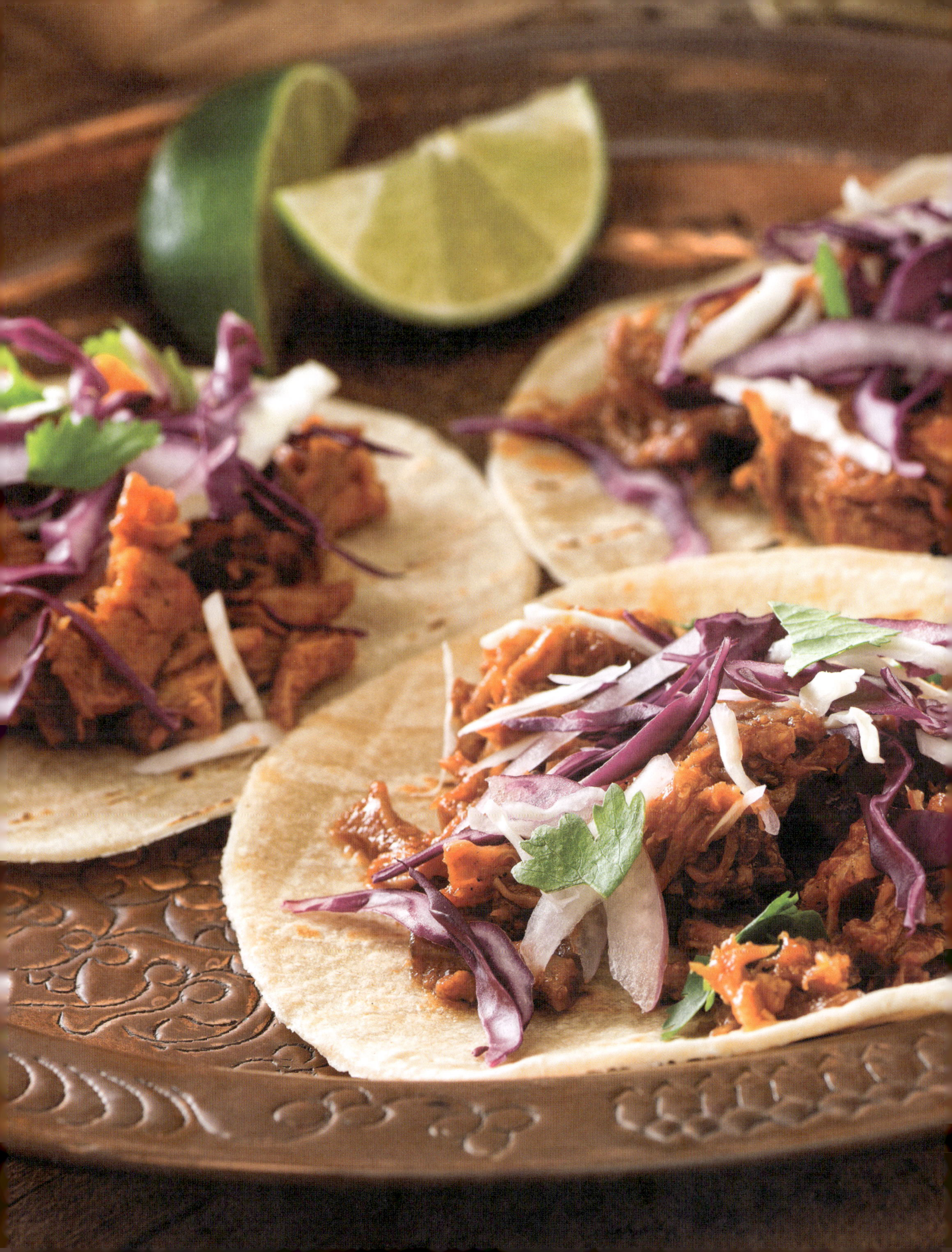

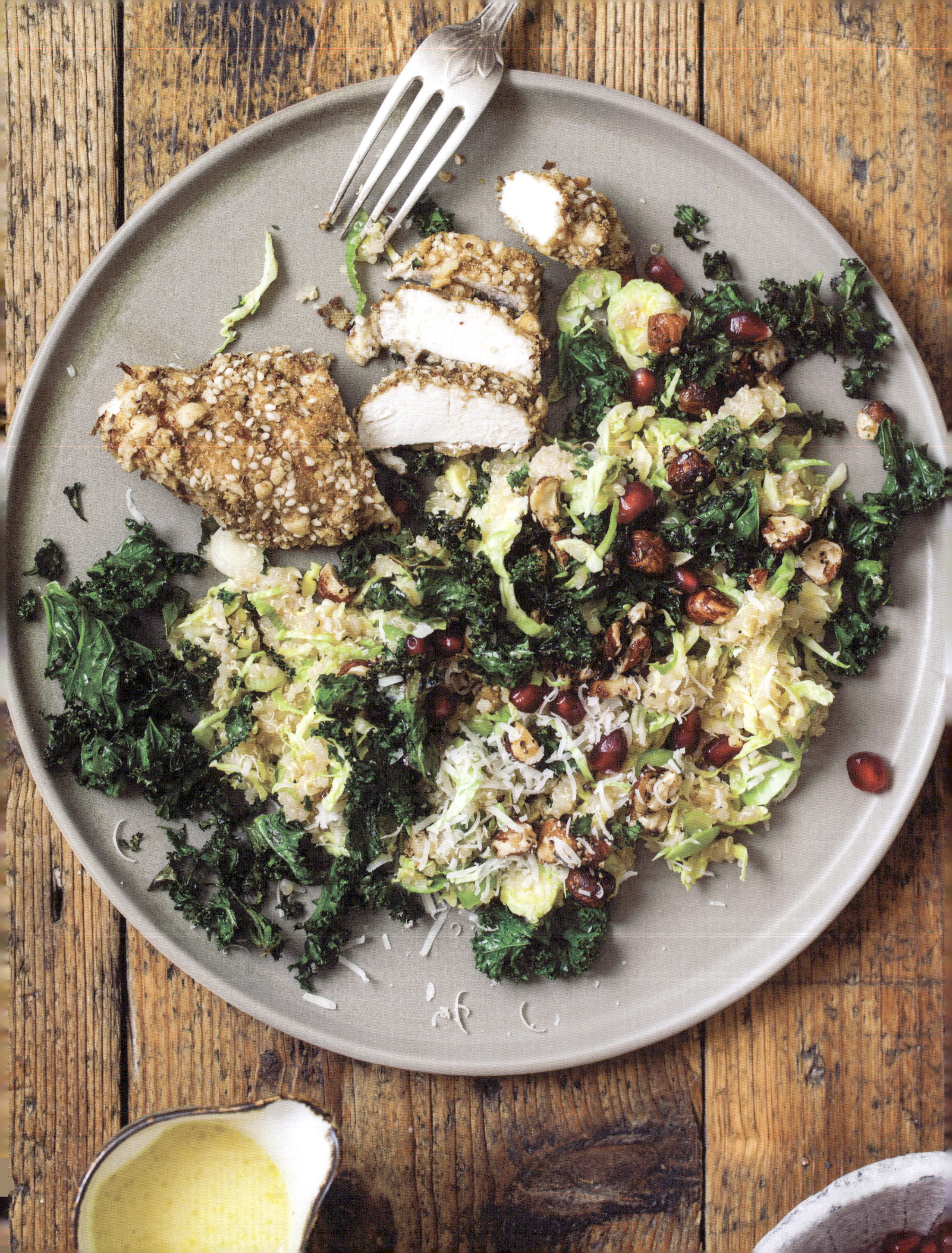

Dukkah-Crusted Chicken with Kale Salad

1 tbsp olive oil

2 tsps lemon zest

¼ cup (30g) dukkah

Salt and pepper to taste

4 chicken breasts

Olive oil cooking spray

300g kale leaves, washed and roughly torn

300g Brussels sprouts, thinly sliced

¼ cup (25g) pomegranate seeds

¼ cup (30g) toasted hazelnuts

¼ cup (25g) Parmesan, grated

DRESSING

2 tbsps fresh lemon juice

¼ cup (60ml) olive oil

1 tsp Dijon mustard

1 small clove garlic, minced

¼ tsp salt

⅛ tsp pepper

Preheat air fryer to 170°C.

Combine olive oil, lemon zest, dukkah and salt and pepper in a small bowl. Rub all over chicken.

Spray air fryer basket with cooking spray.

Place chicken in basket and cook for 20 minutes or until cooked through. Set aside to rest.

Combine kale, Brussels sprouts, pomegranate seeds and hazelnuts in a large bowl.

Place the dressing ingredients in a small bowl or sealable jar with a lid. Stir or shake to combine. Pour over the salad and toss well.

Arrange the salad onto serving plates with the cooked chicken. Sprinkle with Parmesan to serve.

SERVES 4

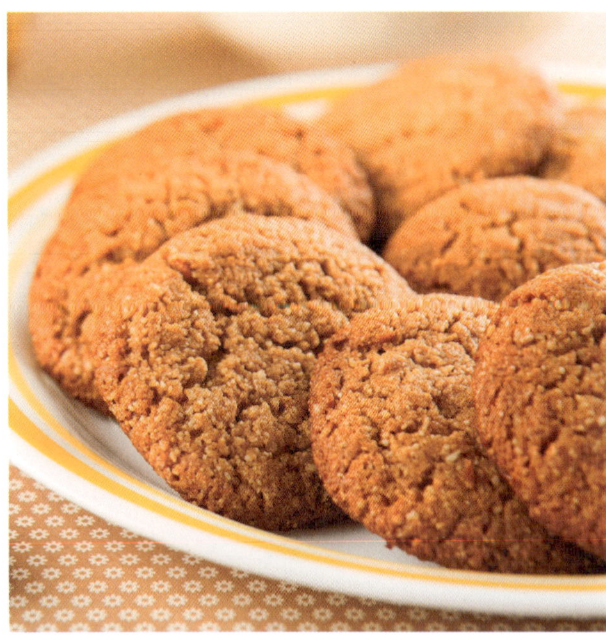

Gluten-Free Ginger Biscuits

1 cup (120g) almond meal

¼ cup (30g) tapioca flour

½ cup (80g) coconut sugar

¾ tsp bicarbonate of soda

¼ tsp salt

½ tbsp ground cinnamon

½ tbsp ground ginger

1 egg

2 tbsps molasses

1 tbsp maple syrup

¼ cup (60ml) melted coconut oil

¼ tsp vanilla extract

In a bowl combine almond meal, tapioca flour, coconut sugar, bicarb, salt and spices. Mix well.

In a separate bowl, whisk together egg, molasses, maple syrup, coconut oil and vanilla. Pour wet ingredients into dry ingredients and stir to combine.

Form dough into a ball. Wrap in plastic wrap and refrigerate for 25 minutes.

Roll dough into 12 balls then press gently to flatten.

Cooking in batches if necessary, arrange biscuits in air fryer basket. Cook for 6-8 minutes at 160°C.

MAKES 12

Gluten-Free Churros

⅔ cup (80g) almond meal

¼ cup (25g) coconut flour

1 tbsp psyllium husk powder

1 tsp xanthan gum

1 cup (240ml) water

60g butter

2 tbsps maple syrup

⅛ tsp salt

1 tsp vanilla extract

2 eggs, beaten

Avocado oil cooking spray

TO COAT

2 tsps cinnamon

¼ cup (40g) icing sugar or coconut sugar

Line a baking tray with greaseproof paper.

In a large bowl mix together almond meal, coconut flour, psyllium husk and xanthan gum. Set aside.

Heat water, butter, maple syrup and salt in a pan over a low heat until simmering. Add in almond meal mixture, stirring constantly to incorporate. Continue to cook and stir for 2-3 minutes until the dough pulls away from the pan and forms into a ball. Remove from heat and return to bowl.

Allow to cool for 5 minutes then add vanilla. Mix well. Add one egg at a time, mixing until fully incorporated.

Once cool enough to handle, transfer dough to a piping bag with a star-shaped nozzle. Pipe churros onto prepared baking tray into 10cm lengths.

Refrigerate for 1 hour.

Preheat air fryer to 180°C.

Carefully transfer churros to air fryer basket and spray with cooking spray. Ensure there is space between each one. Cook in batches or use a double layer accessory if necessary.

Cook for 10-12 minutes until golden brown and crisp.

Combine cinnamon and sugar of choice in a shallow dish.

Immediately transfer baked churros to the cinnamon sugar dish and toss to coat.

Serve warm.

MAKES 12

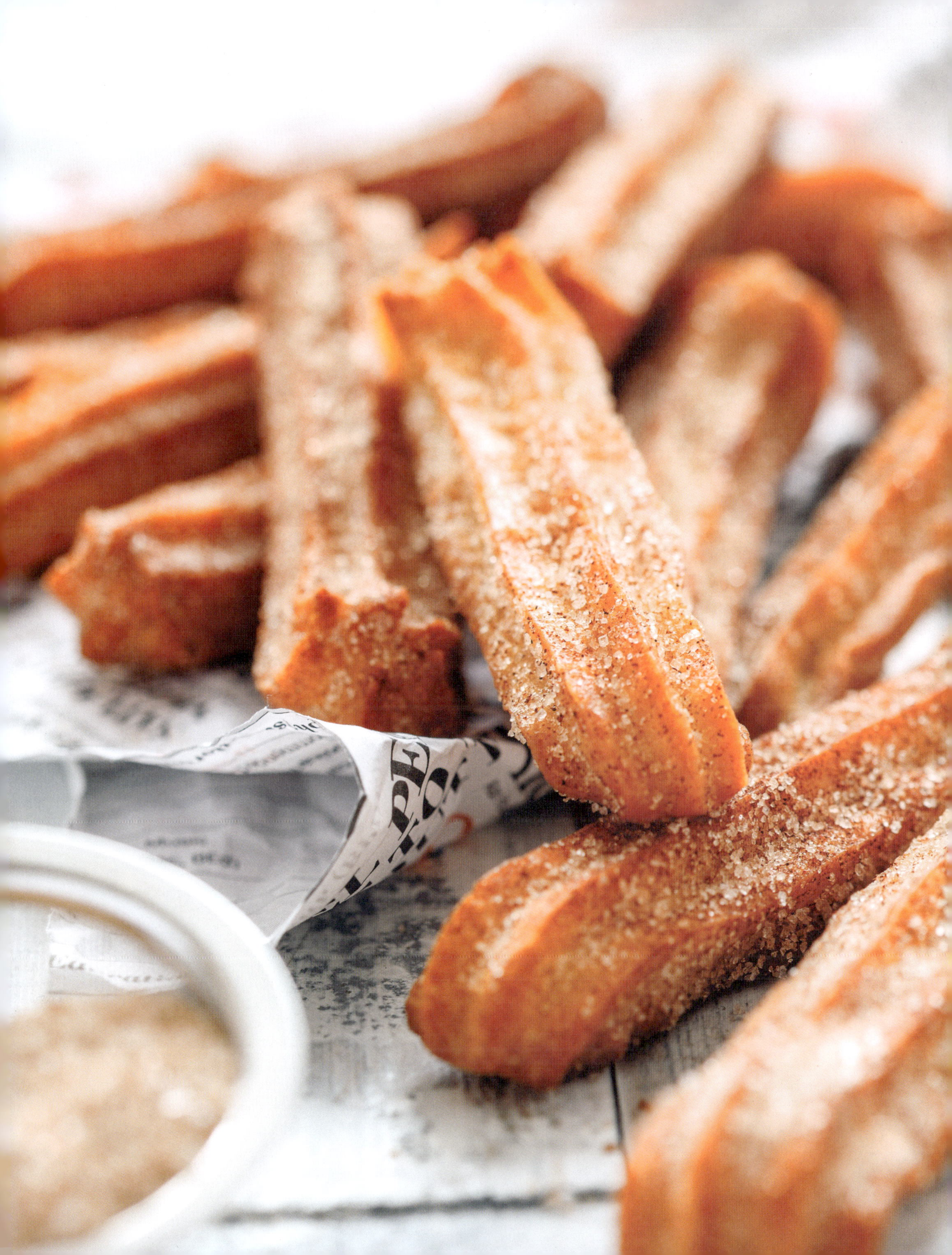

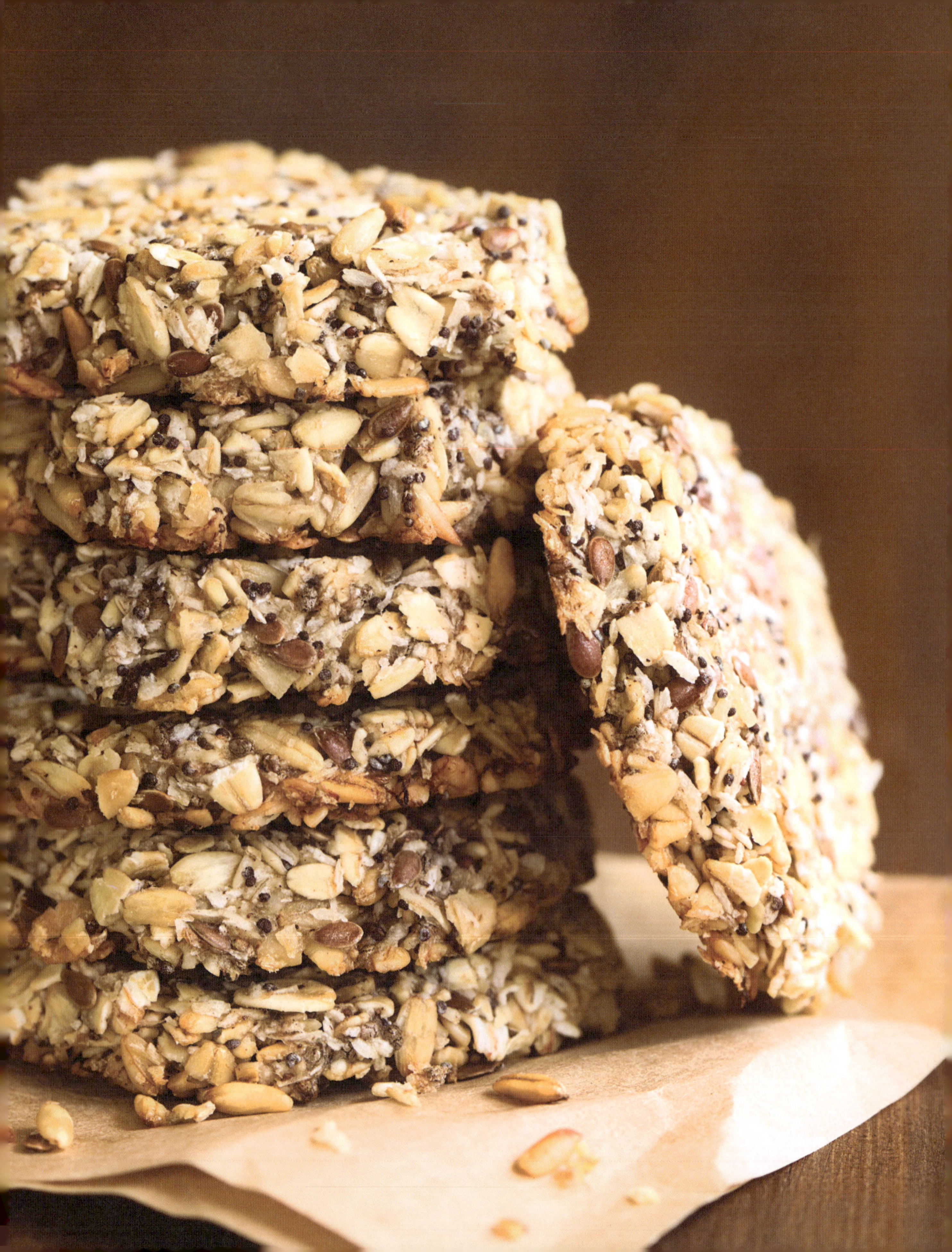

Vegan Banana, Oat and Seed Cookies

¾ cup mashed banana (about two large bananas)

2 cups (180g) gluten-free oats

½ cup (45g) desiccated coconut

1 tsp cinnamon

¼ cup (80g) maple syrup

¼ cup (60ml) olive or avocado oil

2 tbsps pepitas

2 tbsps sunflower seeds

1 tbsp flaxseed

1 tbsp chia seeds

2 tsps poppy seeds

Preheat air fryer to 120°C.

Place all the ingredients in a mixing bowl. Stir well to combine.

Line air fryer basket with greaseproof paper.

Working in batches, drop 2-tablespoon portions of mixture onto the greaseproof paper leaving space in between each one. Use damp hands to flatten slightly.

Cook in the air fryer for 25-30 minutes or until firm to the touch and light golden.

Set aside to cool and repeat with remaining mixture.

MAKES 16

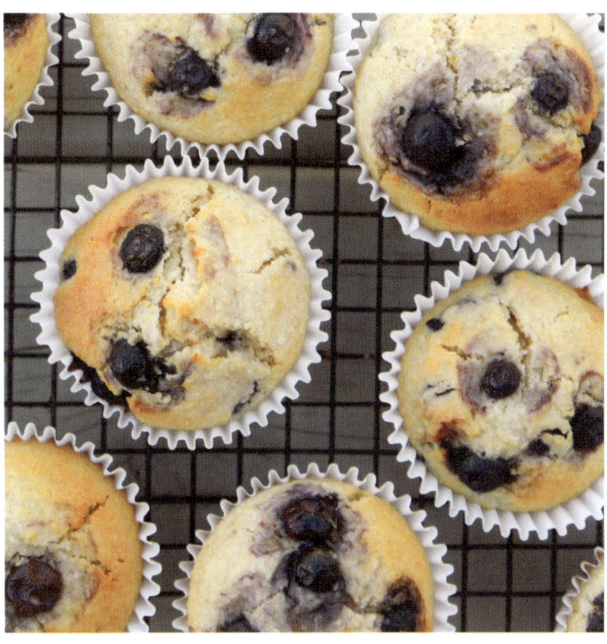

Gluten-Free Blueberry Muffins

2½ cups (300g) almond meal

½ cup (80g) coconut sugar

1½ tsps gluten-free baking powder

¼ tsp salt

⅓ cup (80ml) coconut oil or butter, melted

⅓ cup (80ml) unsweetened almond milk

3 large eggs

½ tsp vanilla extract

¾ cup (75g) blueberries

Muffin tray or silicone moulds

Preheat air fryer to 180°C.

In a large bowl, stir together almond meal, sugar, baking powder and salt.

Mix in coconut oil or butter, almond milk, eggs and vanilla extract. Fold in blueberries.

Pour into silicone moulds or paper liners in muffin tray.

Working in batches, place in air fryer basket and cook for 15-20 minutes until an inserted skewer comes out clean.

MAKES 12

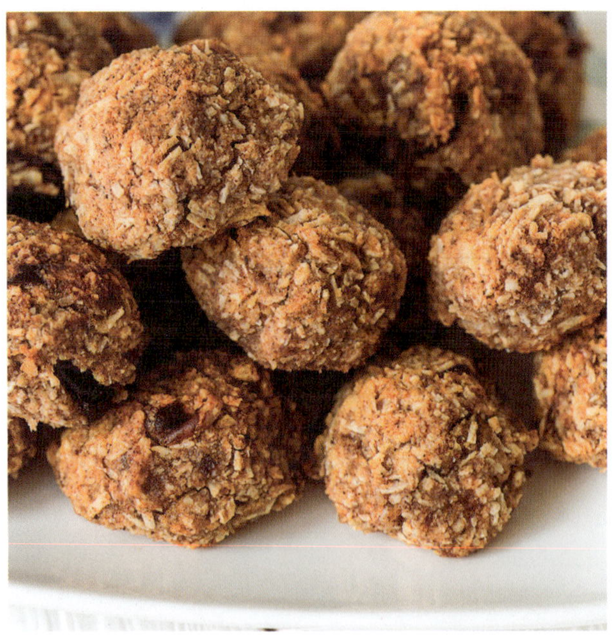

Gluten-Free Apple Cookies

1 apple

1 cup (115g) blanched almond meal

¼ tsp ground cinnamon

⅛ tsp salt

Core and cut apple into chunks. Place in a food processor and blend into a puree, scraping down sides as needed.

Place almond meal in a medium bowl. Add the apple puree, cinnamon and salt. Mix well.

Line air fryer basket with greaseproof paper.

Working in batches, use a tablespoon to scoop small mounds of dough onto the greaseproof paper. Space evenly apart.

Bake in the air fryer at 160°C for 12-15 minutes until golden brown and firm to the touch.

Transfer to a cooling rack and cool completely. Repeat with remaining dough.

MAKES 12

Gluten-Free Doughnuts

1 cup (120g) almond meal

¼ cup (40g) coconut sugar

2 tsps baking powder

1 tsp cinnamon

⅛ tsp salt

60g butter, melted

¼ cup (60ml) almond milk

2 large eggs

½ tsp vanilla extract

150g dark chocolate

¼ cup (30g) pistachios, chopped

Doughnut pan or individual doughnut tins

Preheat air fryer to 150°C.

Grease doughnut pan well.

In a large bowl, stir together almond meal, sugar, baking powder, cinnamon and salt.

In a small bowl, whisk together melted butter, almond milk, egg and vanilla extract. Whisk the wet mixture into the dry mixture.

Working in batches, pour batter into doughnut pan, filling moulds three-quarters of the way.

Bake in the air fryer for about 16-20 minutes until golden brown.

Remove from pan and place on a wire rack to cool.

Melt chocolate in a small bowl in a microwave or over a pan of simmering water on a low heat.

Dip the cooked doughnuts into the chocolate then sprinkle with pistachios to serve.

MAKES 6

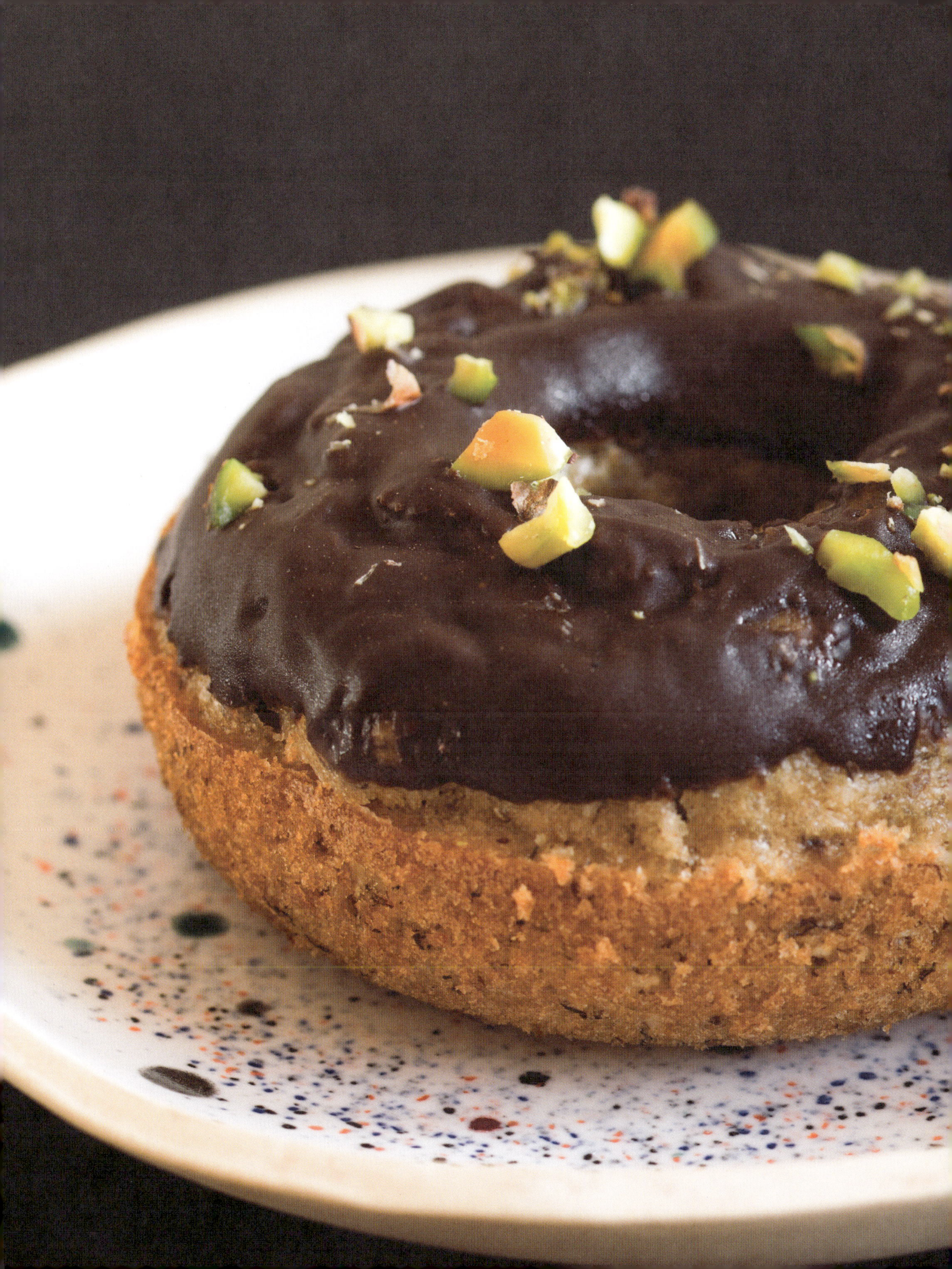

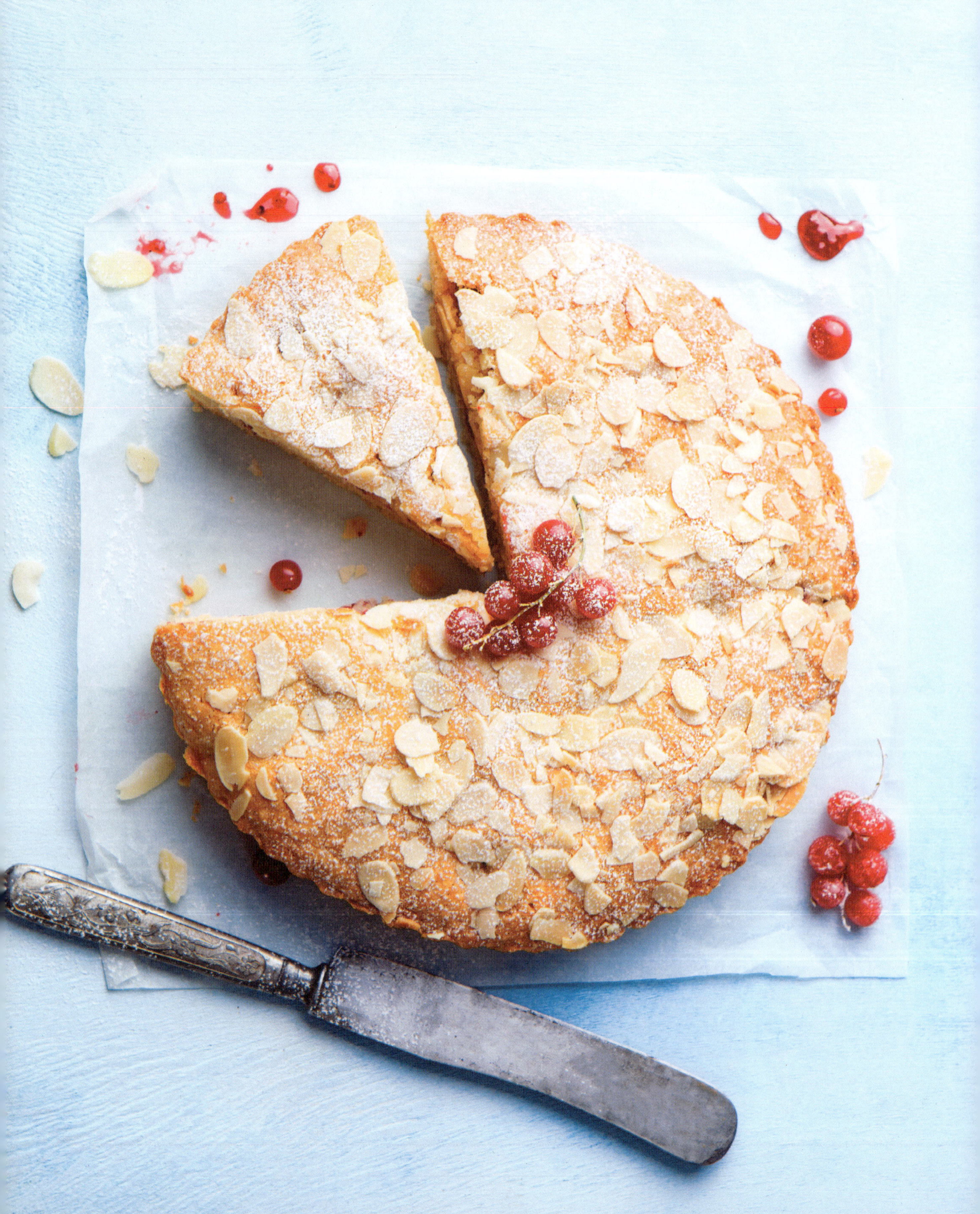

Gluten-Free Bakewell Tart

JAM

1 cup (125g) raspberries

1½ tbsps chia seeds

2 tbsps agave syrup

2 tbsps water

BASE

1 cup (90g) gluten-free oat flour

3 tbsps agave syrup

2 tbsps butter or coconut oil, melted

FRANGIPANE

1 cup (120g) almond meal

1 tsp baking powder

Pinch of salt

1 egg

3 tbsps agave syrup

3 tbsps butter or coconut oil, melted

1 tbsp milk of choice

2 tbsps flaked almonds for topping

Cake tin

Grease and line cake tin with greaseproof paper.

Place ingredients for jam in a small pan over low heat. Bring to a simmer, stirring and mashing raspberries, then leave to cool for 5 minutes to thicken.

Mix together base ingredients, then press into the prepared cake tin. Spread with chia jam.

Combine ingredients for frangipane in a large bowl and mix well. Pour on top of jam and sprinkle with flaked almonds.

Preheat air fryer to 160°C.

Place cake tin in air fryer and bake for around 20-25 minutes until golden.

Leave to cool completely before removing from cake tin.

SERVES 6

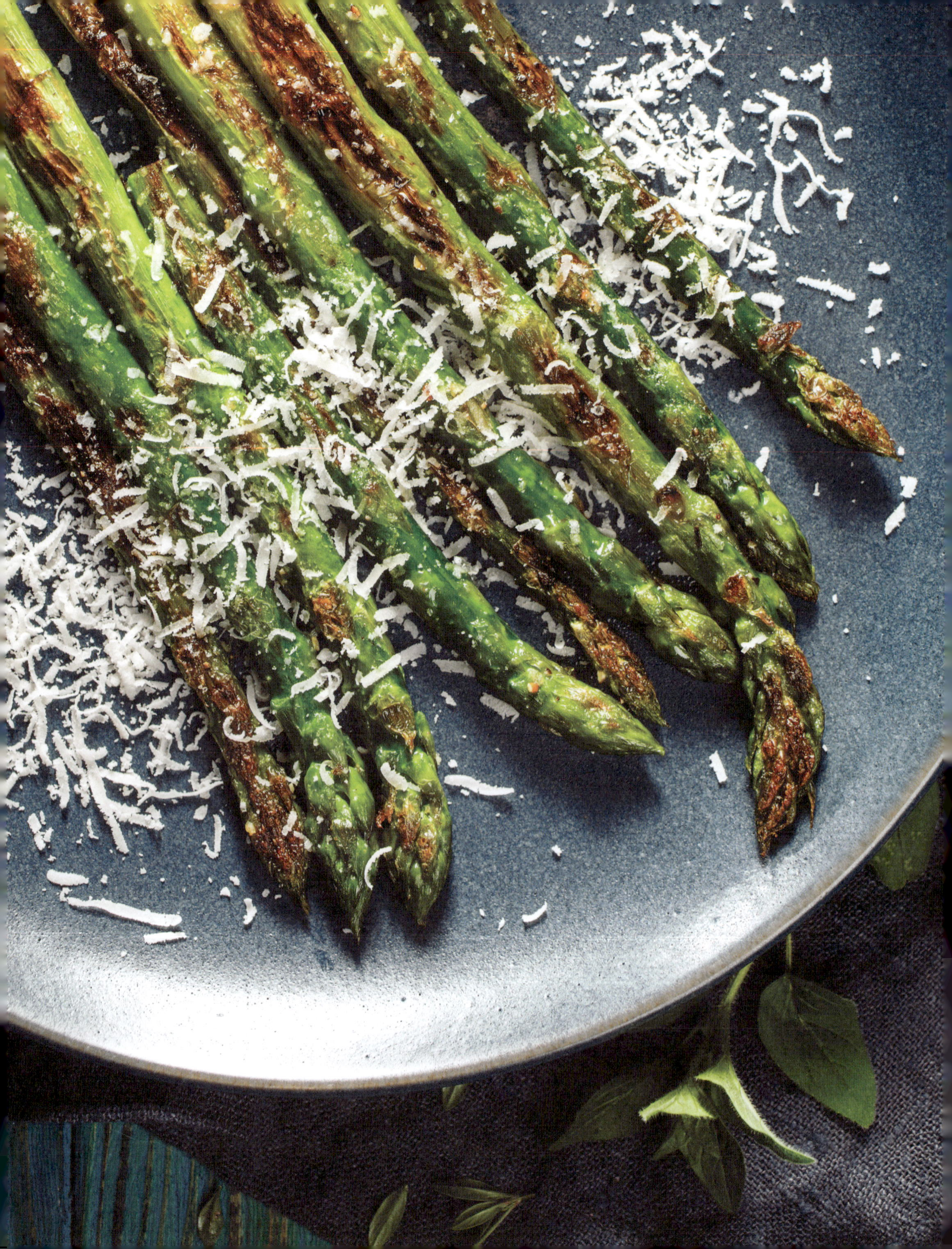

Vegetarian

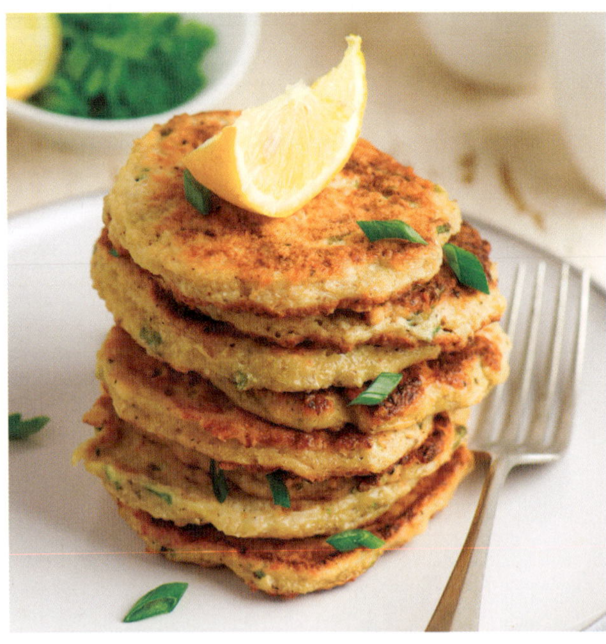

Cauliflower Hash Browns

3½ cups (350g) cauliflower, grated

1 onion, finely chopped

1 egg

½ cup (45g) chickpea flour (besan)

1 cup (125g) Cheddar cheese, grated

½ tsp paprika

1 tsp salt

Pepper to taste

Place grated cauliflower in a clean tea towel and twist to squeeze out moisture.

Place the cauliflower in a large bowl and add onion, egg, flour, cheese, paprika, salt and pepper. Mix until well combined.

Shape the mixture into eight patties and freeze for at least 1 hour.

Preheat air fryer to 200°C.

Spray air fryer basket with oil. Arrange patties in one layer in air fryer basket, Cook in batches or use a double layer accessory if necessary.

Cook for 10 minutes, turning halfway through the cooking process.

SERVES 4

Cheese Souffle

Olive oil spray

¼ cup (30g) panko breadcrumbs

30g butter

½ cup (60g) plain flour

1¼ cups (310ml) milk

½ cup (60g) Cheddar cheese, grated

¼ cup (30g) Parmesan cheese, grated

½ tsp ground nutmeg

4 large eggs, separated

4 ramekins or souffle dishes

Preheat air fryer to 165°C.

Spray four small souffle dishes or ramekins with olive oil spray and sprinkle with breadcrumbs.

Heat butter in a small saucepan, over medium-low heat. When melted add flour and stir until smooth. Add the milk a little at a time, whisking to remove any lumps. Bring to a simmer, stirring constantly until sauce thickens.

Remove sauce from heat and whisk in cheeses and nutmeg. Add egg yolks and beat until smooth.

In a separate bowl, whisk egg whites until stiff peaks form. Use a metal spoon to gradually fold egg whites into the sauce.

Divide mixture between dishes. Use a knife to flatten the tops.

Place dishes in air fryer basket. Cook for 18-20 minutes, until cheese is puffed up and golden brown.

SERVES 4

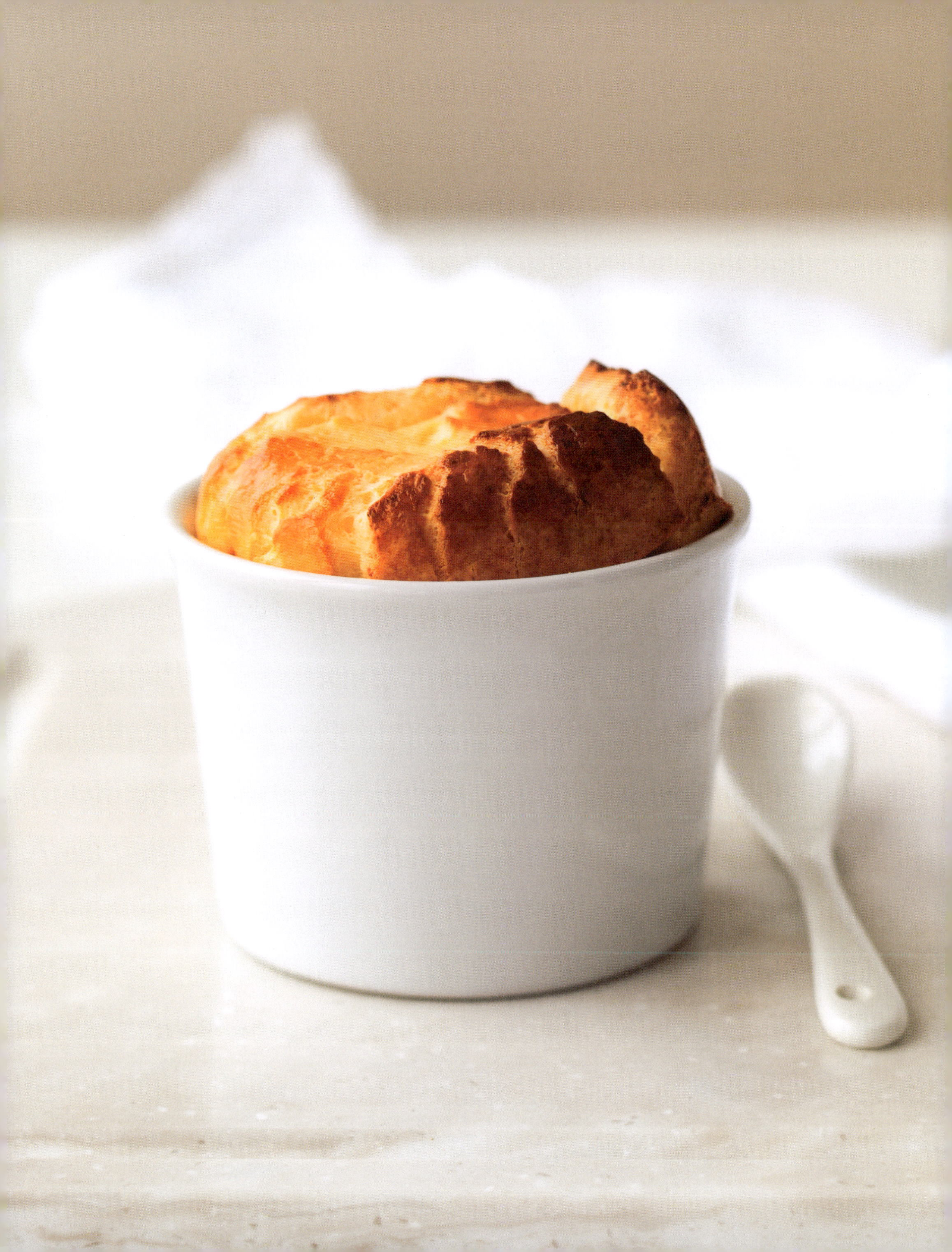

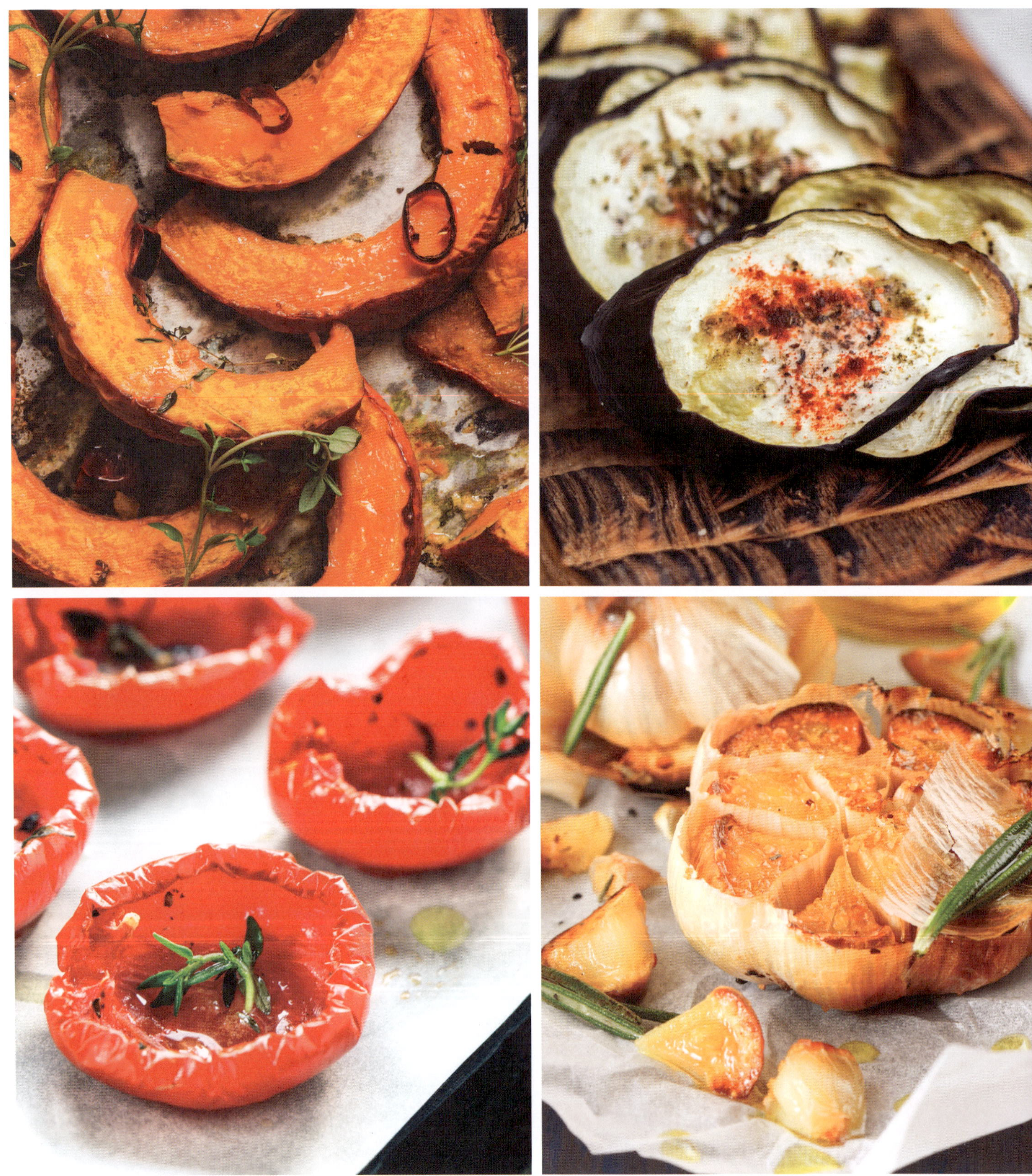

Spiced Roasted Pumpkin

800g pumpkin

3 cloves garlic, chopped

1 red chilli, sliced

6 sprigs thyme

3 lemons, zested

4 tbsps olive oil

Salt and pepper to taste

Cut the pumpkin into 1cm-thick slices.

Preheat air fryer to 180°C.

In a large bowl place garlic, chilli, thyme, lemon zest, olive oil, salt and pepper. Add the pumpkin slices and toss to coat thoroughly.

Arrange slices in air fryer basket making sure there is space between each slice. Cook in batches or use a double layer accessory if necessary.

Cook for 10-12 minutes until pumpkin is tender.

SERVES 2

Spiced Eggplants

1 large eggplant

1 tbsp olive oil

1 clove garlic, minced

Salt and pepper to taste

1 tsp paprika

⅛ tsp cayenne pepper (optional)

Preheat air fryer to 150°C.

Slice eggplant into 1cm-thick sections. Place in a large bowl with olive oil and garlic. Season generously with salt and pepper. Toss well to coat.

Arrange eggplant slices in air fryer basket. Sprinkle with spices.

Cook for 10 minutes or until soft in the centre and crisp around the edges.

SERVES 2

Sun-Dried Tomatoes

500g tomatoes

2 tbsps olive oil

Salt and pepper to taste

3-4 thyme sprigs, broken into 2cm pieces

Cut the tomatoes in half and scoop out the seeds.

Place tomatoes in a large bowl with olive oil, salt and pepper and toss to coat.

Arrange tomatoes in air fryer basket and top each one with a small piece of thyme.

Cook at 115°C for 45 minutes or until required doneness is reached.

SERVES 4

Fresh Roasted Garlic

4 large whole garlic bulbs

2 tbsps olive oil

½ tsp salt

1 sprig rosemary

Preheat air fryer to 200°C.

Remove the outer paper skin from the garlic. Cut off the top 1cm to reveal the garlic cloves.

Place each garlic bulb in a square of aluminium foil.

Drizzle with olive oil, sprinkle with salt and scatter with rosemary leaves.

Wrap the garlic in the foil and place into the air fryer basket.

Cook for 20-30 minutes until soft and golden brown.

SERVES 2

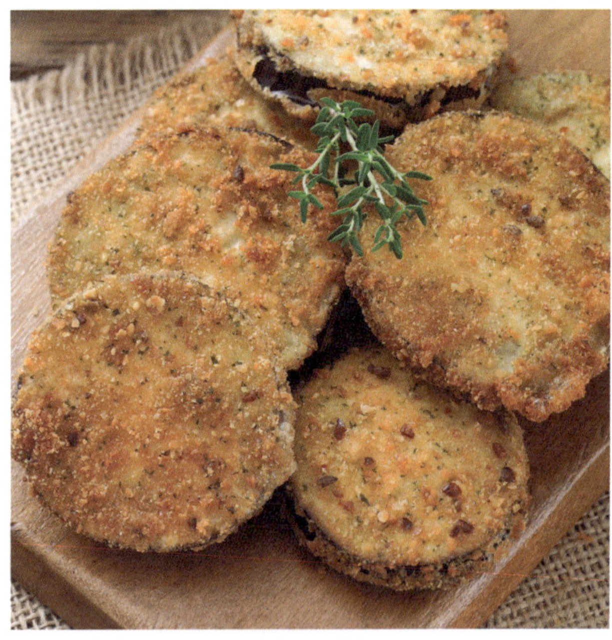

Eggplant Schnitzel

1 large eggplant, cut into 1½cm-thick slices

Salt and pepper to taste

3 tbsps plain flour

1 egg, beaten

½ cup (60g) breadcrumbs

1 tbsp thyme, chopped

3 tbsps Parmesan cheese, finely grated

Olive oil spray

Sprinkle eggplant slices generously with salt and set aside for 15 minutes.

Meanwhile place flour in one shallow dish and season with salt and pepper. Place beaten egg in another dish and finally mix together breadcrumbs, thyme and Parmesan in a third dish.

Pat dry eggplant then dip each slice first into the flour, then egg, then breadcrumb mix and coat evenly.

Preheat air fryer to 180°C.

Spray eggplant with cooking spray and arrange in one layer in air fryer basket. Cook in batches or use a double layer accessory if necessary. Cook for 8-10 minutes until golden brown.

SERVES 4

Falafel

2 x 400g cans chickpeas, drained and rinsed

¼ cup (10g) fresh parsley, chopped

¼ cup (10g) fresh coriander, chopped

2 tsps ground cumin

1 tsp paprika

2 cloves garlic, minced

1 small onion, finely diced

3 tbsps plain flour

1 tbsp lemon juice

1 tsp salt

Olive oil cooking spray

6 pitta breads

Rocket, grated carrot, cucumber, tomato and red onion to serve

TAHINI SAUCE

1¼ cups (310ml) Greek yoghurt

¼ cup (60g) tahini

2 tbsps fresh lemon juice

Combine chickpeas, herbs, spices, garlic, onion, flour, lemon juice and salt in a food processor. Blend into a rough paste.

Shape mixture into tablespoon-sized balls.

Preheat air fryer to 175°C.

Spray air fryer basket with cooking spray.

Cooking in batches, arrange falafel in air fryer basket and spray with cooking spray. Cook for 8 minutes then flip over and cook for another 6 minutes until golden brown and crispy. Repeat with remaining falafel.

Combine ingredients for sauce in a small bowl. Mix well.

Serve falafel hot in pitta bread with salad and tahini sauce.

SERVES 6

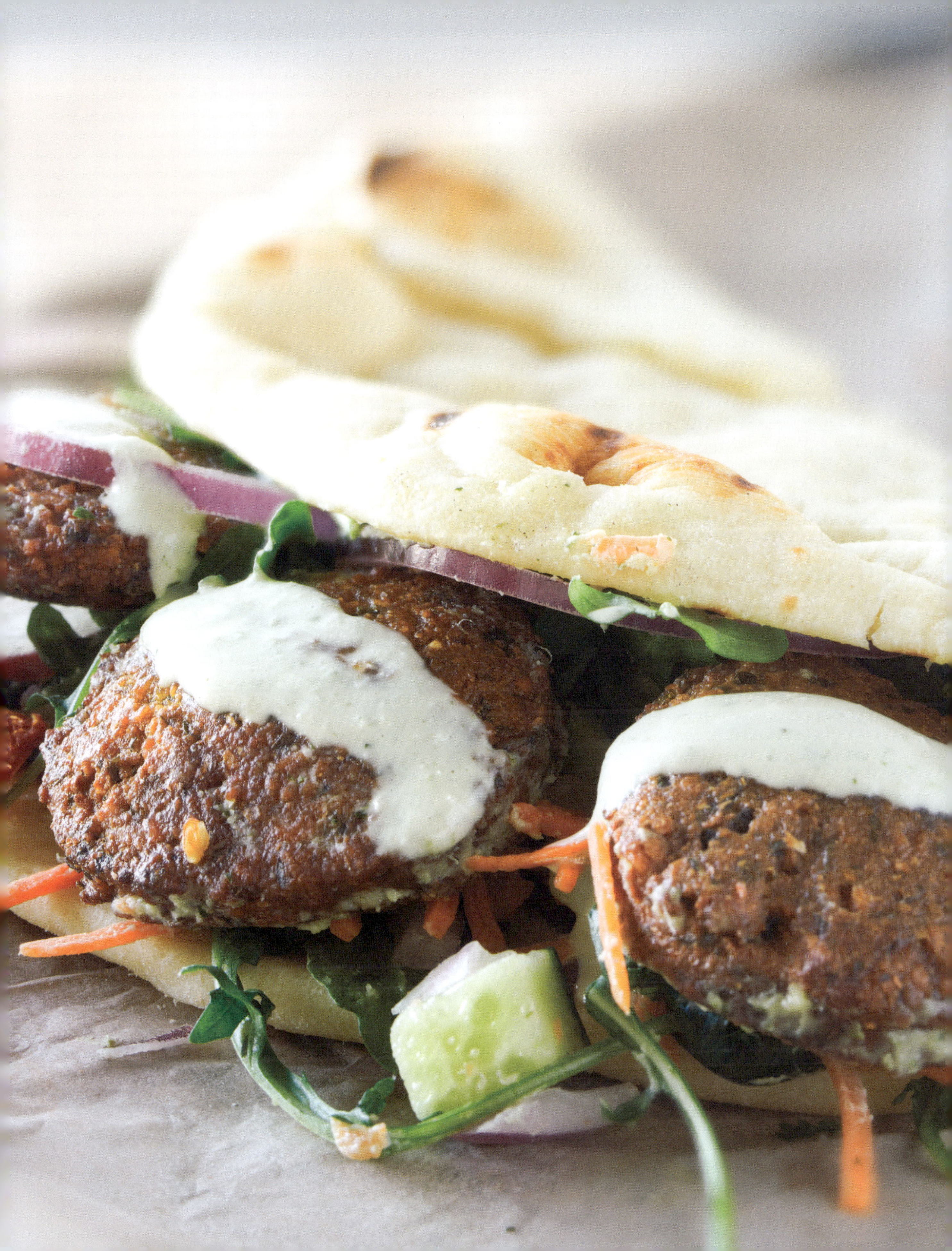

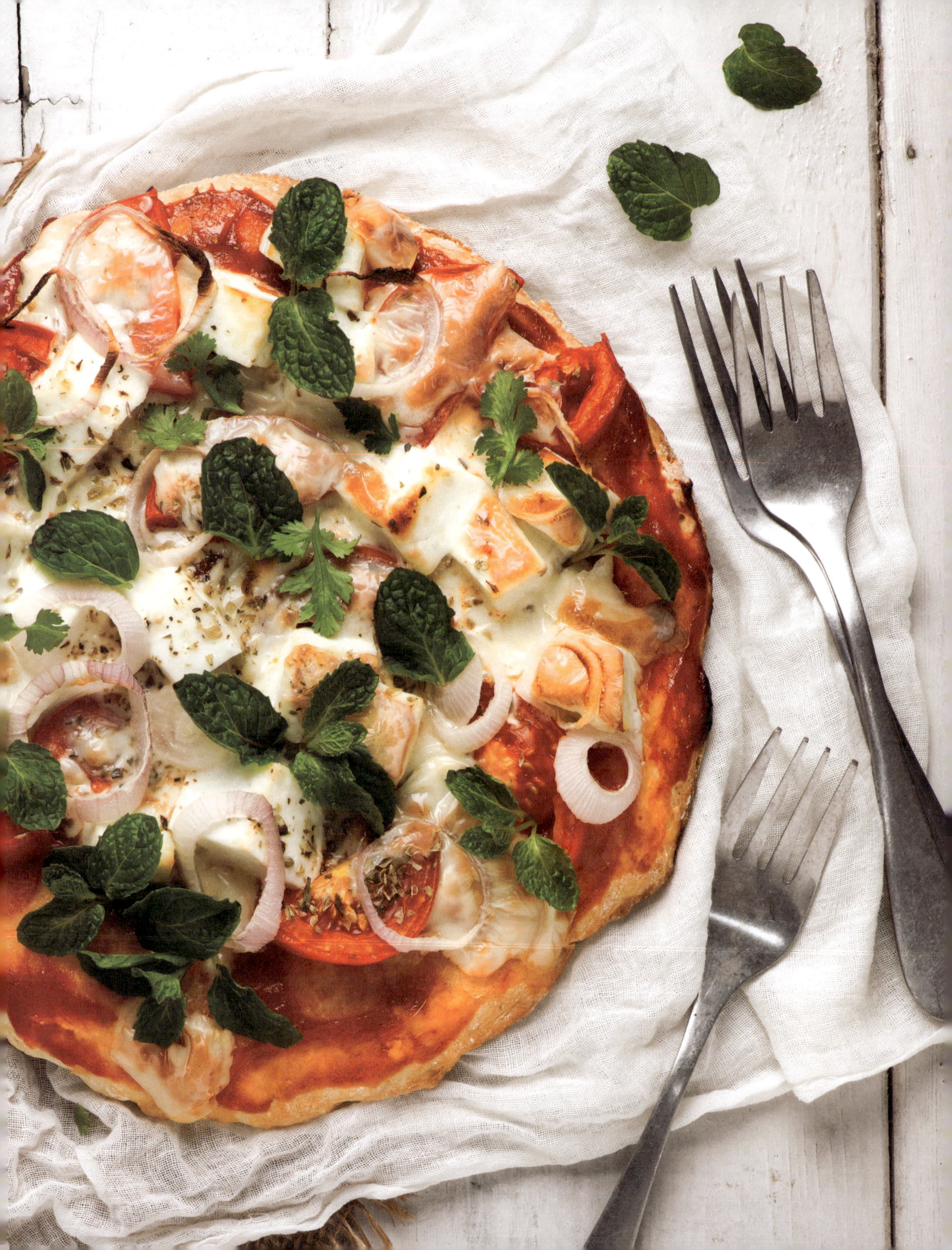

Vegetarian Pizza

DOUGH

2 cups (250g) baker's (or plain) flour

1 x 7g sachet dry active yeast

1 tsp caster sugar

1 tsp salt

¾ cup (200ml) warm water

1 tbsp olive oil + extra to grease

TOPPING

1 tbsp olive oil

¼ cup (60g) pizza sauce

150g fresh buffalo mozzarella, cubed

1 tomato, cut into eighths

1 tsp dried oregano

½ red onion, sliced

Mint leaves to garnish

Salt and pepper to taste

Sift flour into a large bowl. Stir in yeast, sugar and salt. Make a well in the centre and pour in water and oil. Bring the dough together with your hands, then turn out onto a lightly floured surface. Clean the bowl for reuse.

Knead for 5 minutes until the dough is smooth.

Lightly grease the bowl with oil, then add dough and cover with a tea towel or plastic wrap. Set aside in a warm place to prove for 1 hour, until doubled in size.

Knock back the dough by punching it to remove air and divide into two balls.

Preheat air fryer to 190°C. Spray air fryer basket with cooking spray.

Roll out one ball of pizza dough to the size of air fryer basket. Carefully transfer to air fryer and brush with olive oil.

Spread with pizza sauce. Top with mozzarella, tomatoes, oregano and onion.

Bake for 7 minutes until crust is crispy and cheese is melted. Top with mint leaves and season with salt and pepper.

Repeat with second ball of pizza dough.

SERVES 2

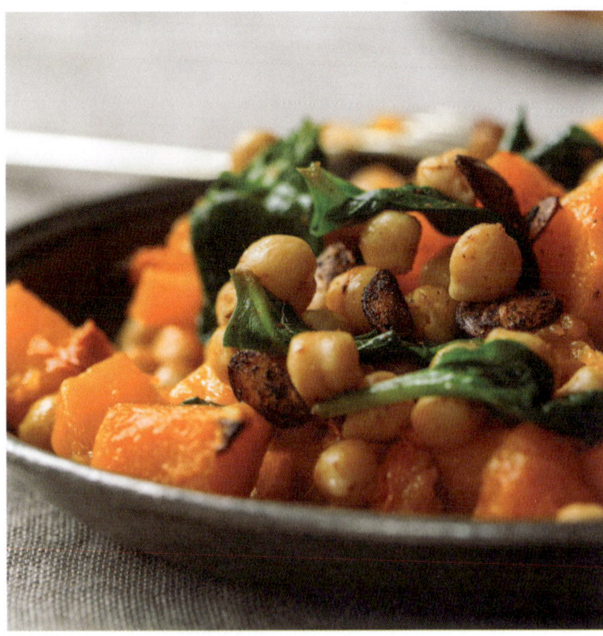

Roast Butternut Pumpkin with Chickpeas

4 cups (540g) butternut pumpkin, cubed

1 x 400g can chickpeas, drained and rinsed

4 cloves garlic, thinly sliced

1 tsp paprika

2 tbsps olive oil

Salt and pepper to taste

1 cup (30g) baby spinach leaves

Olive oil cooking spray

Place pumpkin and chickpeas in a large bowl with garlic, paprika and olive oil. Season with salt and pepper and toss to coat.

Add to air fryer basket and cook at 200°C for 20-25 minutes, until just tender, shaking halfway through.

Add the spinach leaves to air fryer basket and toss to combine. Return to air fryer and cook for 2 minutes to wilt.

SERVES 2

Grilled Portobello Mushroom Burger

2 tbsps olive oil

1 tbsp tamari

1 clove garlic, minced

1 tsp salt

4 large portobello mushrooms, wiped clean and stems removed

1 red capsicum, sliced

4 wholemeal burger buns

2 tbsps mayonnaise

Handful rocket leaves, washed and dried

80g blue cheese, crumbled

Preheat air fryer to 180°C.

Mix together 1 tablespoon oil, tamari, garlic and salt. Brush each mushroom generously with the mixture.

Spray the air fryer basket with cooking spray. Place the mushrooms in the basket, stem-side down.

Cook for 8-10 minutes until tender. Set aside and keep warm.

Place the capsicum in a bowl with remaining oil and toss to coat.

Place capsicum in air fryer basket and cook for 7 minutes until tender.

To assemble, spread each burger bun with mayonnaise, then cover with rocket leaves, top with a portobello mushroom, crumble over some blue cheese and layer with sliced capsicum. Finish with burger bun top and serve immediately.

SERVES 4

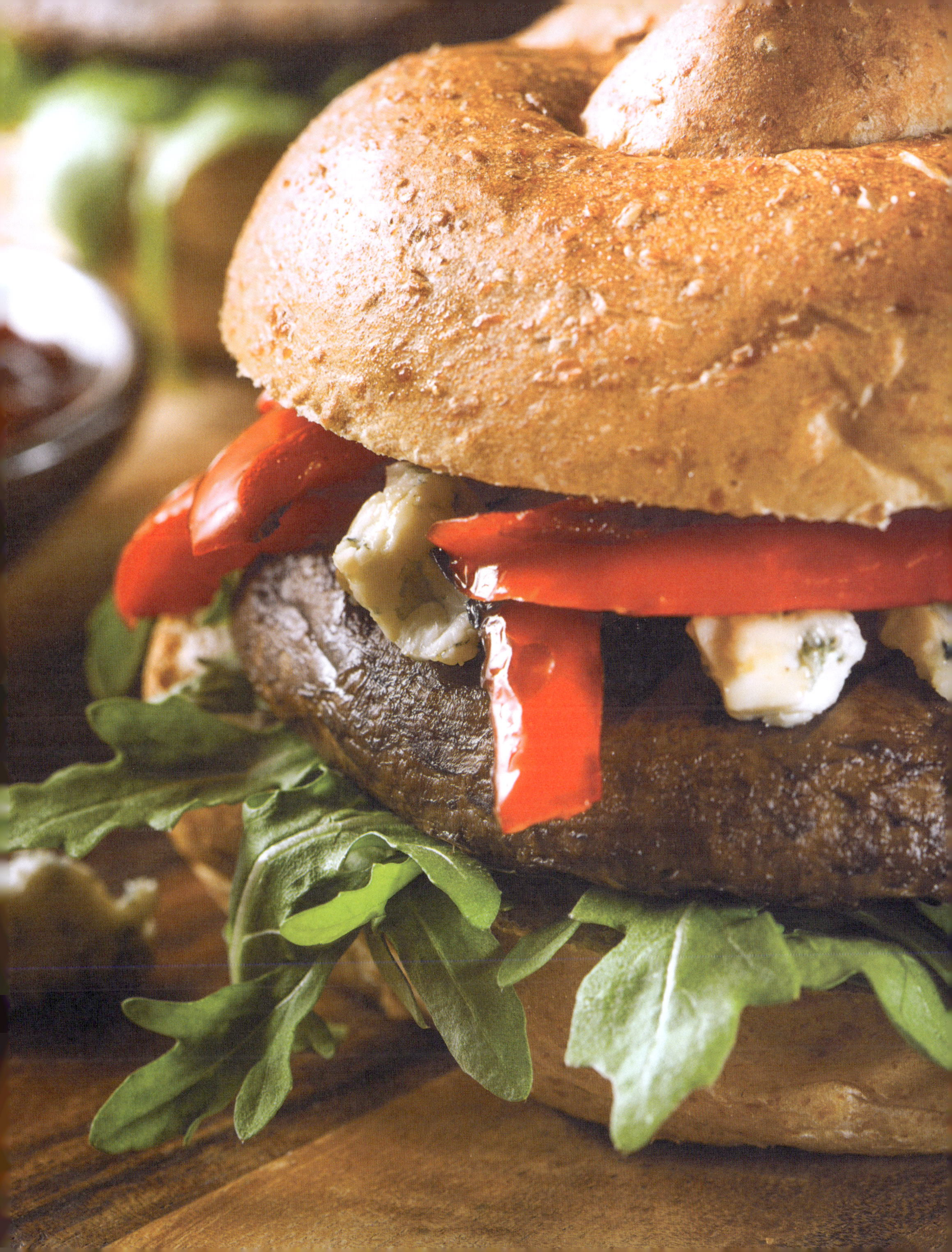

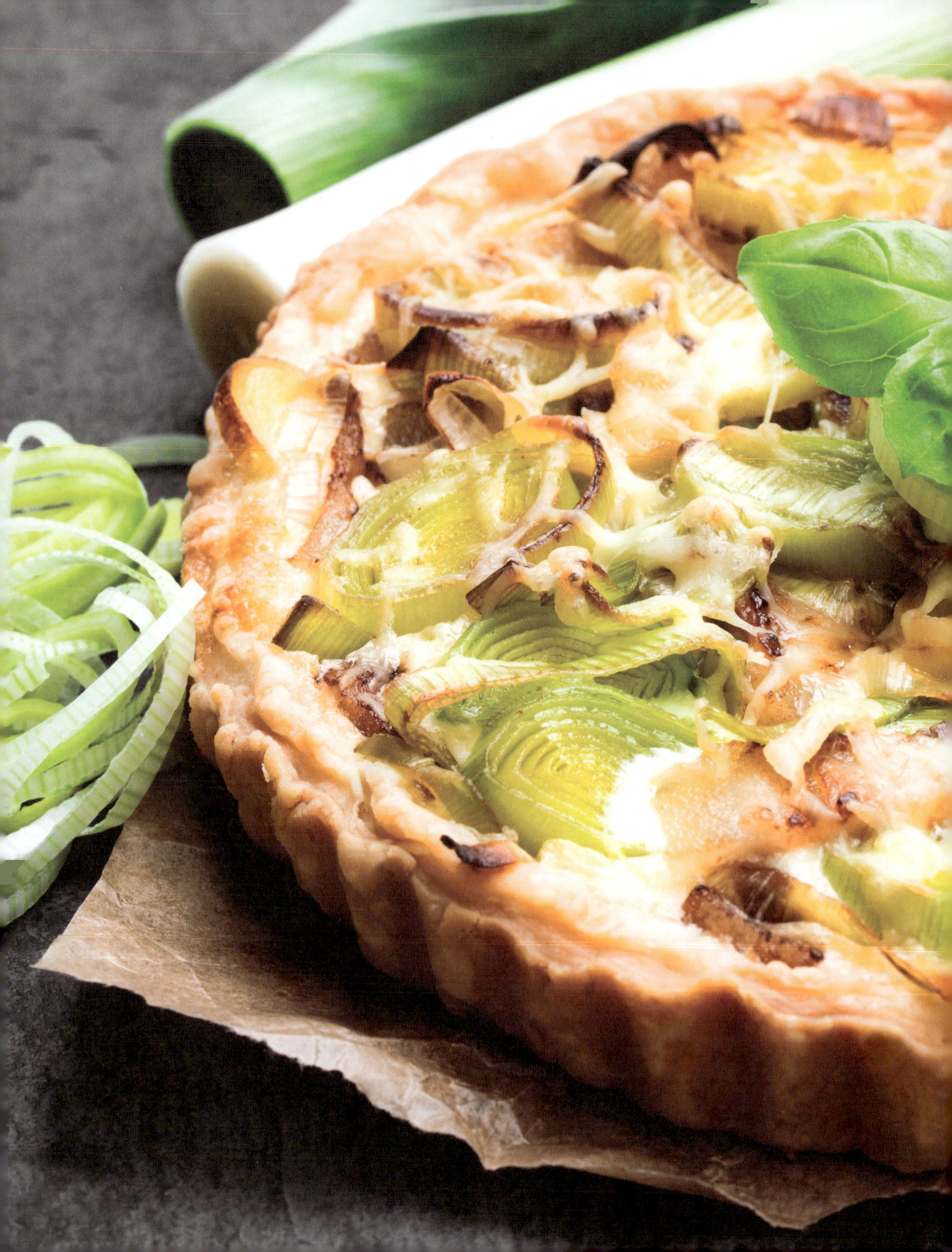

Leek and Mushroom Tart

25g butter

3 leeks, sliced and washed

150g chestnut mushrooms, sliced

1 egg

¾ cup (180ml) thickened cream

¾ cup (100g) Gruyère cheese, coarsely grated

PASTRY

1½ cups (190g) plain flour

100g cold butter, diced

6 tbsps cold water

Cake tin

For the pastry place flour and butter in a large bowl. Rub together with your fingertips until crumbly. Add water 1 tablespoon at a time, mixing with a knife. Bring pastry together, wrap in plastic wrap and chill for 1 hour.

Heat butter in a pan over medium heat. Add leeks and cook for 10 minutes, add mushrooms and cook for a further 5 minutes until soft. Set aside.

In a large bowl mix together egg, cream and half of the cheese. Add leeks and mushrooms. Stir to combine.

Roll out pastry, transfer to a flan dish or cake tin that fits into your air fryer. Trim the edges and prick with a fork.

Place into air fryer and cook at 160°C for 10-15 minutes.

Pour filling into pastry, top with remaining cheese. Cook for 15-20 minutes at 160°C until set and golden brown.

SERVES 4

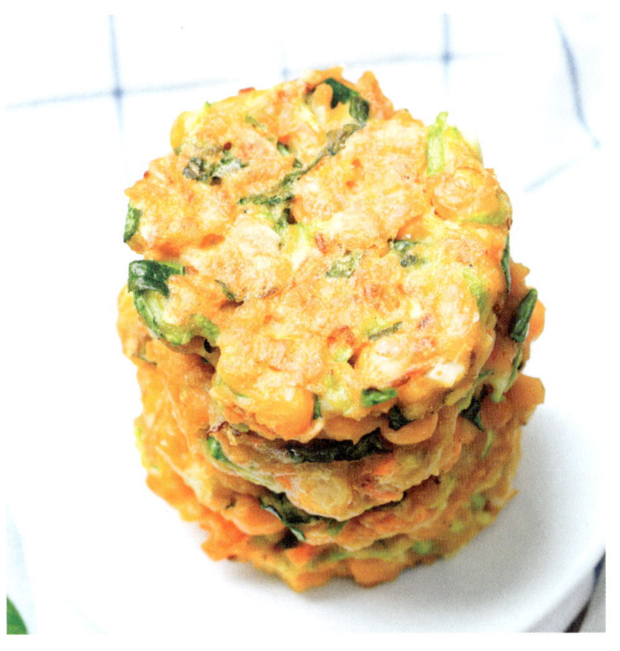

Zucchini Chickpea Patties

1 large zucchini, grated

1 x 400g can chickpeas, drained and rinsed

3 spring onions, chopped

1 tsp garlic powder

3 tbsps ground coriander

½ tsp chilli powder

1 tsp ground cumin

Salt and pepper to taste

Avocado or olive oil cooking spray

Preheat air fryer to 200°C.

Place grated zucchini in a clean tea towel with chickpeas and squeeze to remove any excess liquid.

Place zucchini and chickpeas in a large bowl with spring onions, garlic powder, spices and seasoning. Use your hands to combine, then shape mixture into patties.

Arrange patties in air fryer. Spray with cooking spray.

Cook for 12 minutes, turning halfway, until golden brown.

SERVES 2

Apple, Pumpkin and Blue Cheese Galette

SHORTCRUST PASTRY

1½ cups (185g) plain flour

¼ tsp salt

125g butter, chilled

2-4 tbsps ice water

FILLING

750g pumpkin, cut into 2cm-thick slices

Olive oil cooking spray

Salt and pepper to taste

1 red onion, thickly sliced

25g butter

4 sprigs thyme

1 tbsp Dijon mustard

1 apple, thinly sliced

80g crumbled blue cheese

1 egg, beaten

To make pastry, combine flour and salt in a large bowl. Add butter and rub with fingertips until it resembles coarse crumbs. Gradually add water until the mixture begins to hold together. Gather dough into a ball and flatten into a thick disc. Wrap in plastic wrap and refrigerate for 30 minutes.

Preheat air fryer to 180°C.

Place pumpkin slices in air fryer basket. Spray with cooking spray and season with salt and pepper. Cook for 10 minutes until tender.

Meanwhile, combine onion, butter and half the thyme in a frying pan over medium heat. Fry gently for 10 minutes until onion is soft and translucent.

Roll out pastry on a large sheet of greaseproof paper to a circle 10cm larger than air fryer basket. Leaving a 5cm rim around the edge, spread the pastry with mustard, then spoon over cooked onion. Add pumpkin and apple slices and sprinkle over blue cheese and remaining thyme. Fold over edges of pastry. Brush folded edges with egg.

Cook for 20 minutes until golden brown.

SERVES 3

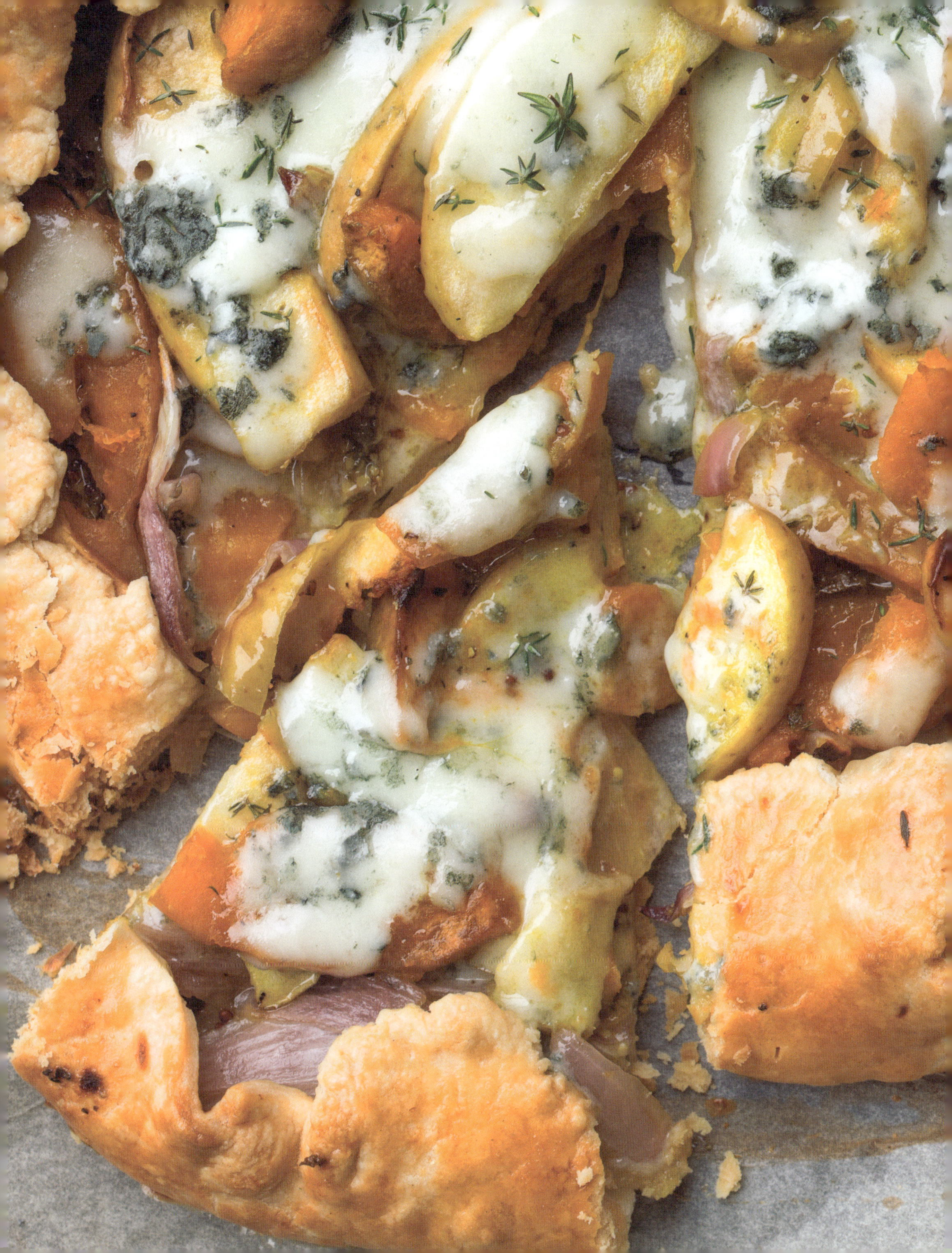

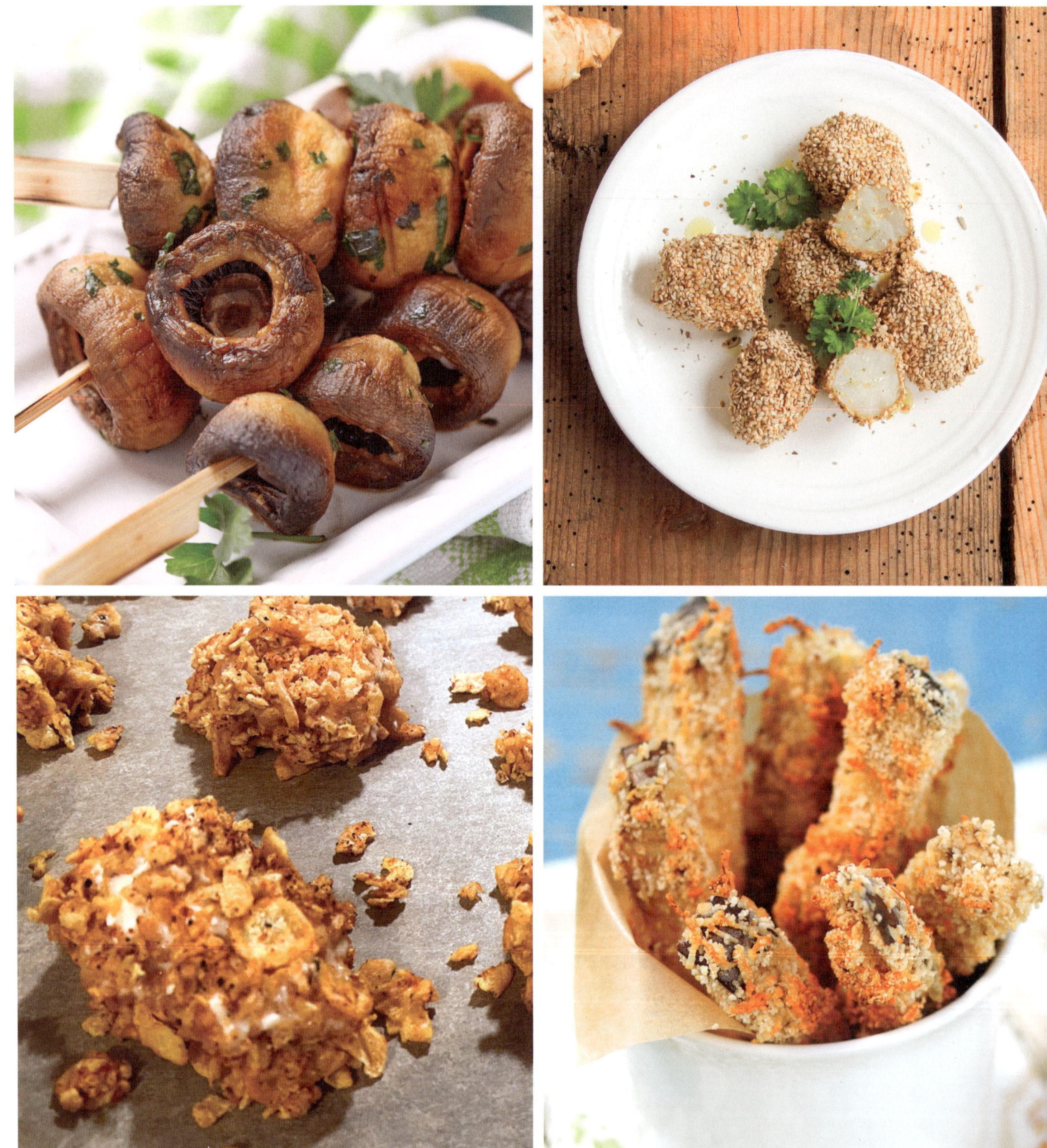

Mushroom Kebabs

250g button mushrooms

1 tbsp olive oil

1 tbsp balsamic vinegar

2 cloves garlic, minced

1 tbsp fresh parsley, chopped

Salt and pepper to taste

Skewers

Mix all the ingredients together in a glass bowl and allow to marinate for at least 30 minutes, stirring occasionally.

Preheat air fryer to 200°C.

Thread the mushrooms onto skewers and place in air fryer basket.

Cook for 5 minutes, then turn the skewers and cook for a further 5-6 minutes, until mushrooms are soft and tender.

SERVES 2

Sesame Jerusalem Artichokes

500g Jerusalem artichokes

¾ cup (185ml) olive oil

2 cloves garlic, minced

½ tsp salt

2 egg whites

1 cup (160g) sesame seeds

Preheat air fryer to 155°C.

Scrub Jerusalem artichokes and cut into 3cm pieces. Place in a large bowl with olive oil, garlic and half the salt. Toss to coat. Arrange in one evenly spaced layer in air fryer.

Cook for 15 minutes. Remove from air fryer. Set aside to cool.

Whisk together egg whites and remaining salt in a shallow dish. Place sesame seeds in another dish.

When cool enough to handle dip Jerusalem artichokes first into egg white then into sesame seeds.

Return to air fryer and cook for 15-20 minutes at 155°C until golden brown and cooked through.

SERVES 2

Crumbed Tofu

350g block firm tofu

1 tbsp tapioca flour

1 tsp garlic powder

1 tsp onion powder

Salt and pepper to taste

¾ cup (185ml) almond milk

3 tbsps wholemeal flour

1 cup (30g) cornflakes

Drain tofu and press dry with a tea towel or paper towels. Tear into 3cm pieces.

In a bowl combine tapioca, garlic powder, onion powder, salt and pepper. Add tofu pieces and toss to coat well.

In a small bowl whisk together almond milk and flour. In another bowl place cornflakes.

Quickly dip tofu first into milk then roll into cornflakes to coat. Arrange on greaseproof paper in air fryer. Cook in batches or use a double layer accessory if necessary.

Cook at 190°C for 15 minutes, flipping halfway through.

SERVES 2

Crispy Eggplant Fries

1 large eggplant

1¼ cups (155g) panko breadcrumbs

½ cup (50g) Parmesan cheese, grated

1 tsp Italian seasoning

Salt and pepper to taste

1 egg, beaten

Olive oil spray

Cut eggplant into 10cm-long, 2cm-thick fries.

Combine panko with Parmesan and Italian seasoning in a shallow dish. Season with salt and pepper. Place beaten egg in another dish.

Dip each eggplant fry first into the beaten egg and then into the breadcrumbs and gently press to coat.

Preheat air fryer basket to 200°C. Spray air fryer basket with cooking spray.

Evenly space eggplant fries in air fryer basket, Cook in batches or use a double layer accessory if necessary. Spray eggplant with cooking spray, then cook fries for 14 minutes until crispy. Sprinkle with salt to serve.

SERVES 4

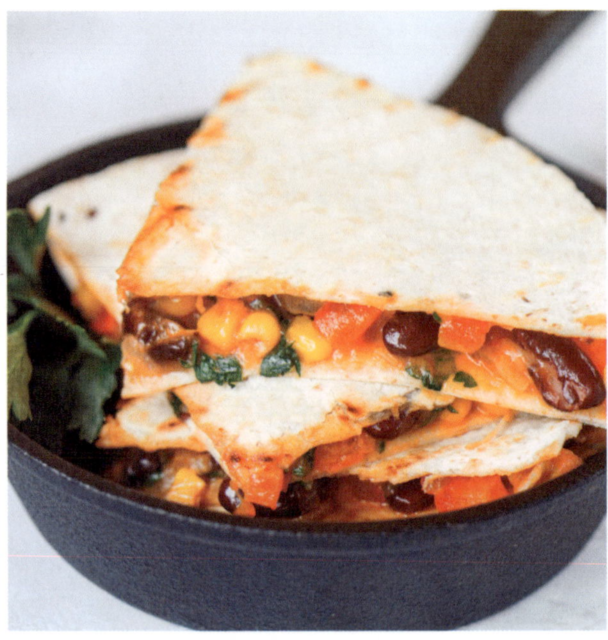

Vegetarian Quesadilla

4 large flour tortillas

1 cup (125g) Cheddar cheese, grated

1 red capsicum, sliced

1 tomato, chopped

1 cup (175g) corn kernels

1 x 400g can black beans, drained and rinsed

2 tbsps coriander, chopped

Cooking spray

Preheat air fryer to 200°C.

Place tortillas on a work surface. Sprinkle 2 tablespoons grated cheese over half of each tortilla. Top cheese with capsicum slices, tomato, corn, black beans and coriander. Sprinkle evenly with remaining cheese. Fold tortillas over to form half-moon shaped quesadillas. Lightly coat quesadillas with cooking spray and secure with toothpicks.

Spray air fryer basket with cooking spray. Carefully place two quesadillas in the basket and cook for 10 minutes, turning halfway through, until cheese is melted and vegetables are tender. Repeat with remaining quesadillas.

SERVES 4

Broccoli and Cheese Quiche

Cooking spray

1 sheet frozen shortcrust pastry, thawed

½ head of broccoli, broken into florets

½ cup (60g) cheese, grated

2 eggs

½ cup (125ml) milk

2 tbsps double cream

Salt and pepper to taste

Cake tin

Preheat air fryer to 160°C.

Lightly spray a 16cm quiche pan or cake tin with cooking spray.

Gently press pastry into tin, lining base and sides. Trim edges with a sharp knife.

Arrange broccoli in the pastry case.

Mix together cheese, eggs, milk and cream in a large bowl. Season with salt and pepper. Pour over broccoli.

Place tin into air fryer basket and cook for 18-20 minutes until filling is set and pastry is golden brown.

SERVES 2

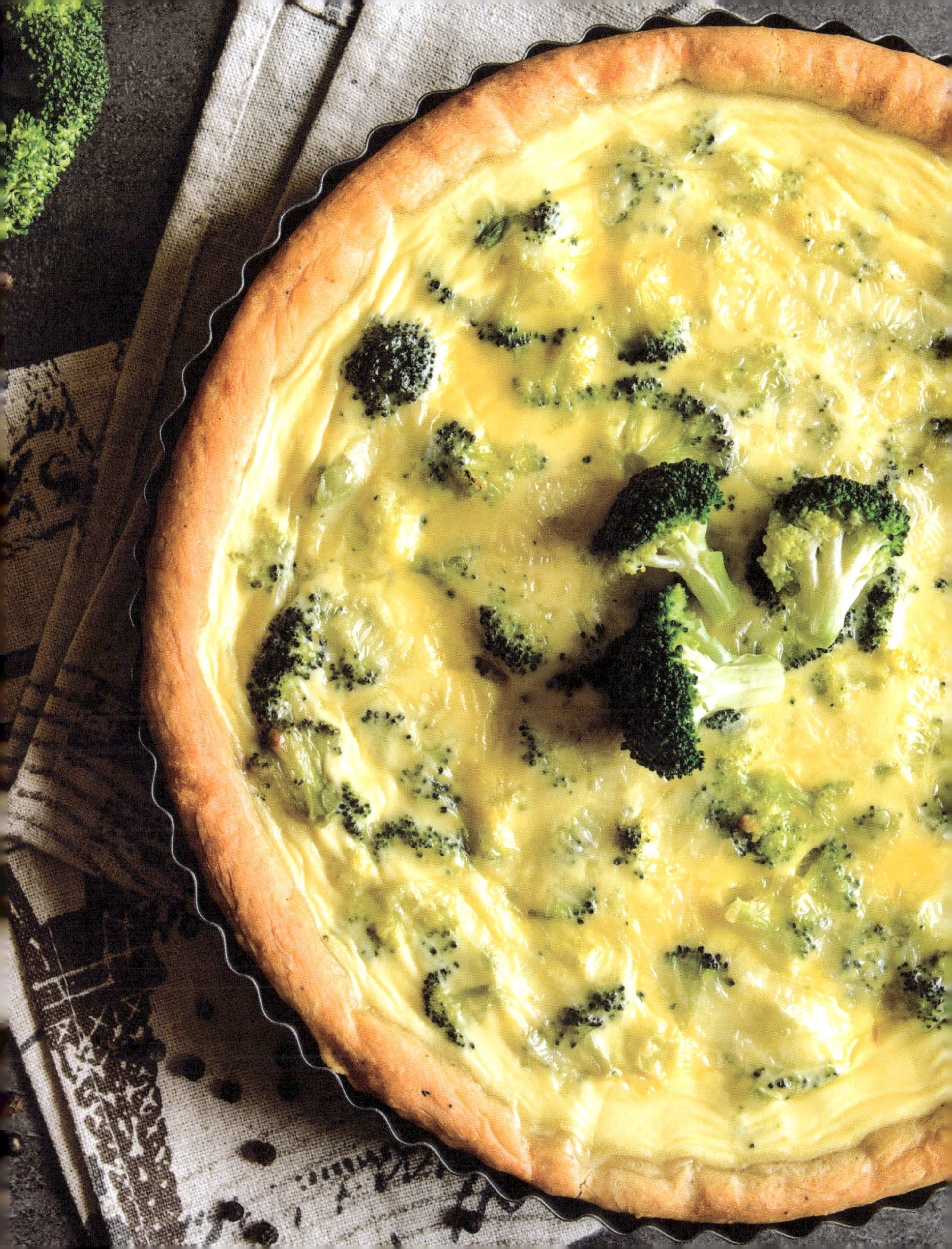

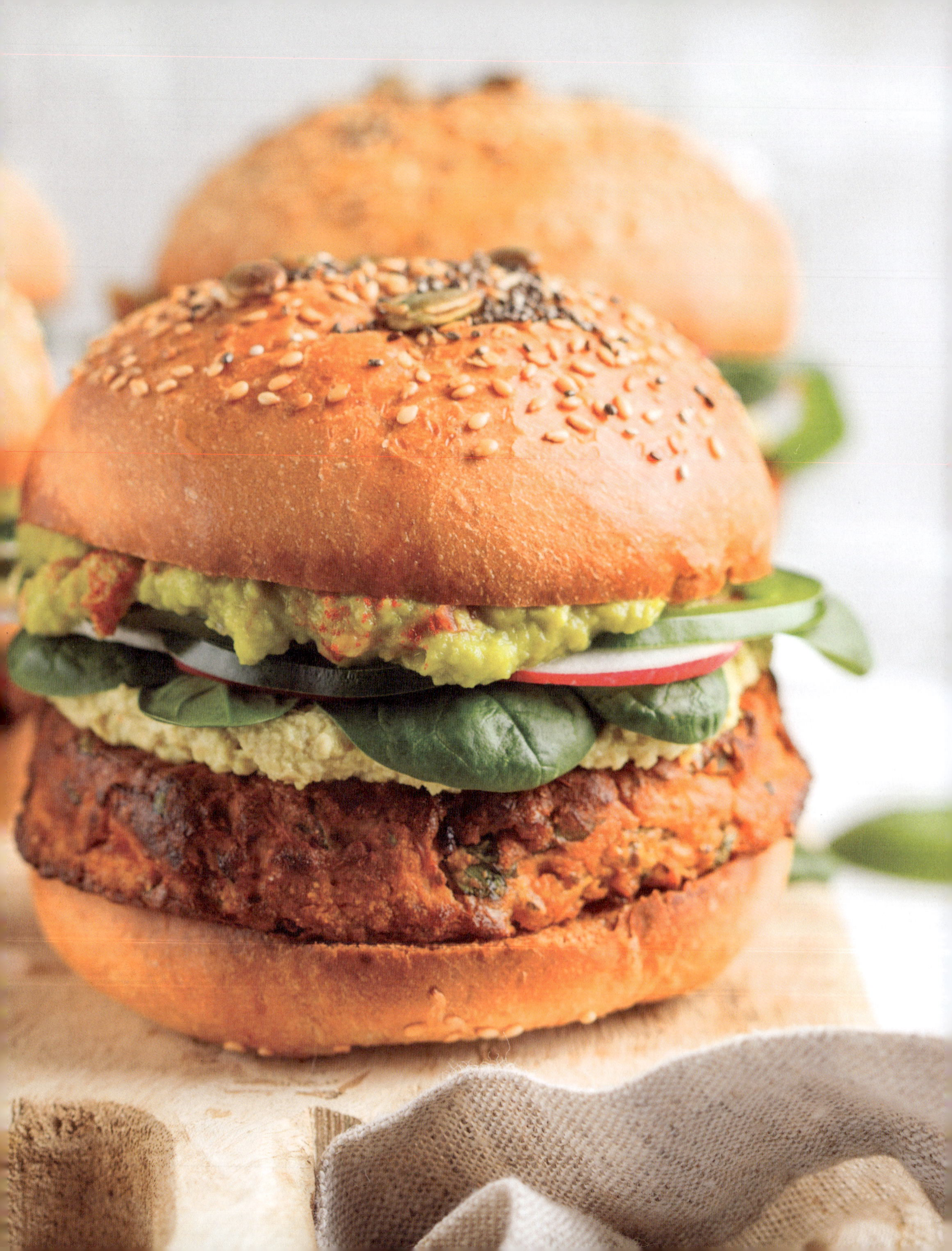

Sweet Potato Burger

1 x 400g can cannellini beans, drained and rinsed
1½ cups (250g) cooked mashed sweet potato
⅔-1 cup (165g) cooked brown rice
2 spring onions, finely diced
⅓ cup (40g) walnuts, very finely chopped
2 tsps ground cumin
½ tsp paprika
Salt and pepper to taste
Cooking spray
2 large avocados
1 tsp lemon juice
1 clove garlic, minced
3 tbsps mayonnaise
½ cup (15g) salad leaves
½ green capsicum, sliced
½ red onion, sliced
¼ tsp chilli powder
4 burger buns

Place cannellini beans in a mixing bowl and partially mash with a fork. Add sweet potato and ⅔ cup rice, spring onion, walnuts and spices. Season with salt and pepper and mix to combine. Add more rice if the mixture feels too wet.

Form mixture into four patties and place on a greaseproof-paper-lined plate. Refrigerate for 30 minutes to set.

Preheat air fryer to 175°C.

Spray air fryer basket with cooking spray.

Arrange patties in air fryer, spray with cooking spray and cook for 5-7 minutes, flip over and cook for another 2-4 minutes until cooked through.

Meanwhile scoop flesh from avocados and place in a medium bowl. Add lemon juice, garlic and a pinch of salt. Mash with a fork.

Spoon half of mashed avocado into another bowl and mix with mayonnaise.

Place burgers in burger buns and spread with avocado mayonnaise mix. Top with salad leaves, capsicum and onion. Spoon over mashed avocado, sprinkle with chilli powder and finish with bun lid.

SERVES 4

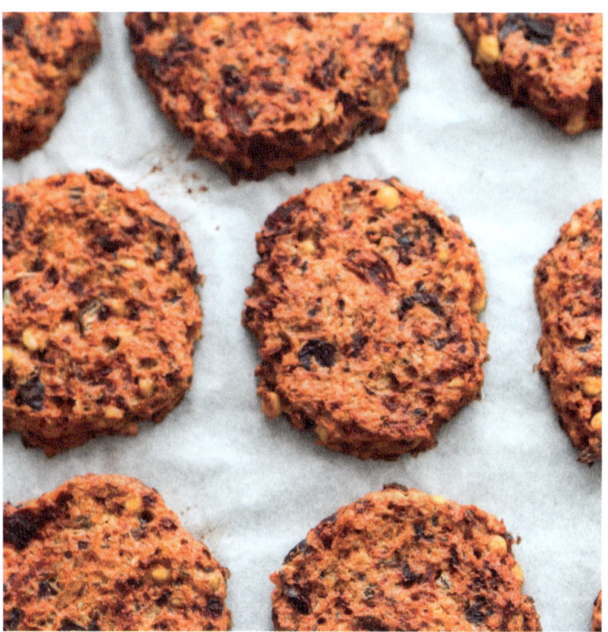

Beetroot and Chickpea Patties

1 x 400g can chickpeas, drained and rinsed
2 medium cooked beetroots, diced
1 onion, diced
2 cloves garlic, peeled
½ cup (45g) oats
⅓ cup (20g) nutritional yeast
1 tsp smoked paprika
¼ cup (5g) fresh parsley
Salt and pepper to taste

Add chickpeas, beetroot, onion, garlic, oats, nutritional yeast, paprika, parsley, salt and pepper to a food processor. Pulse to combine, maintaining a chunky texture.

Preheat air fryer to 180°C.

Shape mixture into eight patties.

Spray air fryer basket with olive oil spray.

Arrange patties in air fryer leaving space between each one. Cook in batches or use a double layer accessory if necessary. Cook for 15-20 minutes, turning halfway through cooking.

SERVES 4

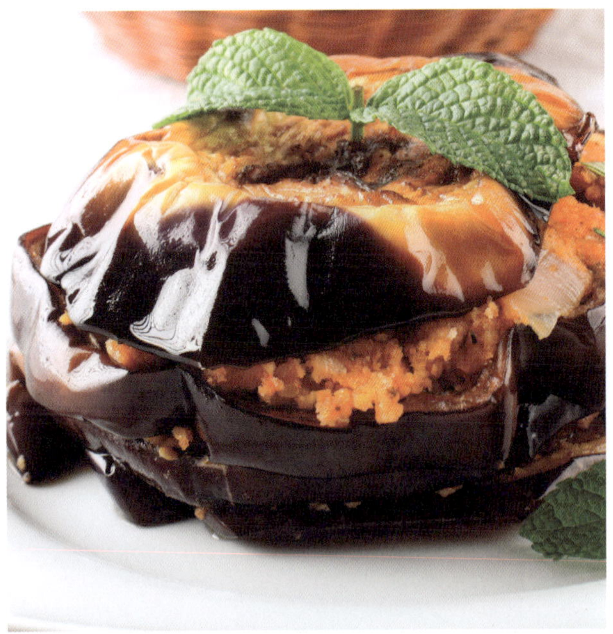

Eggplant Parmesan

2 tbsps olive oil

1 small onion, finely chopped

1 clove garlic, minced

1 x 400g can chopped tomatoes

Salt and pepper to taste

1 large eggplant, sliced into 2cm-thick slices

Olive oil cooking spray

½ cup (50g) Parmesan cheese, grated

½ cup (60g) breadcrumbs

Heat oil in a large pan over medium-high heat, add onion and cook, stirring, for 3-5 minutes until soft and translucent. Add garlic and cook for 1 minute more, until fragrant. Add chopped tomatoes and season with salt and pepper. When bubbling, reduce heat and simmer for 10 minutes.

Meanwhile spray eggplant with olive oil spray. Place in air fryer and cook for 5 minutes at 180°C. Flip the eggplant and cook for another 3 minutes.

Spread eggplant with the cooked tomato sauce. Sprinkle with Parmesan and top with breadcrumbs.

Cook for a further 3-4 minutes or until cheese is melted and breadcrumbs are golden brown.

Arrange the eggplant Parmesan in two stacks to serve.

SERVES 2

Sun-Dried Tomato Arancini

1 tbsp olive oil

1 onion, finely diced

1 cup (155g) Arborio rice

4 cups (1L) vegetable stock

Salt and pepper to taste

1 cup (100g) Parmesan cheese, grated

⅓ cup (40g) mozzarella cheese, grated

⅓ cup (20g) sun-dried tomatoes packed in oil, finely chopped

⅓ cup (15g) fresh basil, roughly chopped

1 cup (125g) plain flour

1½ cups (185g) breadcrumbs

2 eggs, beaten

Heat oil in a large pan over medium heat. Add onions and saute until soft. Add rice and fry for 1 minute.

Add stock, ½ cup at a time, stirring until liquid is absorbed before adding the next ½ cup. Continue until all liquid is absorbed and rice is soft. Season well with salt and pepper. Stir in Parmesan, mozzarella, sun-dried tomatoes and basil.

Pour risotto into a large dish. Refrigerate for at least 2 hours.

In a shallow dish place the flour. In a small bowl, place the breadcrumbs. In another bowl, place the beaten eggs.

Remove chilled rice from the fridge. Shape into 3cm balls.

Dip each ball into flour, then eggs, then into breadcrumbs. Refrigerate for 45 minutes.

Spray air fryer basket with cooking spray.

Place into air fryer in small batches or use a double layer accessory. Cook at 200°C for 10 minutes, shaking halfway through.

MAKES 18

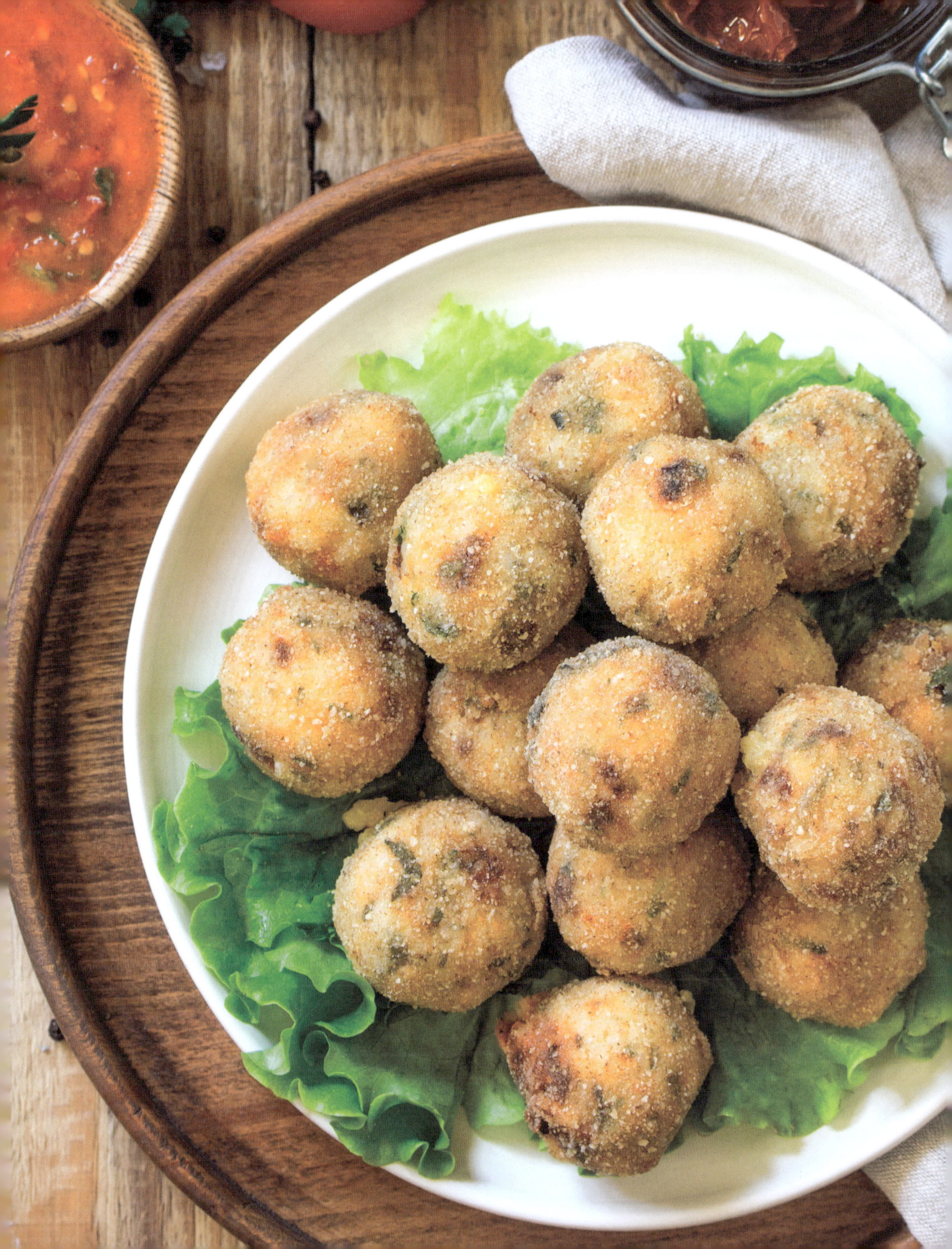

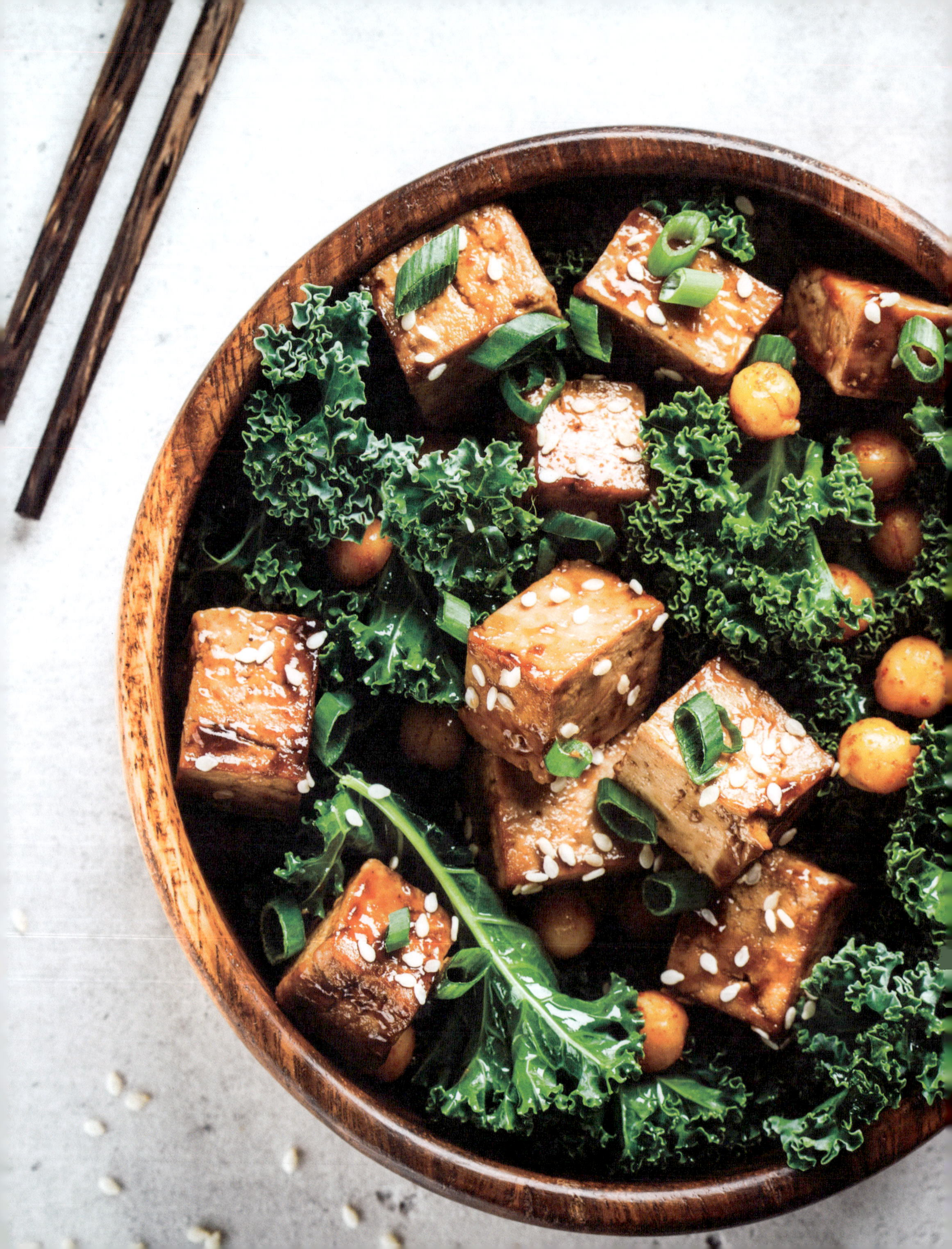

Teriyaki Tofu Salad

¼ cup (60ml) soy sauce

3 tbsps maple syrup

2 tsps apple cider vinegar

3 tbsps water

2 cloves garlic, minced

Small piece of ginger, grated

1 tsp cornflour

1 tsp sesame oil

450g firm tofu, cut into pieces

1 tbsp sesame seeds

1 x 400g can chickpeas, drained and rinsed

1 tbsp olive oil

½ tsp paprika

⅛ tsp salt

¼ tsp garlic powder

¼ tsp onion powder

150g kale, washed and roughly torn

2 spring onions, chopped

Baking pan

Preheat air fryer to 200°C. Line baking pan with greaseproof paper.

In a medium bowl combine soy sauce, maple syrup, vinegar, water, garlic, ginger, cornflour and sesame oil. Mix well.

Add the tofu and toss to coat.

Arrange tofu on lined pan. Place in air fryer and cook for 25-30 minutes, shaking halfway through cooking. Sprinkle with sesame seeds. Set aside and keep warm.

Combine chickpeas with olive oil, paprika and seasonings in a large bowl. Toss to coat then place directly in air fryer basket. Cook for 12-15 minutes at 200°C, shaking halfway through cooking.

Place kale and spring onions in a large bowl. Add tofu and chickpeas. Toss to combine, then serve into bowls.

SERVES 2

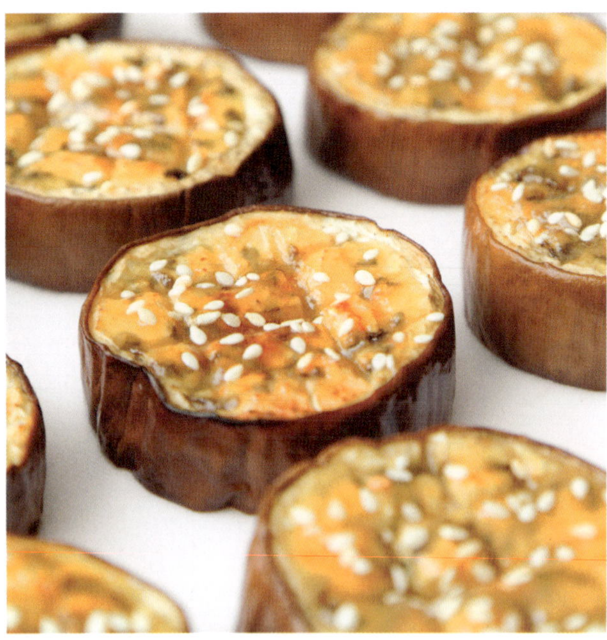

Miso Eggplant Slices

1 large eggplant, cut into 2cm-thick rounds

2 tbsps peanut oil or other neutral flavoured oil

⅓ cup (90g) white miso

2 tbsps mirin

1 tbsp honey or brown sugar

2 tsps rice wine vinegar

1 tbsp sesame seeds

Brush eggplant with oil. Place in air fryer and cook for 5 minutes at 180°C. Flip the eggplant and cook for another 3 minutes.

Mix together miso, mirin, honey or sugar and rice wine vinegar.

Brush miso glaze liberally on top of eggplant slices.

Return to air fryer and cook for 3 minutes.

Sprinkle with sesame seeds to serve.

SERVES 2

Roasted Capsicums

2 tbsps olive oil

1 onion, diced

1 clove garlic, minced

1 tsp dried oregano

250g mushrooms, chopped

2 cups (330g) cooked rice

½ cup (115g) passata

Salt and pepper, to taste

150g goat's cheese, crumbled

4 red capsicums

Heat 1 tablespoon olive oil in a large pan over medium heat. Add onion and cook for 3-5 minutes until soft and translucent. Add garlic and oregano and cook for 1 minute more until fragrant.

Add mushrooms and stir-fry for 4 minutes until tender.

Add cooked rice and passata and cook, stirring, for 2 minutes until heated through. Remove from heat, season with salt and pepper and gently stir through goat's cheese.

Cut tops off capsicums and scoop out seeds. Fill with mixture and replace tops. Drizzle with remaining oil.

Arrange capsicums in air fryer basket and cook for 15 minutes at 180°C.

SERVES 2

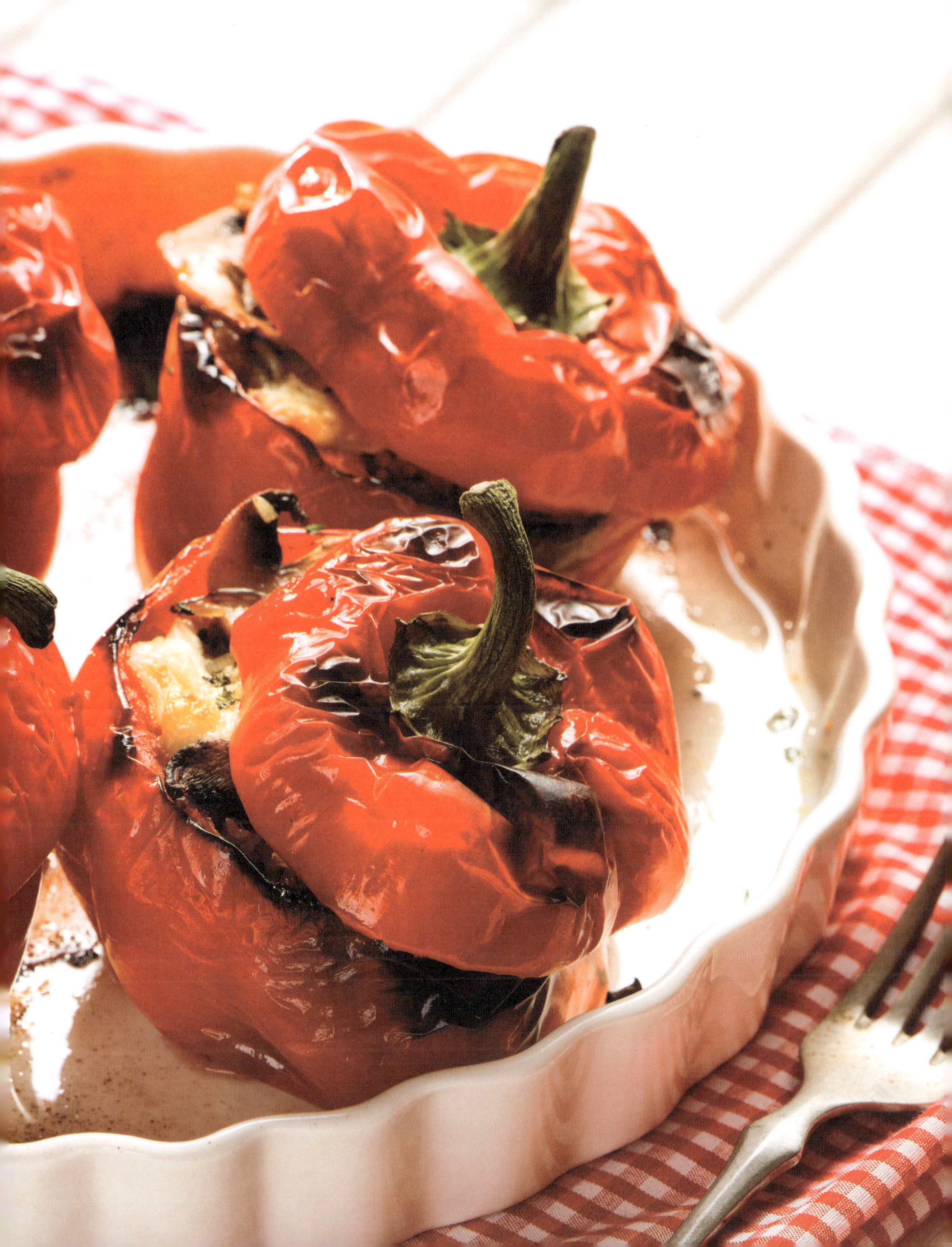

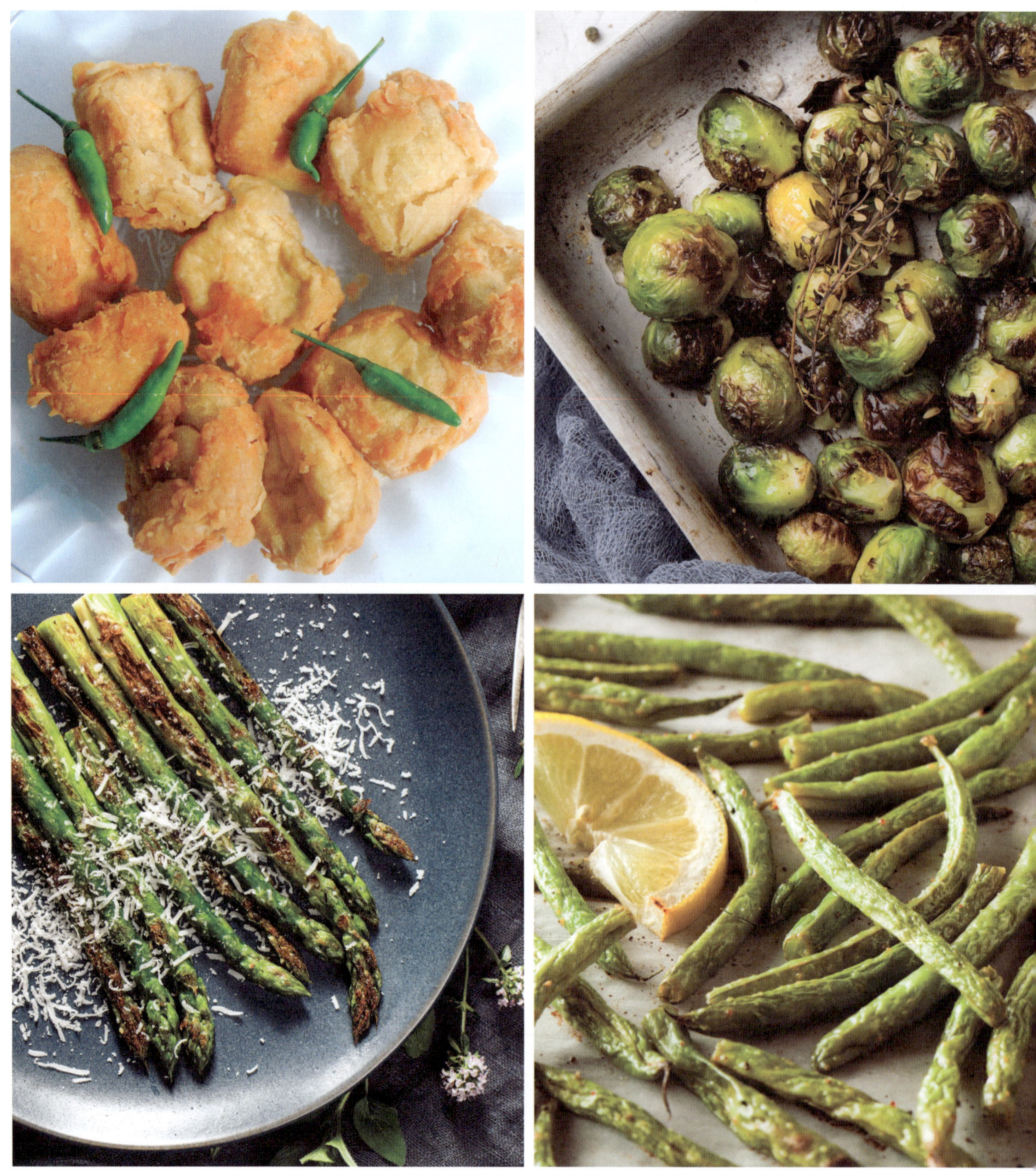

Crispy Tofu

Olive oil or avocado oil cooking spray

½ cup (60g) plain flour

2 eggs, beaten

1 tbsp water

450g semi-firm tofu, dried and cut into 3cm cubes

Salt to taste

Line air fryer basket with greaseproof paper and spray with cooking spray.

Place flour in one bowl, mix eggs and water in another.

Dip each piece of tofu into the flour and then the egg. Then repeat process to dip in the flour and egg once again.

Arrange tofu in air fryer basket. Spray with cooking spray and sprinkle with salt.

Cook at 190°C for 8 minutes, then gently remove the greaseproof paper from beneath the tofu and cook for a further 4 minutes.

SERVES 2

Roasted Brussels Sprouts

750g Brussels sprouts

2 tbsps olive oil

1 tsp garlic powder

1 tsp salt

½ tsp pepper

Preheat air fryer to 200°C.

Place Brussels sprouts, olive oil, garlic powder, salt and pepper in a large bowl and mix well to coat.

Spread Brussels sprouts evenly in the air fryer basket. Cook for 15-18 minutes, shaking the basket halfway through, until Brussels sprouts are crisp and tender.

SERVES 4

Parmesan Asparagus

500g fresh asparagus

1 tbsp olive oil

⅛ tsp salt

⅛ tsp pepper

¼ cup (25g) Parmesan cheese, grated

Trim off the woody ends of asparagus.

Place on a large plate and drizzle with olive oil and season with salt and pepper.

Toss well to coat.

Arrange asparagus in air fryer basket. Cook for 7 minutes at 200°C.

Serve asparagus onto a large serving plate and sprinkle with grated Parmesan.

SERVES 2

Lemony Green Beans

500g fresh green beans

2 tbsps olive oil

½ tsp garlic powder

1 lemon, sliced

Salt and pepper, to taste

In a large bowl, combine green beans, olive oil, garlic powder and lemon slices. Season with salt and pepper. Toss well to combine.

Place the seasoned green beans mixture in air fryer basket.

Cook at 180°C for 10-14 minutes, until cooked to your liking, shaking every 4 minutes.

SERVES 4

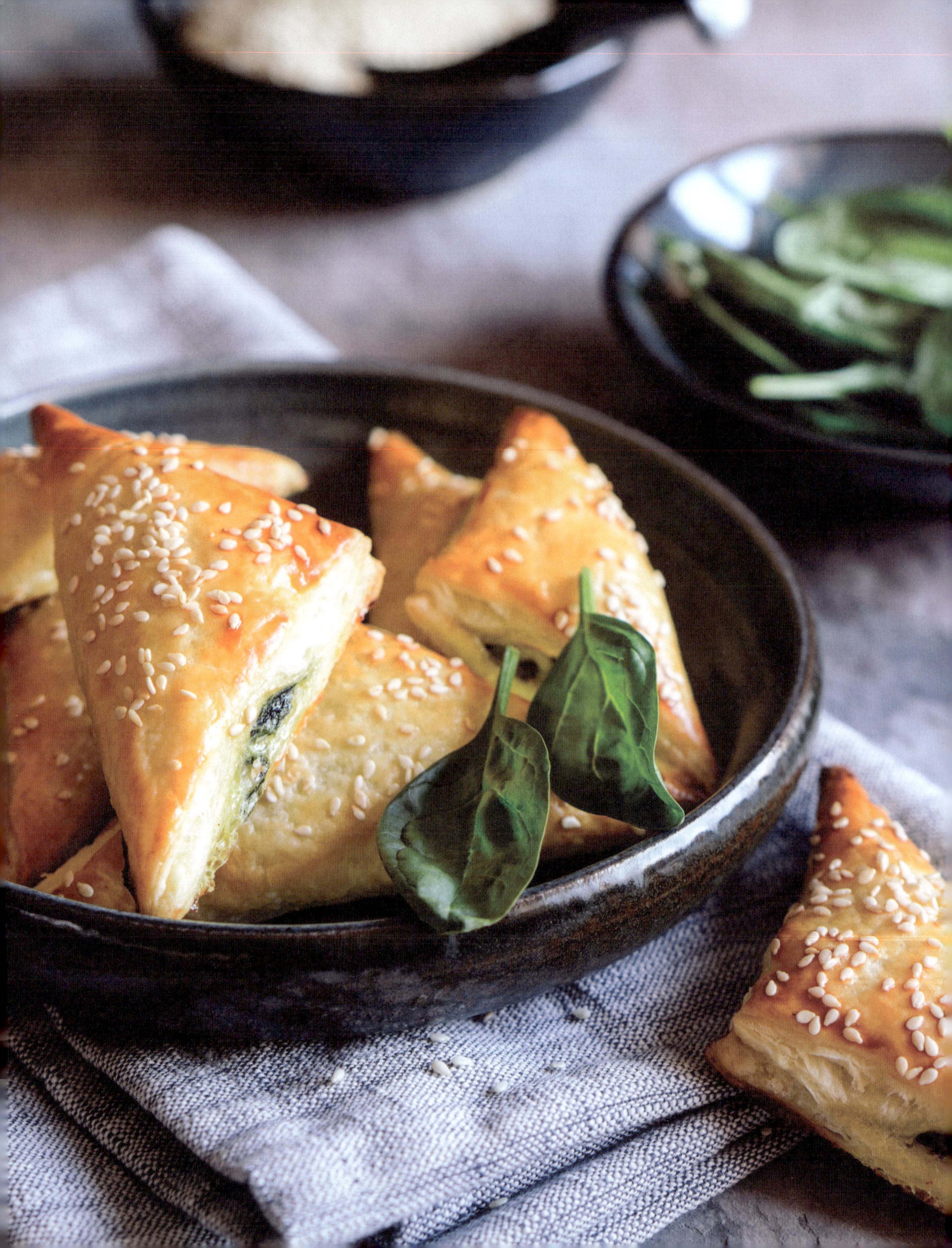

Spanakopita Triangles

300g baby spinach leaves

100g feta cheese, crumbled

2 tbsps Parmesan cheese, finely grated

1 large egg white

1 tsp lemon zest

1 tsp dried oregano

Salt and pepper to taste

8 sheets frozen filo pastry, thawed

3 tbsps olive oil

Cooking spray

1 tbsp sesame seeds

Rinse spinach then wilt in a large pan over high heat, stirring, for 3-5 minutes. Drain spinach and squeeze out excess moisture.

In a large bowl stir together spinach, feta, Parmesan, egg white, lemon zest, oregano, salt and pepper.

Lay one sheet of filo pastry on a dry surface. Brush with olive oil. Add another sheet of filo pastry on top and repeat the oiling process. Continue until there is a stack of four oiled sheets. Repeat process on a new stack with remaining four sheets.

Cut each stack into four equal strips using a pizza cutter.

Add a spoonful of spinach mix to the corner of each strip and begin folding over the layers of pastry, creating a triangle with each fold and brushing each fold with oil. Repeat this process for the remaining strips.

Lightly coat air fryer basket with cooking spray. Arrange filo triangles seam-side down in air fryer basket. Cook in batches or use a double layer accessory if necessary. Spray tops with cooking spray. Cook at 190°C for 6 minutes, flip over and sprinkle with sesame seeds. Spray once more. Cook for a further 6 minutes, until golden brown and crispy.

MAKES 8

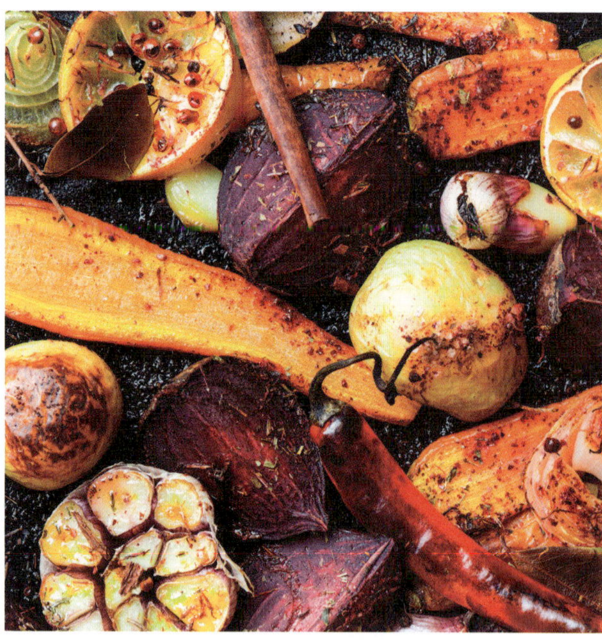

Spiced Roasted Vegetables

4 small carrots, halved lengthways

2 medium beetroots, peeled and quartered

4 baby onions

2 whole chillies

1 whole garlic bulb, cut horizontally

1 lemon, sliced

1 tbsp olive oil

1 cinnamon stick

½ tsp salt

½ tsp pink peppercorns

1 tsp paprika

Preheat air fryer to 190°C.

Place all ingredients in a bowl and toss to coat with oil and seasonings.

Arrange in the air fryer basket and cook for 15-20 minutes or until tender.

SERVES 2

Stuffed Mushrooms

8 whole mushrooms

1 tbsp olive oil

½ small onion, chopped

1 clove garlic, minced

300g baby spinach, chopped

¼ cup (35g) toasted pine nuts, roughly chopped + more to serve

¼ cup (30g) breadcrumbs

Salt and pepper to taste

Olive oil cooking spray

Parmesan cheese, grated, to serve

Parsley leaves, to serve

Remove stems from mushrooms, chop finely and set aside.

Heat oil in a large pan over medium heat and cook onion for 3-5 minutes until soft and translucent. Add garlic and cook for 1 minute until fragrant.

Add mushroom stems and cook for 4 minutes until tender. Add spinach to the pan and cook, stirring, for 2 minutes until spinach wilts.

Add pine nuts and breadcrumbs, season with salt and pepper and stir to combine. Remove from heat.

Spoon mixture into each mushroom cap, then spray with cooking spray. Arrange in air fryer basket.

Cook for 6-8 minutes at 180°C.

Sprinkle with Parmesan and pine nuts and top with parsley to serve.

SERVES 2

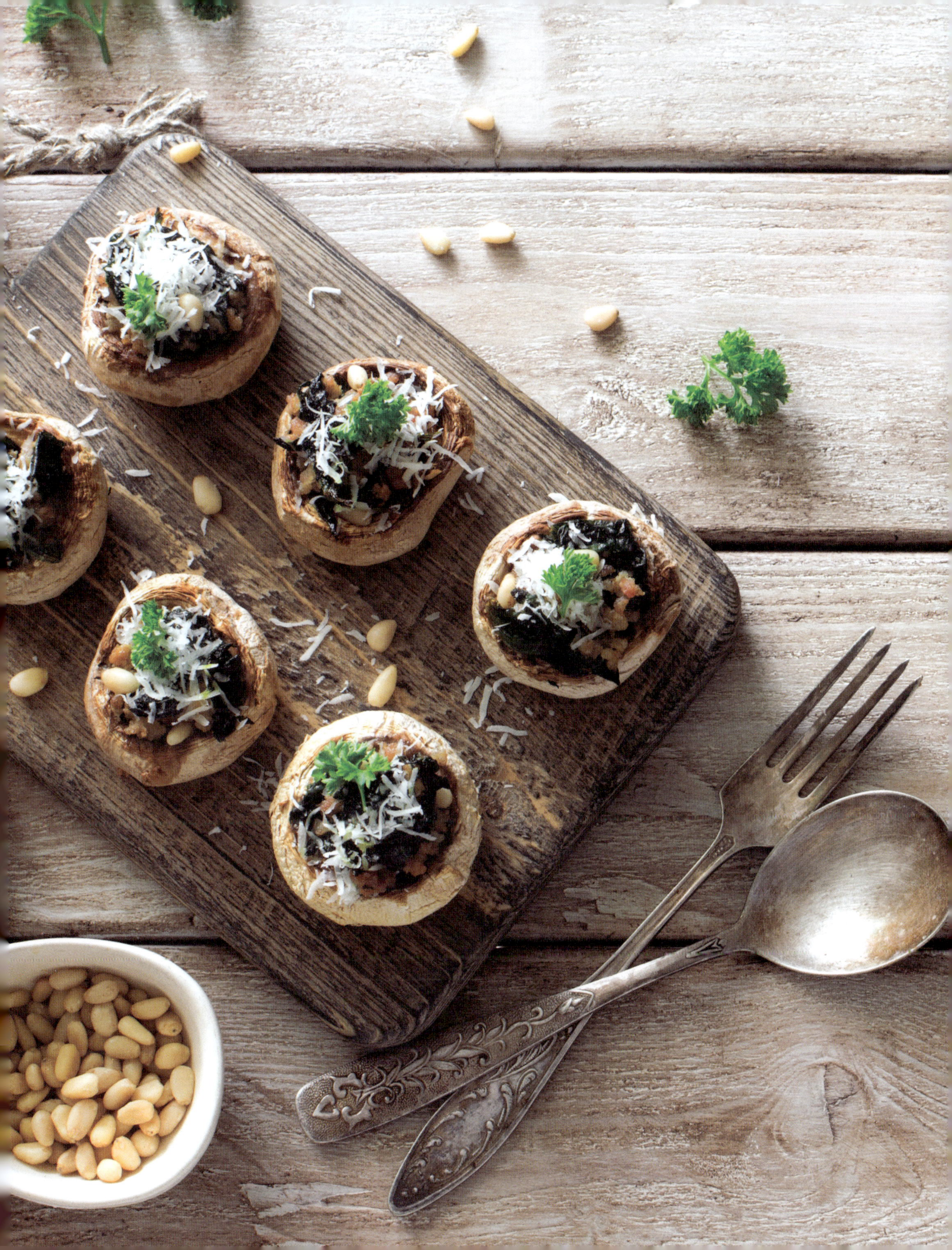

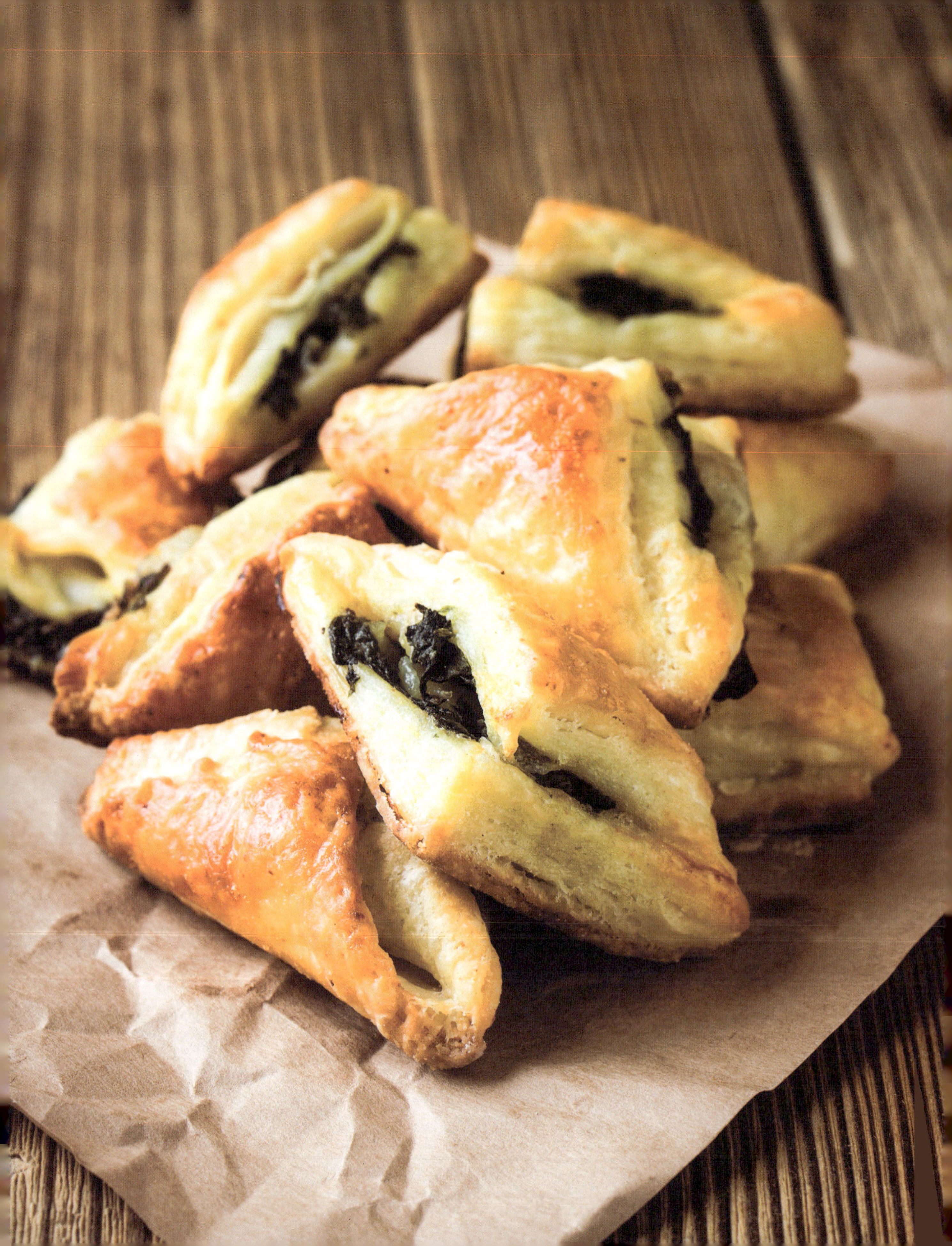

Spinach and Cheese Puffs

300g baby spinach, washed and chopped

1 clove garlic, minced

1½ cups (375g) ricotta

1 cup (125g) mozzarella, grated

⅔ cup (80g) Parmesan cheese, grated

¼ tsp ground nutmeg

Salt and pepper to taste

1-2 sheets puff pastry

1 egg, beaten

Add spinach, garlic, ricotta, cheeses and nutmeg to a bowl. Season with salt and pepper and stir to combine.

Cut the puff pastry into 9 even squares. (Use the second sheet if you have leftover filling.)

Place a tablespoon of spinach mixture into one corner of each square, then fold over pastry to make a triangle. Brush each triangle with beaten egg.

Evenly space the triangles in air fryer basket. Cook in batches or use a double layer accessory if necessary. Cook for 15 minutes at 170°C until golden brown and crispy.

SERVES 3

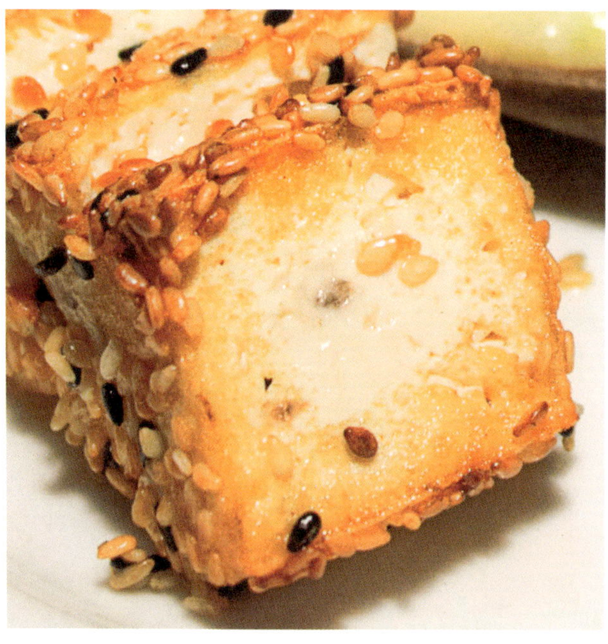

Sesame Coated Tofu

350g firm tofu, dried

2 tbsps tamari

1 tsp toasted sesame oil

1 tsp rice wine vinegar

1 tsp maple syrup

1 clove garlic, minced

Small piece of ginger, grated

1 egg

⅓ cup (60g) white and black sesame seeds

Olive oil spray

Cut tofu into 2cm-wide rectangles, the length of the block.

In a small bowl, whisk together tamari, sesame oil, vinegar, maple syrup, garlic and ginger. Add tofu and toss to coat. Marinate in the fridge for 1 hour.

Place egg in one bowl, sesame seeds in another. Dip tofu into egg then sesame seeds, coating each side. Spray with cooking spray.

Cook for 10 minutes at 200°C, flipping halfway, until crisp. Slice into 1cm-thick squares to serve.

SERVES 2

Vegan Black Bean Burger

BURGER PATTIES

2 x 400g cans black beans, drained and rinsed

1 cup (125g) wholemeal breadcrumbs

½ red onion, finely chopped

¼ cup (20g) broccoli, chopped

½ cup (115g) mashed avocado

Salt and pepper to taste

1 tsp ground cumin

½ tsp chilli powder

Olive oil or avocado oil cooking spray

TO SERVE

4 burger buns

2 tbsps vegan mayonnaise

½ cup (15g) mixed salad leaves

1 beef tomato, sliced

Pat dry the rinsed black beans with a clean tea towel.

When dry, place beans in a large bowl with the remaining burger patty ingredients. Mash together with a fork, then form into four patties.

Place the patties on a plate lined with greaseproof paper and refrigerate for 30 minutes.

Preheat air fryer to 175°C.

Spray air fryer basket with cooking spray.

Arrange patties in air fryer, spray with cooking spray and cook for 5-7 minutes, flip over and cook for another 2-4 minutes until cooked through.

To assemble the burgers spread the burger buns with vegan mayonnaise, then fill with salad leaves, tomato slices and black bean patties.

SERVES 4

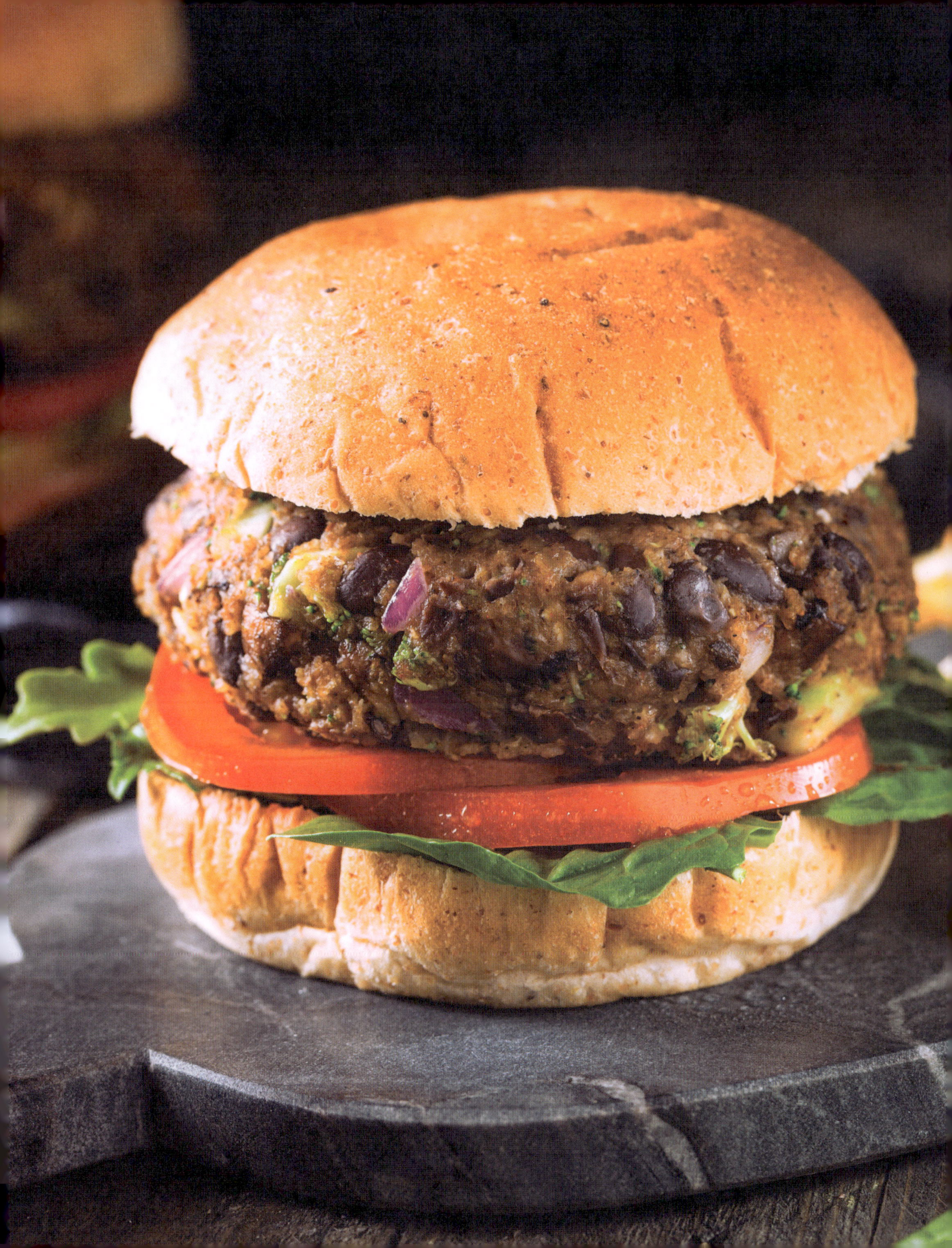

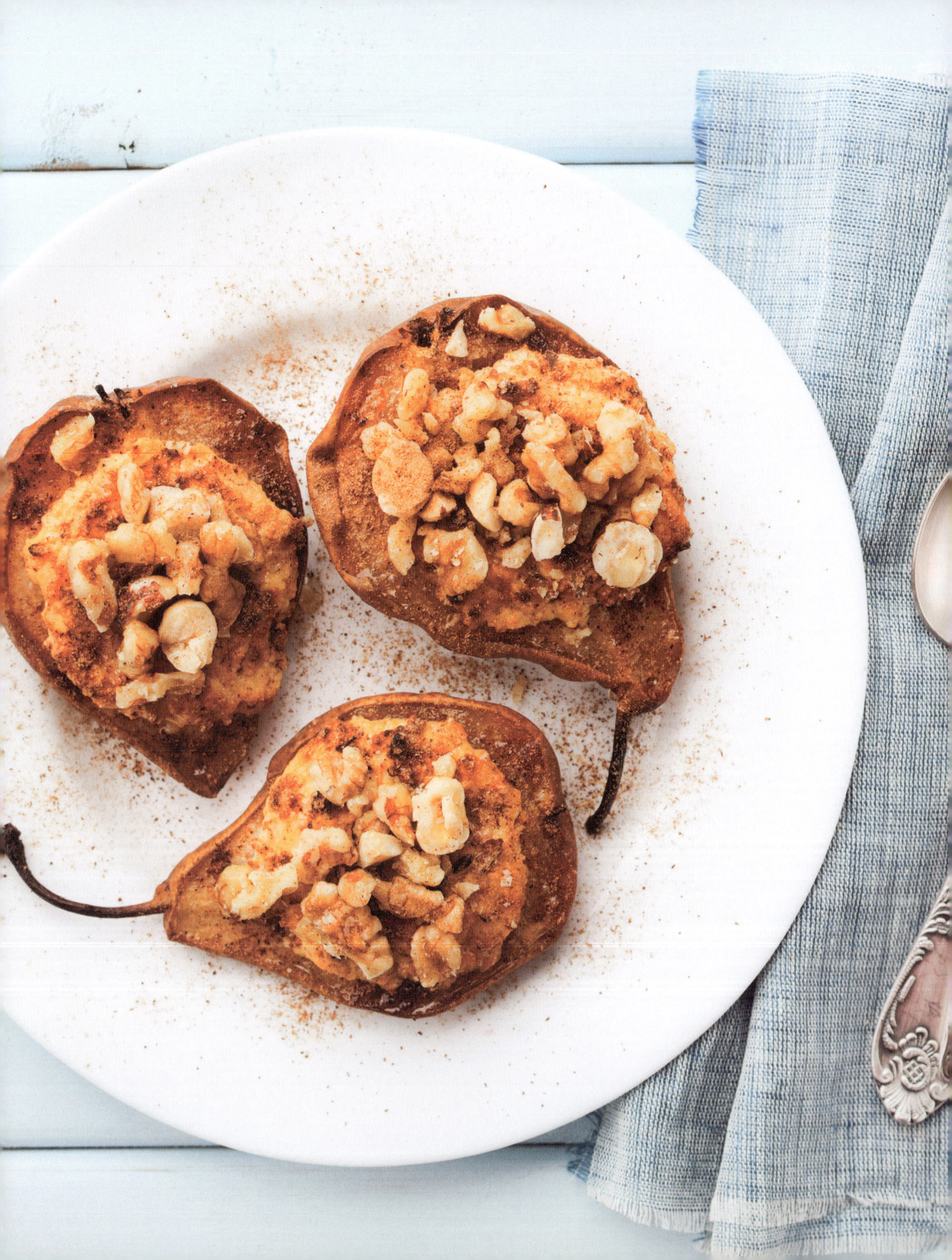

Low-Sugar Desserts

Peach and Blueberry Cobbler

4 peaches, sliced

1 cup (100g) blueberries

1 tbsp coconut sugar

1 tsp ground cinnamon

1 tbsp butter, cubed

TOPPING

2 tbsps almond meal

80g butter

⅓ cup (30g) oats

¼ cup (20g) coconut flakes

½ cup (80g) coconut sugar

¼ tsp cinnamon

Cake tin or pie dish

Grease cake tin or pie dish.

Arrange peaches and blueberries in the dish. Sprinkle with sugar, cinnamon and salt, and dot with butter.

Place almond meal and butter in a large bowl. Cut through the butter with a knife until the mixture resembles coarse crumbs. Add oats, coconut flakes, sugar and cinnamon. Stir to combine.

Sprinkle topping over peach filling.

Preheat air fryer to 175°C.

Place dish into air fryer and bake for 18-20 minutes until fruit is bubbling and topping is crisp and golden brown.

SERVES 4

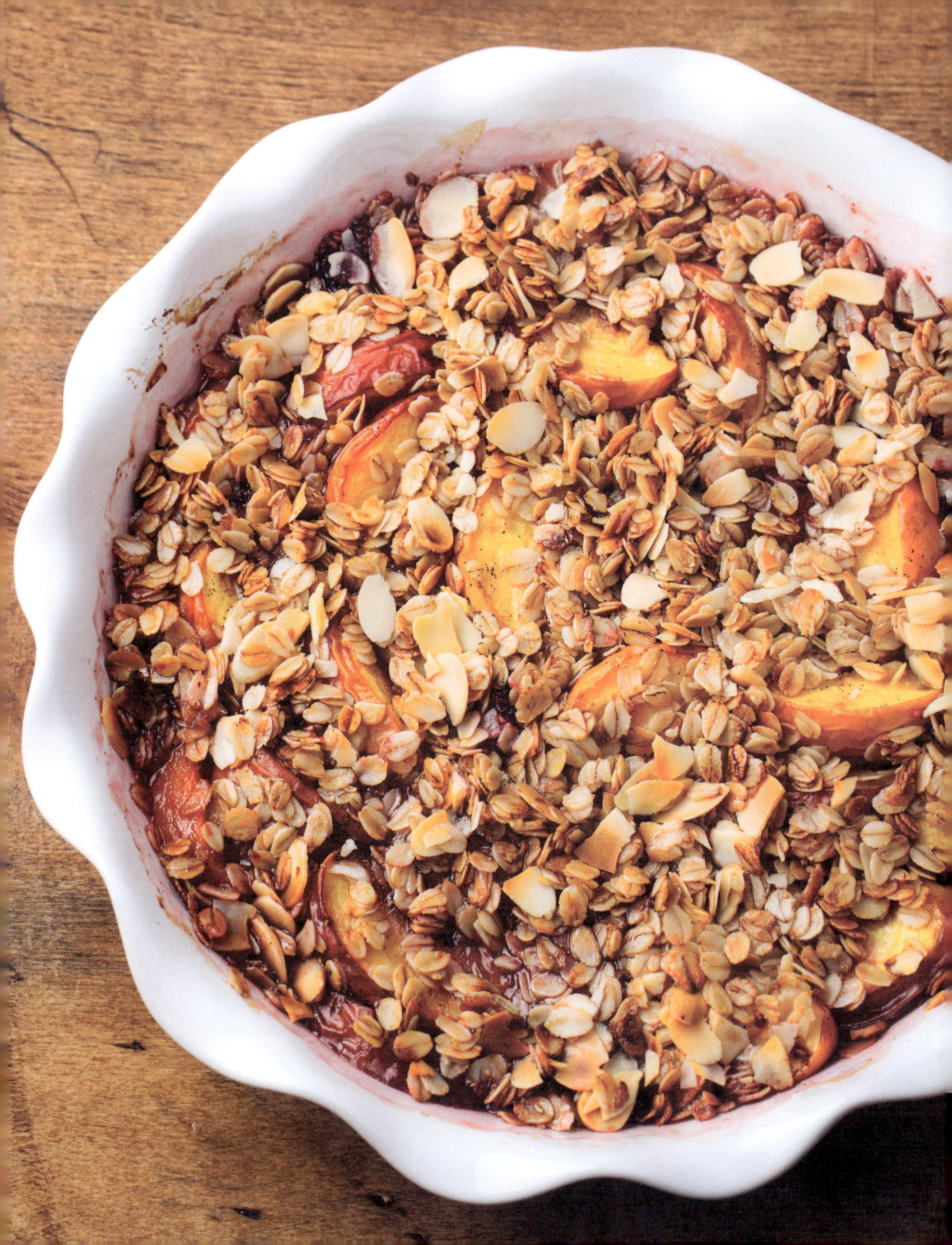

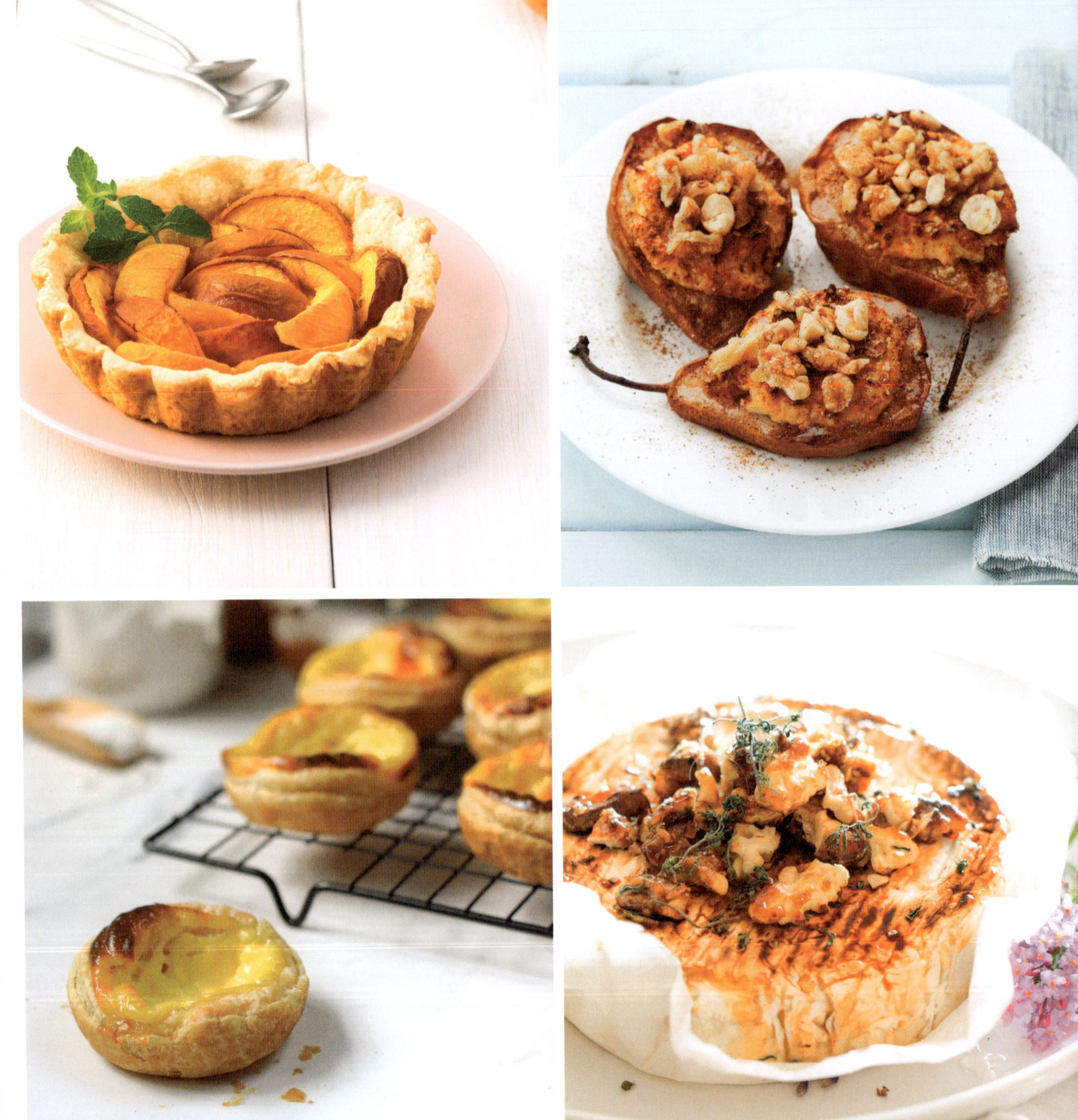

Peach Tart

2 sheets shortcrust pastry

8 peaches, sliced

4 tbsps butter, melted

1 tsp ground cinnamon

4 ramekins or small flan tins

Cut the pastry to fit into four ramekins or small flan tins. Trim the edges and prick with a fork.

Arrange the peaches in the flan tins. Drizzle with melted butter and sprinkle with cinnamon.

Working in batches, cook at 150°C for 15-20 minutes, until peaches are soft and pastry is golden brown.

SERVES 4

Baked Pears with Ricotta

2 tbsps butter, melted

1 tsp vanilla powder

½ tsp cinnamon + ½ tsp to serve

2 pears, cut in half and cored

½ cup (125g) ricotta cheese

1 tbsp maple syrup

¼ cup (30g) toasted walnuts, chopped

Baking pan

Pre-heat air fryer to 175°C.

Combine melted butter, vanilla and cinnamon. Mix well. Baste pears all over with butter mixture and place cut-side down in baking pan.

Bake for 10 minutes, then baste pears once again and cook for a further 2 minutes.

Transfer pears to a serving plate and baste once more.

Combine ricotta and maple syrup in a bowl. Mix well. Spoon ricotta on top of the pears. Sprinkle with walnuts and dust with extra cinnamon to serve.

SERVES 2

Portuguese Tarts

2 sheets puff pastry

2 tbsps honey

½ cup (135ml) milk

3 eggs

1 tsp cinnamon

Muffin tray or silicone moulds

Use a large round cookie cutter or cut around a coffee mug to create 12 even circles of pastry. Press into silicone cupcake moulds or a greased muffin tray. You will need to cook in batches or use a double layer accessory.

Combine honey and milk in a small pan over medium heat. Bring to a boil, stirring regularly. Set aside to cool.

Whisk the eggs and cinnamon in a medium bowl.

When milk is cool, whisk into eggs.

Pour filling into pastry cases, ensuring you don't fill more than three-quarters full.

Cook in air fryer at 150°C for 15 minutes. Reduce temperature to 130°C and cook for a further 3 minutes.

Repeat with remaining mixture.

MAKES 12

Baked Camembert

1 x 250g Camembert

2 tsps honey

Pinch of salt

3 thyme sprigs

¼ cup (30g) toasted walnuts

Remove any packaging then return the Camembert to its wooden box, or place on greaseproof paper in a small ovenproof dish.

Score a deep cross or a crosshatch pattern on the top rind of the cheese. Drizzle with 1 teaspoon honey and sprinkle with salt and the leaves of one sprig of thyme.

Place in the air fryer and cook at 160°C for 8-10 minutes until soft and gooey.

Remove from the air fryer. Scatter with nuts and drizzle over remaining honey. Top with thyme sprigs to serve.

SERVES 4

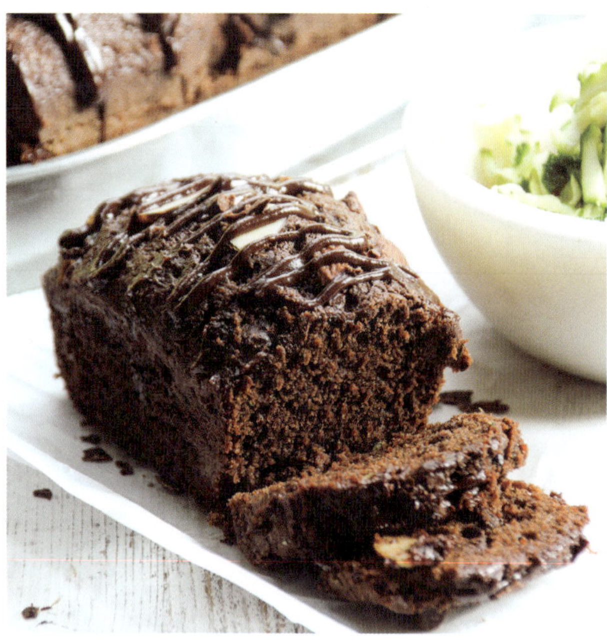

Chocolate Zucchini Bread

½ cup (60g) plain flour

¼ cup (30g) cocoa powder

½ tsp bicarbonate soda

¼ tsp salt

1 egg

¼ cup (80g) maple syrup

4 tbsps butter, melted

½ tsp vanilla extract

¾ cup (170g) packed zucchini, grated

½ cup (80g) chocolate chips

70g chocolate, melted, to serve

Flaked almonds, to serve

Mini loaf pan

Preheat air fryer to 150°C. Grease and line loaf pan with greaseproof paper.

In one bowl, whisk together flour, cocoa powder, bicarb and salt. In another bowl, combine egg, maple syrup, melted butter and vanilla. Whisk until smooth. Add dry ingredients to wet mixture and stir to combine. Fold in zucchini and chocolate chips. Transfer to loaf pan.

Cook for 30-35 minutes, or until an inserted skewer comes out clean.

Drizzle with melted chocolate and sprinkle with flaked almonds to serve.

SERVES 8

Clafoutis with Blueberries

4 large eggs

1 cup (250ml) milk of choice

¼ cup (90g) honey or maple syrup

1 tsp pure vanilla extract

¼ tsp salt

½ cup (60g) almond meal

¼ cup (30g) tapioca flour

1 cup (125g) mixed berries

4 ramekins

Preheat the oven to 180°C.

Combine eggs, milk, honey, vanilla, salt, almond meal and tapioca flour in a food processor. Blend until smooth.

Pour mixture into 4 ramekins then add a handful of berries to each one.

Place in air fryer and cook for about 30-32 minutes until set.

Allow to cool, then place in the fridge to chill before serving.

SERVES 4

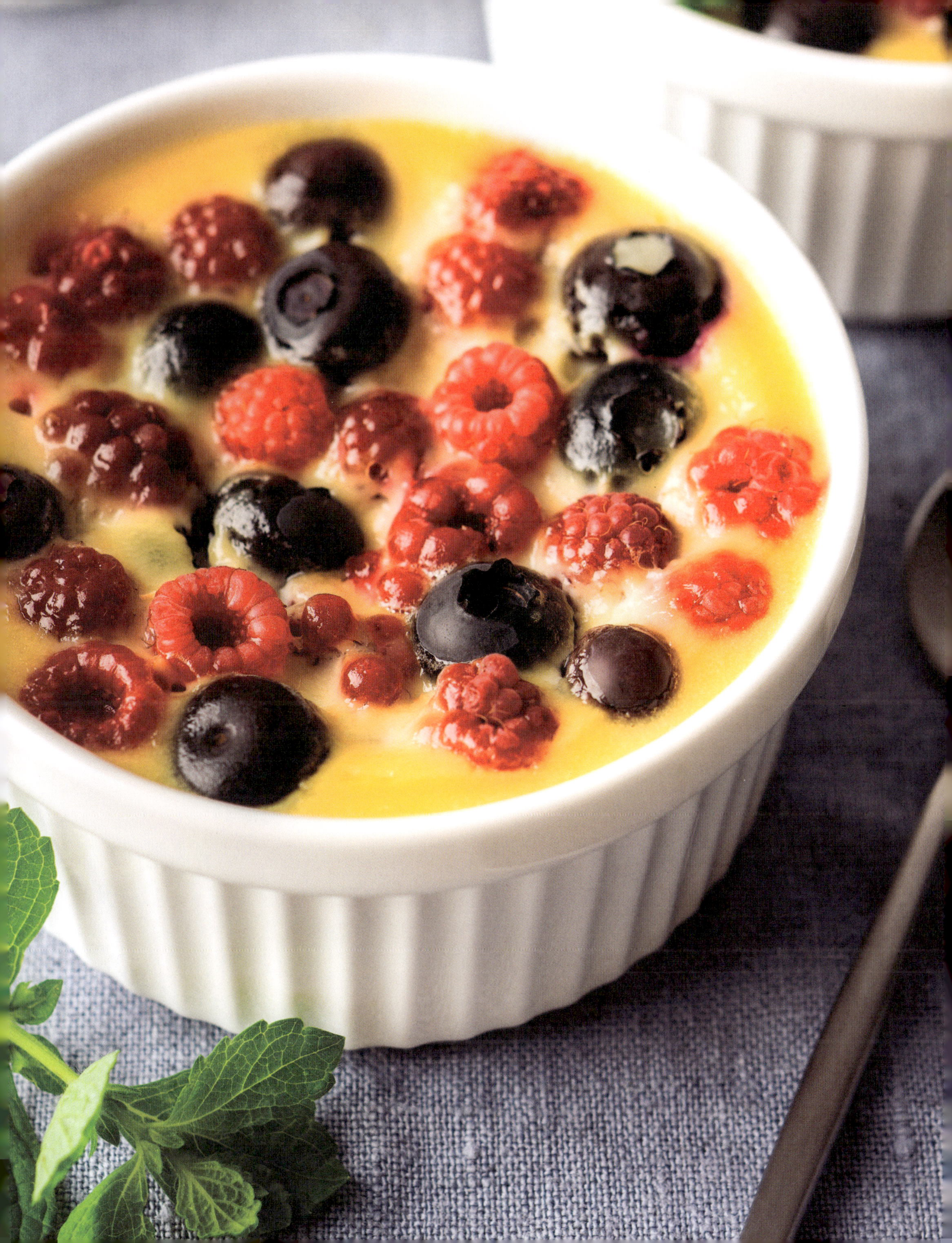

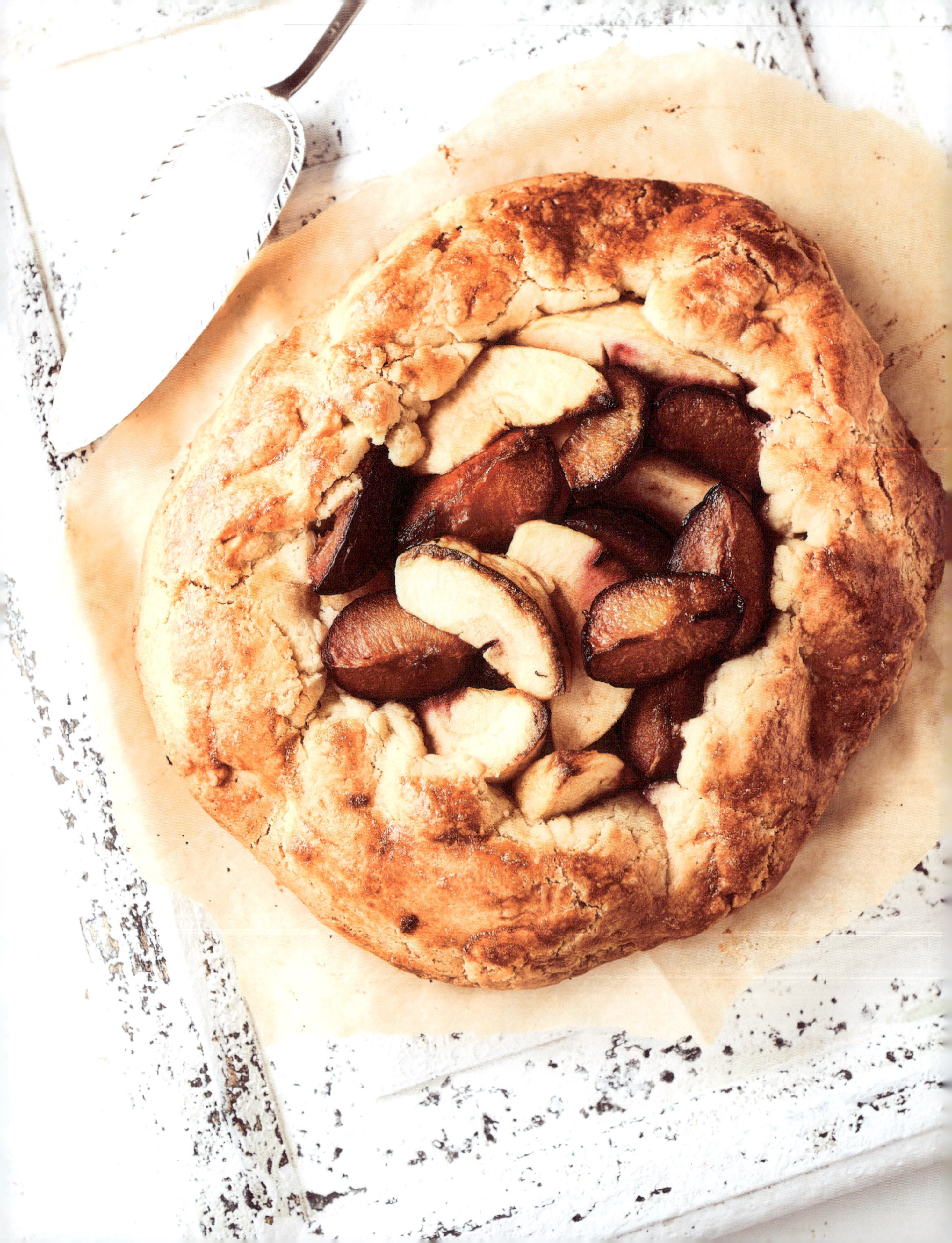

Plum and Apple Galette

¾ cup (90g) almond meal

¼ cup (30g) tapioca flour

2 tsps coconut sugar

⅛ tsp salt

75g cold butter, diced

2 eggs

2 apples, sliced

4 plums, sliced

Juice and zest from 1 orange

1 tbsp maple syrup

½ tsp vanilla extract

½ tsp cinnamon

2 tsps cornflour

In a food processor, combine almond meal, tapioca flour, coconut sugar, salt and butter and pulse until a breadcrumb consistency is reached.

Add one egg and pulse again until the dough comes together. Form into a flattened disc, wrap in plastic wrap and place in refrigerator for 30 minutes to chill.

Place apple and plum slices in a large bowl with orange juice and zest, maple syrup, vanilla, cinnamon and cornflour. Toss to coat.

Remove dough from fridge. Place dough between two sheets of greaseproof paper. Roll out to roughly 16cm in diameter. Remove top sheet of paper.

Add the fruit to the centre of the dough, leaving about 5cm around the edge. Fold the edges of the dough over the fruit to create the galette.

Beat the other egg and brush it over the dough.

Preheat the air fryer to 160°C. Use the bottom sheet of greaseproof paper to lift the galette into air fryer. Bake for 12-15 minutes until golden brown and cooked through.

Use the greaseproof paper to remove the galette from the air fryer and allow it to cool slightly before serving.

SERVES 3

Sliced Plum and Almond Tart

ALMOND CRUST

¾ cup (90g) almond meal

¼ cup (30g) tapioca flour

1 tbsp maple syrup

⅛ tsp salt

75g cold butter, diced

1 egg

1 tsp cinnamon

FILLING

6-8 plums, sliced

1 tbsp maple syrup

1 tsp vanilla bean paste

½ tsp cinnamon

2-3 star anise

3 tbsps almond meal

2 tbsps milk

¼ cup (30g) flaked almonds, toasted

In a food processor, combine almond crust ingredients and pulse until the dough comes together. Form into a flattened disc, wrap in plastic wrap and place in refrigerator for 30 minutes to chill.

In a bowl combine the plums, maple syrup, vanilla bean paste, cinnamon and star anise. Stir gently to combine. Set aside to marinate for 10 minutes.

Remove dough from fridge. Place dough between two sheets of greaseproof paper. Roll out to roughly 16cm in diameter. Remove top sheet of paper.

Sprinkle the almond meal into the centre of the pastry leaving a 2cm border. Top with fruit and any juice from the bowl. Brush the crust edges with milk.

Use greaseproof paper to lift tart into air fryer. Cook at 160°C for 25-30 minutes until crust is golden brown and fruit is soft.

Sprinkle with flaked almonds, cut into pieces and serve.

SERVES 6

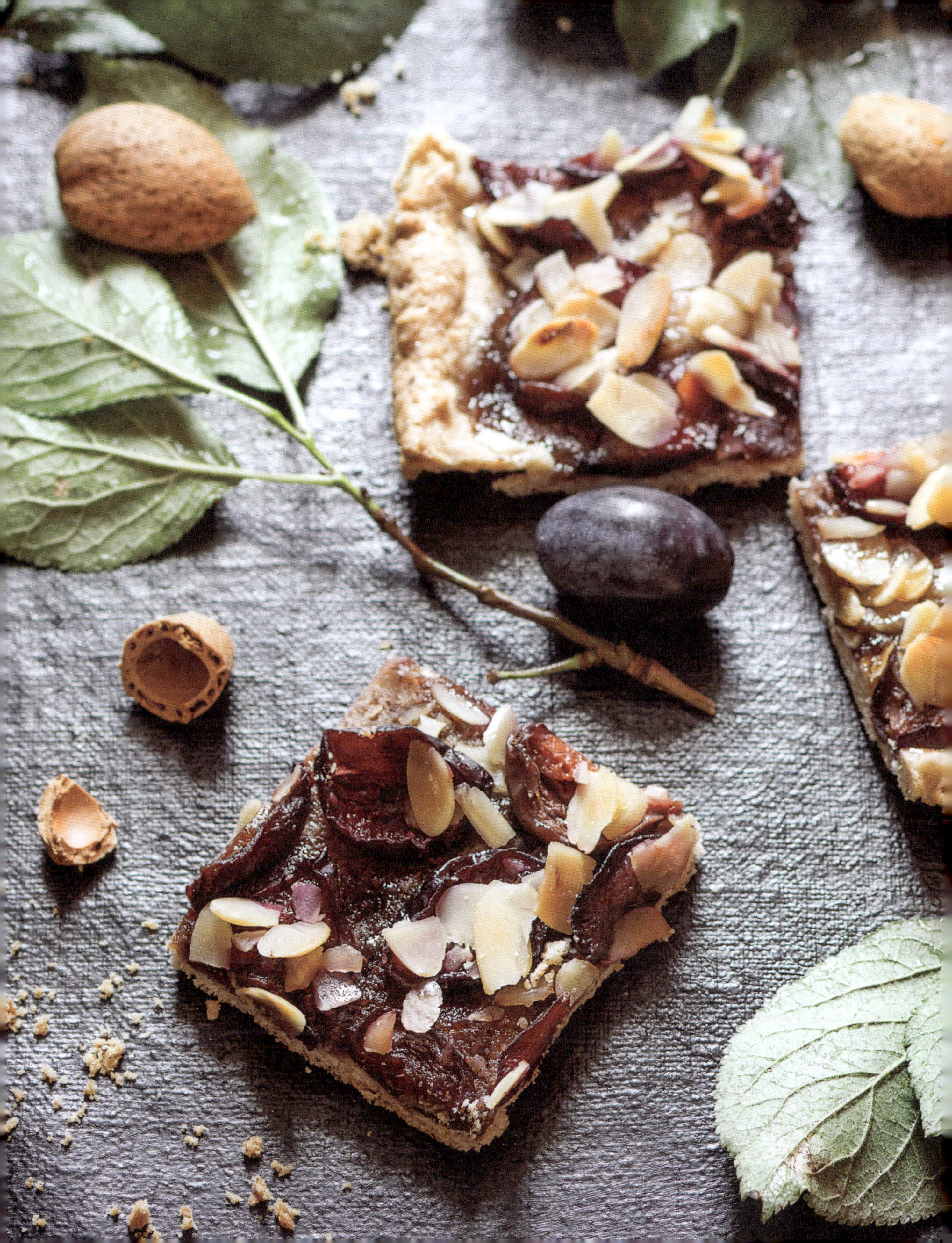

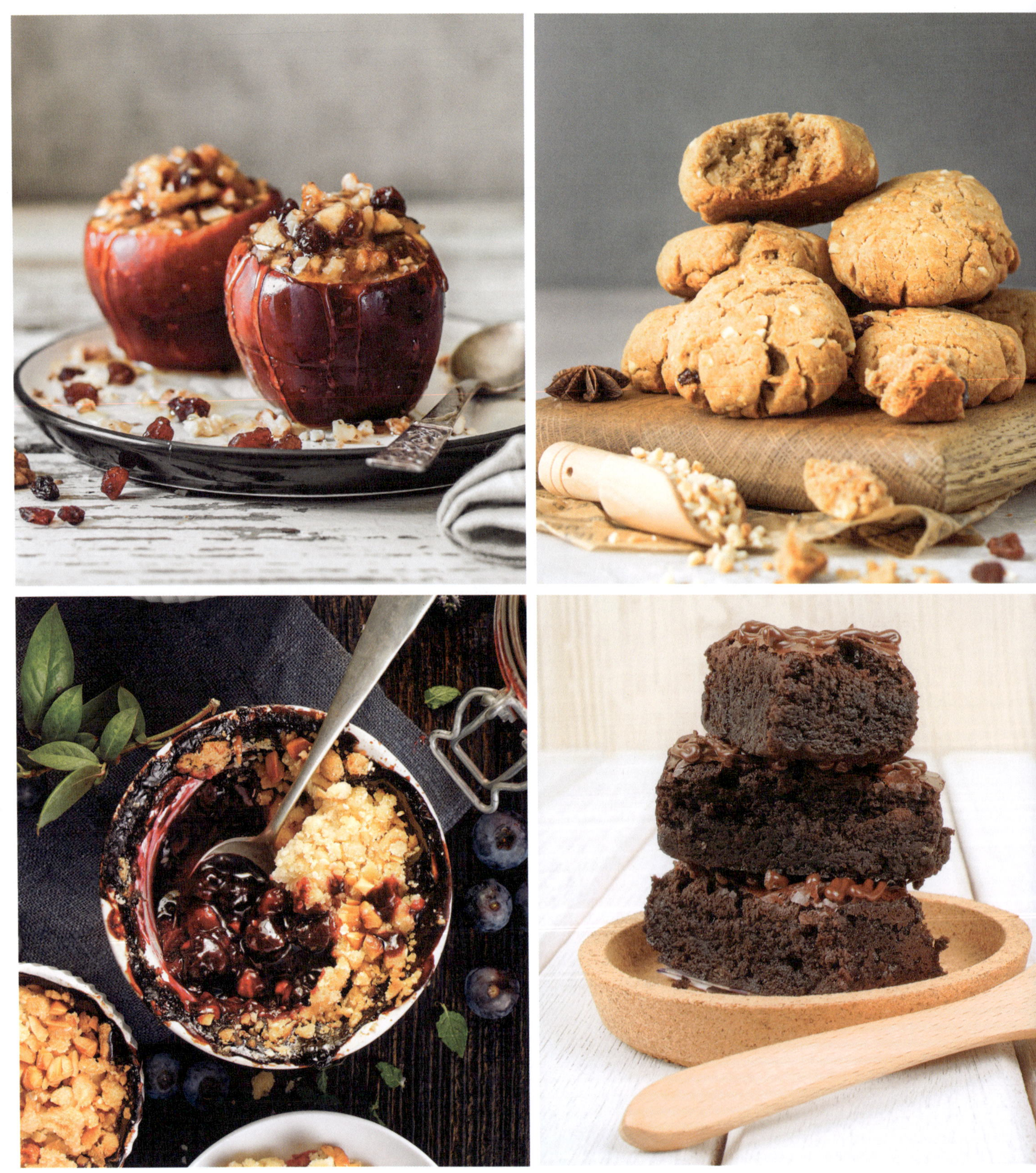

Baked Apples

4 apples

⅓ cup (50g) raisins

⅓ cup (40g) walnuts, chopped

1 tsp cinnamon

4 tbsps butter, softened

Baking pan

Cut off the tops of the apples, then core using a sharp knife or corer.

Place the raisins, walnuts and cinnamon in a small bowl and stir briefly. Add the butter and mix to combine.

Spoon the filling into the centre of the apples.

Place apples in the baking pan and place in the air fryer.

Cook for 20 minutes at 175°C.

Allow to cool slightly before serving.

SERVES 4

Buckwheat Raisin Biscuits

1 cup (120g) buckwheat flour

½ cup (80g) coconut sugar

⅓ cup (80ml) coconut oil, melted

2 tbsps water

1 tsp vanilla extract

½ tsp salt

½ tsp bicarbonate of soda

1 tsp apple cider vinegar

½ cup (80g) raisins

½ cup (60g) almonds, chopped

In a large bowl, stir together buckwheat flour, coconut sugar, oil, water, vanilla, salt and bicarb. Mix in vinegar.

Fold in raisins and almonds then form dough into a ball. Wrap in plastic wrap and refrigerate for 25 minutes.

Roll dough into 12 balls then press gently to flatten.

Cooking in batches if necessary, arrange biscuits in air fryer basket. Cook for 6-8 minutes at 160°C.

MAKES 12

Blueberry Crumble

1½ cups (150g) blueberries

¼ cup (30g) plain flour

¼ cup (20g) oats

2 tbsps butter

2 tbsps coconut sugar or rapadura

½ tsp cinnamon

2 ramekins

Preheat air fryer to 180°C.

Place blueberries in ramekins or a small ovenproof dish.

In a large bowl, combine the flour, oats and butter with your fingertips until the mixture resembles breadcrumbs. Add sugar and cinnamon. Mix well

Spoon the crumble mixture over the fruit. Cook for 15 minutes until golden brown.

SERVES 2

Black Bean Brownies

1 x 440g can black beans, drained and rinsed

2 eggs

3 tbsps coconut oil, melted

¾ cup (90g) cocoa powder

¼ tsp salt

1 tsp vanilla extract

½ cup (80g) coconut sugar

1½ tsps baking powder

1 cup (150g) chocolate chips, melted, to serve

Cake tin

Grease and line cake tin. Preheat air fryer to 160°C.

Place all the ingredients except the chocolate chips into a food processor and pulse until smooth.

Pour mixture into cake tin and place in air fryer. Cook for 18-20 minutes until crisp outside and soft in the centre.

Melt chocolate chips in a microwave or small saucepan over a low heat. Pour over cooked brownie.

Cool slightly before cutting brownie into squares to serve.

MAKES 10

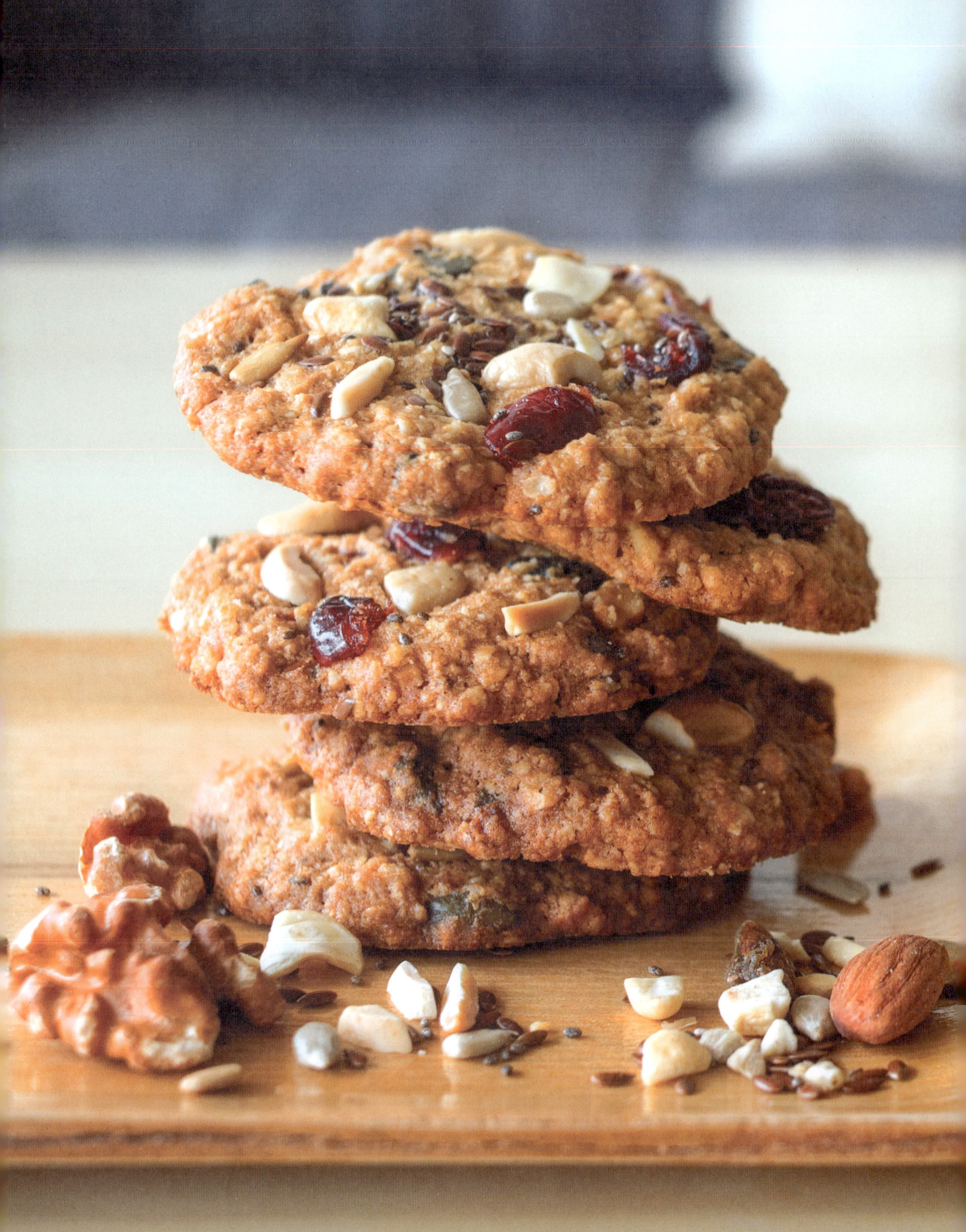

Cranberry, Nut and Seed Biscuits

2 cups (240g) almond meal

½ tsp salt

1 tsp bicarbonate of soda

⅓ cup (80ml) butter, melted

⅓ cup (105g) maple syrup

1 large egg

1 tsp vanilla extract

½ cup (80g) dried cranberries

½ cup (60g) nuts, roughly chopped (cashews, walnuts and almonds)

1 tsp chia seeds

1 tsp flaxseed

1 tbsp sunflower seeds

Cake tin or baking pan

Preheat air fryer to 155°C. Line cake tin or baking pan with greaseproof paper.

In a medium bowl, combine almond meal, salt and bicarb.

In another bowl, whisk together melted butter, maple syrup, egg and vanilla extract.

Add dry ingredients to the wet mixture and mix to combine. Stir in cranberries, nuts and seeds.

Working in batches, scoop tablespoons of dough into cake tin or baking pan, leaving space between each one. Gently press to flatten slightly.

Place tin into air fryer and cook for 7-10 minutes until edges are slightly golden brown. Set aside to cool.

Repeat with remaining mixture.

MAKES 26

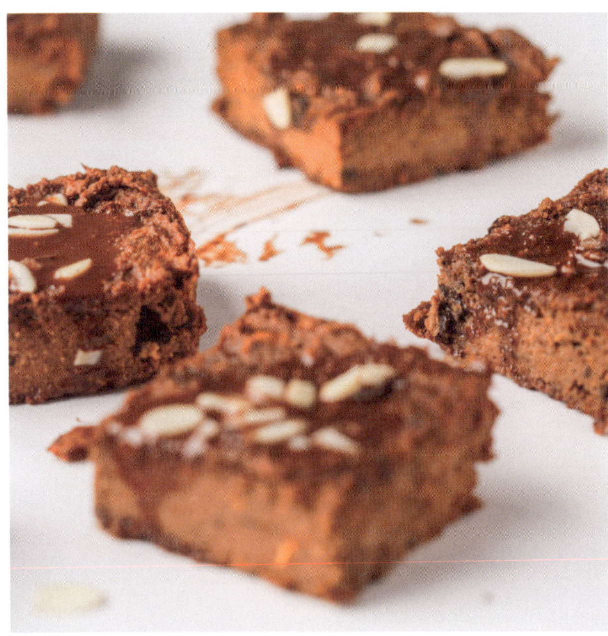

Sweet Potato Brownies

1 medium sweet potato, grated

½ cup (125ml) coconut oil, melted

⅓ cup (115g) honey

2 tsps vanilla extract

½ cup (60g) cocoa powder or raw cacao powder

1 tsp baking powder

1 tsp bicarbonate of soda

3 tbsps coconut flour

1 cup (150g) chocolate chips, to serve

Flaked almonds, to serve

Cake tin

Grease and line cake tin. Preheat air fryer to 160°C.

In a large bowl place grated sweet potato, coconut oil, honey and vanilla extract. Mix well.

Add cocoa, baking powder, bicarb and coconut flour. Stir to combine.

Pour into prepared tin and place in air fryer.

Cook for 20-30 minutes until firm on the outside and soft in the centre.

Melt chocolate chips in a microwave or small saucepan over a low heat. Pour over cooked brownie. Scatter with flaked almonds.

Cool slightly before cutting into squares to serve.

MAKES 10

Pumpkin Pie

1 sheet shortcrust pastry

2¼ cups (500g) mashed cooked pumpkin

½ cup (125ml) thickened cream or coconut cream

2 large eggs

½ cup (155g) maple syrup

1 tsp cinnamon

¼ tsp nutmeg

¼ tsp ground cloves

⅛ tsp ground ginger

¼ tsp salt

Zest of 1 orange

Whipped cream and cinnamon to serve

1 large or 2 small pie dishes

Roll out pastry and cut out circles to line pie dishes. You may need to cook one at a time depending on the size of your air fryer.

Prick pastry case with a fork and place in air fryer. Cook at 160°C for 8-10 minutes.

Combine pumpkin, cream, eggs, maple syrup, spices, salt and orange zest in a large bowl. Mix well then pour into prepared cases.

Place in air fryer and cook at 170°C for 25-30 minutes or until set.

Allow pumpkin pies to cool completely.

Top with whipped cream and cinnamon to serve.

SERVES 2

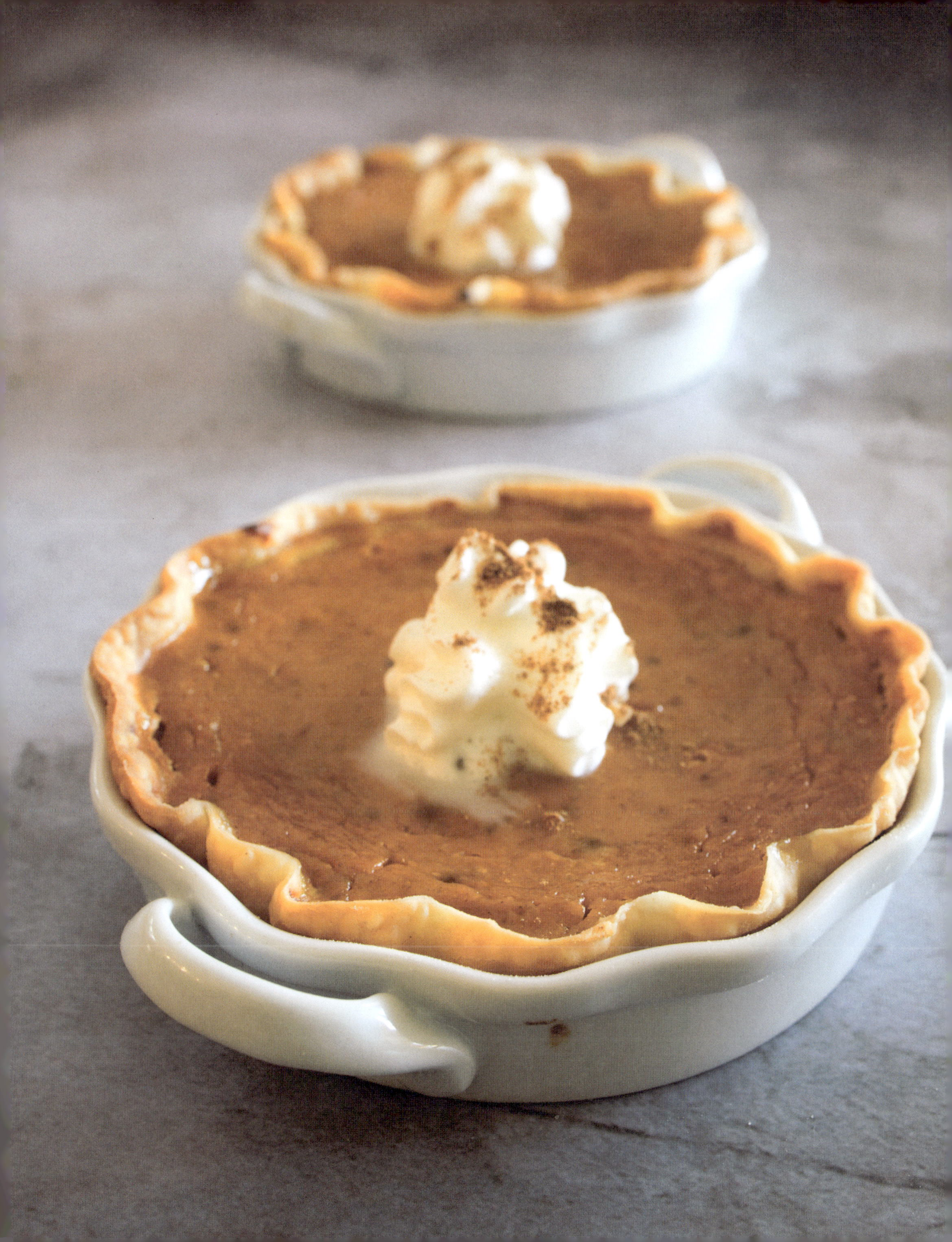

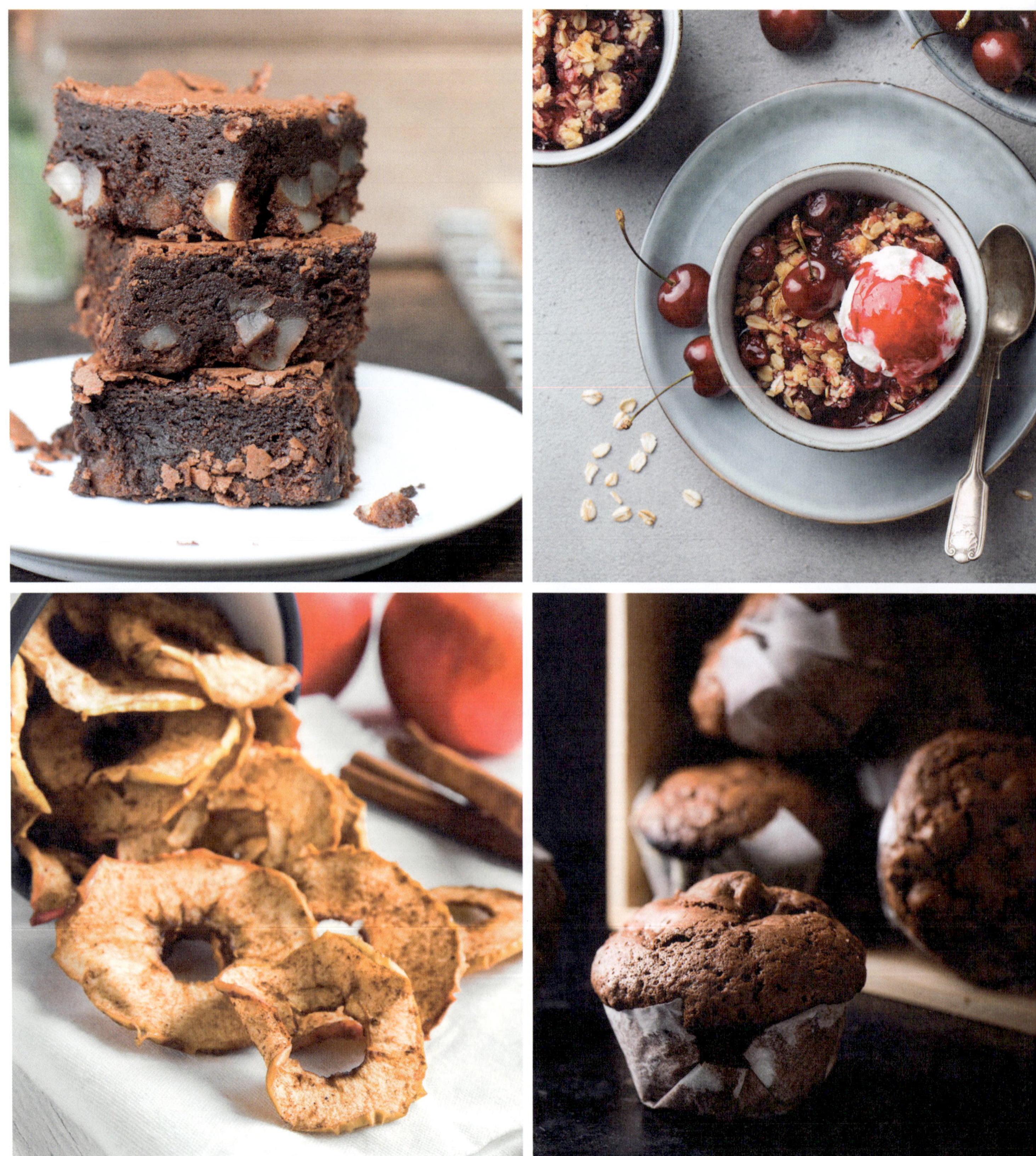

Macadamia Fudge Brownies

⅓ cup (80ml) coconut oil, melted

⅓ cup (105g) maple syrup

1 tsp vanilla extract

2 eggs

¼ cup (65g) macadamia butter

⅔ cup (80g) almond meal

⅓ cup (35g) raw cacao powder

1 tsp baking powder

¼ tsp salt

⅓ cup (40g) macadamias, chopped

Cake tin

Grease and line cake tin with greaseproof paper. Preheat the air fryer to 160°C.

Add coconut oil, maple syrup, vanilla extract, eggs and macadamia butter to a large bowl. Mix well, then add remaining ingredients. Stir well to combine.

Pour batter into cake tin and place in air fryer. Cook for 20-25 minutes. Allow to cool before cutting up.

SERVES 12

Baked Cherry Crunch

3 cups (450g) cherries, halved and pitted

2 tbsps maple syrup

1 tbsp butter, melted

½ tsp almond extract (optional)

4 tbsps granola or toasted muesli

Vanilla ice cream, to serve

2 ramekins

Preheat air fryer to 180°C.

Mix together cherries, maple syrup, butter and almond extract (if using) and divide between ramekins.

Place ramekins into the air fryer and cook for 15 minutes, until cherries are soft, stirring once halfway through cooking.

Sprinkle granola over the cooked cherries.

Cook for a further 2-3 minutes.

Serve warm with ice cream.

SERVES 2

Apple Cinnamon Chips

1 large apple

1 tsp cinnamon

Avocado oil cooking spray

Preheat air fryer to 150°C.

Thinly slice the apple with a mandoline or sharp knife.

Place apple slices in a large bowl and sprinkle with cinnamon. Spray evenly with avocado oil and toss to coat.

Place apple slices in air fryer basket. Cook for 20-25 minutes, shaking every 5 minutes, until apples are completely dried out.

For crispy apple chips increase the temperature to 160°C and cook for a further 5 minutes, shaking every minute and a half.

SERVES 1

Chocolate and Avocado Muffins

150g dark chocolate, chopped

1 large avocado

¼ cup (80g) maple syrup

2 tsps vanilla extract

½ cup (60g) cocoa powder

⅓ cup (40g) almond meal

½ tsp bicarbonate of soda

Muffin tray or silicone moulds

Preheat air fryer to 160°C.

Melt chocolate in a microwave or small bowl over pan of simmering water. Stir until smooth, then set aside.

Place avocado flesh in a food processor with maple syrup and vanilla extract. Blend to a creamy consistency.

Transfer to a bowl and add cocoa powder, almond meal and bicarb. Stir to combine, then mix through melted chocolate.

Spoon mixture into silicone moulds or paper liners inside an air fryer muffin tray. Cook in batches or use a double layer accessory for 10-12 minutes.

MAKES 6

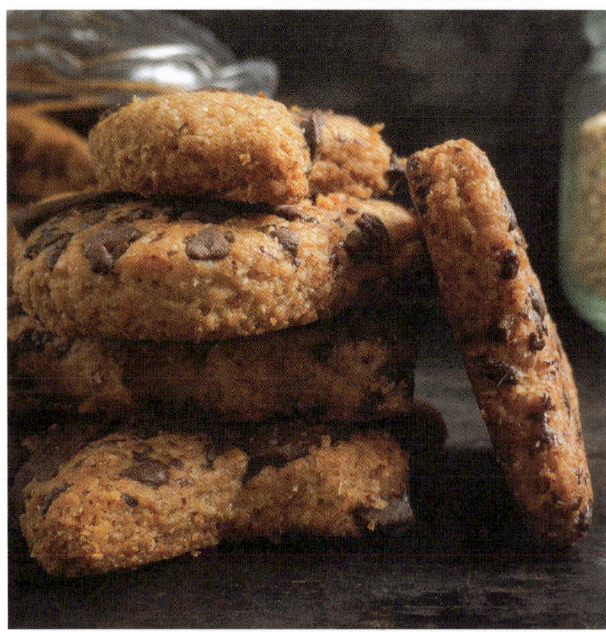

Buckwheat Chocolate Chip Cookies

¾ cup (90g) buckwheat flour

¼ cup (20g) desiccated coconut

½ cup (80g) coconut sugar

½ cup (125ml) coconut oil, melted

1 tsp vanilla extract

¼ tsp salt

½ tsp bicarbonate of soda

1 tsp apple cider vinegar

½ cup (80g) dark chocolate chips

In a large bowl, stir together buckwheat flour, desiccated coconut, coconut sugar, oil, vanilla, salt and bicarb. Then mix in the vinegar.

Fold in chocolate chips then form dough into a ball. Wrap in plastic wrap and refrigerate for 25 minutes.

Roll dough into 12 balls then press gently to flatten.

Cooking in batches if necessary, arrange biscuits in air fryer basket. Cook for 6-8 minutes at 160°C.

Allow to cool for 10 minutes before serving.

MAKES 12

Beetroot Chocolate Cake

125g raw beetroot

2 tbsps milk

1 tsp lemon juice

¾ tsp white wine vinegar

1 tsp vanilla extract

65g unsalted butter, softened

1 large egg

¾ cup (90g) self-raising flour

⅓ cup (50g) rapadura or coconut sugar

2 tbsps cocoa powder

1½ tsps baking powder

Cake tin

Grease and line cake tin with greaseproof paper.

Peel and finely chop the beetroot, place into a food processor with milk and lemon juice, vinegar and vanilla extract. Blend to a fine, smooth puree.

Add butter and egg and pulse to combine. Transfer to a large mixing bowl.

Sift flour, sugar, cocoa powder and baking powder into the beetroot mixture and stir to combine.

Preheat the air fryer to 160°C.

Transfer the batter to the cake tin and use a spatula to smooth the surface.

Put the cake tin in the air fryer basket and slide the basket into the air fryer. Cook for 20-25 minutes until cake is nicely browned and an inserted skewer comes out clean.

Allow the cake cool in the tin for 5 minutes, then turn out onto a wire rack to cool.

SERVES 6

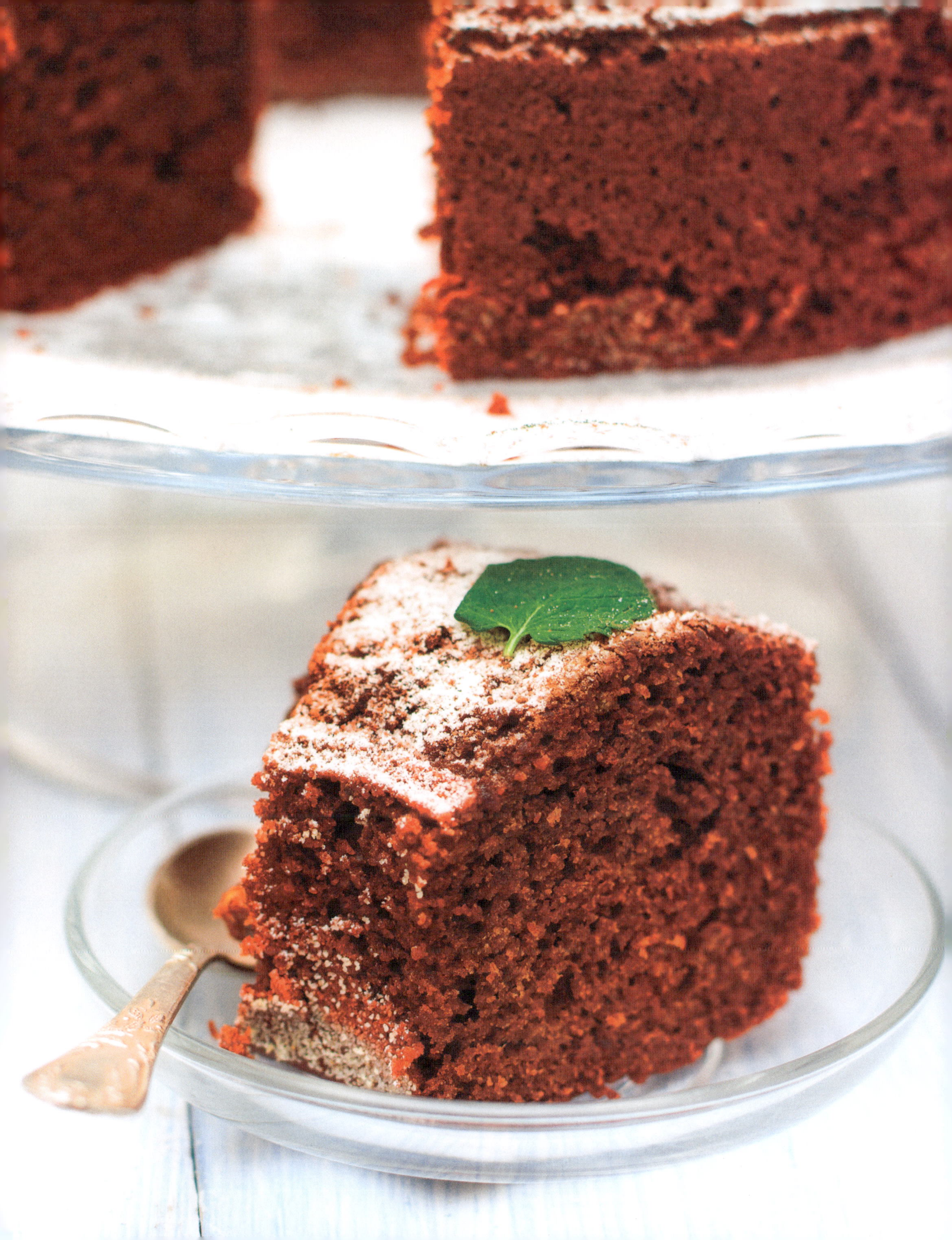

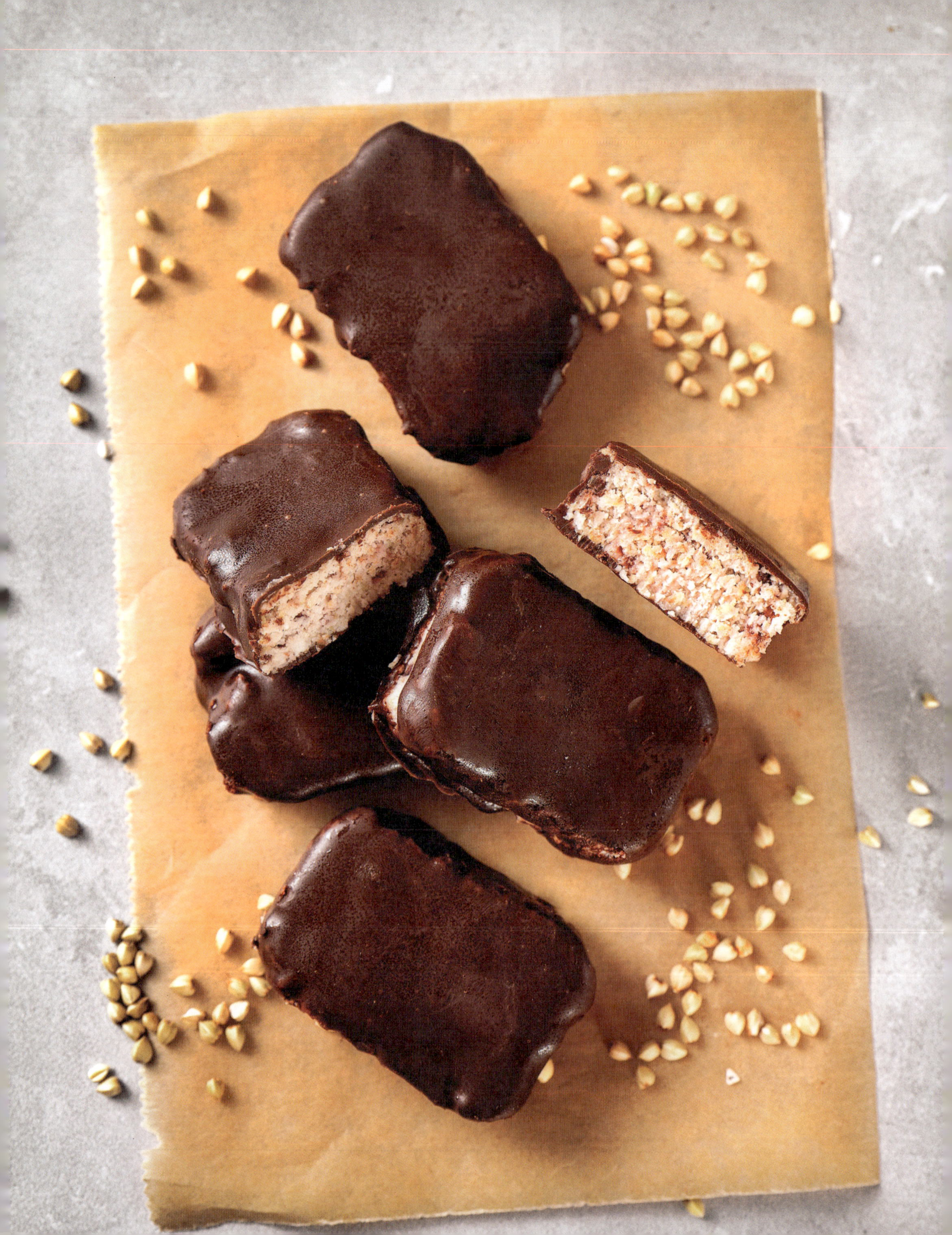

Vegan Buckwheat Bars

⅔ cup (100g) dried cranberries

1 cup (110g) pepitas (pumpkin seeds)

1 cup (90g) desiccated coconut

1 cup (170g) raw activated buckwheat

½ cup (60g) tapioca flour

½ cup (155g) rice malt syrup

⅔ cup (160ml) coconut oil

2 tsps ground flaxseed

1 tsp vanilla powder

1 tbsp cinnamon

150g vegan dark chocolate, chopped

Cake tin

Line cake tin with greaseproof paper.

Place cranberries and pepitas in a food processor and pulse to finely chop.

Add remaining ingredients, except for the chocolate, to the food processor and pulse to combine.

Pour mixture into tin and press down evenly.

Place tin in air fryer and cook for 18-20 minutes at 160°C until golden brown and fragrant.

Allow to cool then cut into bars.

Melt chocolate in a small bowl in a microwave or over a pan of simmering water on a low heat.

Dip each bar into the melted chocolate and turn to coat both sides.

Arrange on a baking tray lined with greaseproof paper and transfer to the fridge to set.

MAKES 14

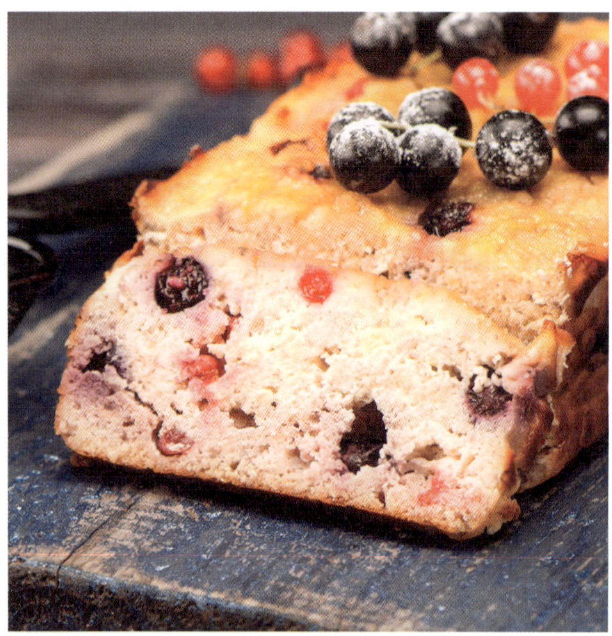

Easy Berry Cake

½ cup (155g) rice malt syrup or maple syrup

150g mascarpone cheese

2 eggs

60g butter, melted

Zest of 1 orange

1 tsp vanilla extract

⅔ cup (80g) plain flour

1 tsp baking powder

⅔ cup (80g) mixed berries

Mini loaf tin

Preheat air fryer to 180°C. Line loaf tin with greaseproof paper.

Combine syrup, mascarpone, eggs, butter, orange zest and vanilla in a large bowl. Mix well.

Add flour and baking powder and stir to combine.

Add berries and gently fold through.

Pour cake batter into prepared tin.

Place tin in air fryer and cook for 30-35 minutes or until an inserted skewer comes out clean.

SERVES 4

Caramelised Nut Clusters

1 sheet shortcrust pastry

1 egg white

¼ cup (80g) maple syrup

¼ tsp cinnamon

¼ cup (30g) macadamia halves

¼ cup (30g) almonds

¼ cup (30g) hazelnuts

¼ cup (30g) cashews

¼ cup (30g) walnuts halves

2 tbsps salted butter, melted

Muffin tray or silicone moulds

Use a pastry cutter to cut out fluted circles. Press into silicone moulds or an air fryer muffin tray.

Place in air fryer and cook for 15-18 minutes at 160°C until golden brown. Remove from air fryer and set aside.

Line the air fryer basket with aluminium foil.

Mix egg white, maple syrup and cinnamon together in a bowl. Add nuts and toss to coat.

Pour melted butter into lined air fryer basket. Add the nuts and spread out evenly.

Cook for 5 minutes at 150°C, then shake basket and cook for a further 5 minutes. Shake basket again and cook for another 2-4 minutes until golden brown.

Remove nuts from air fryer. Spoon into precooked pastry cases and serve.

MAKES 8

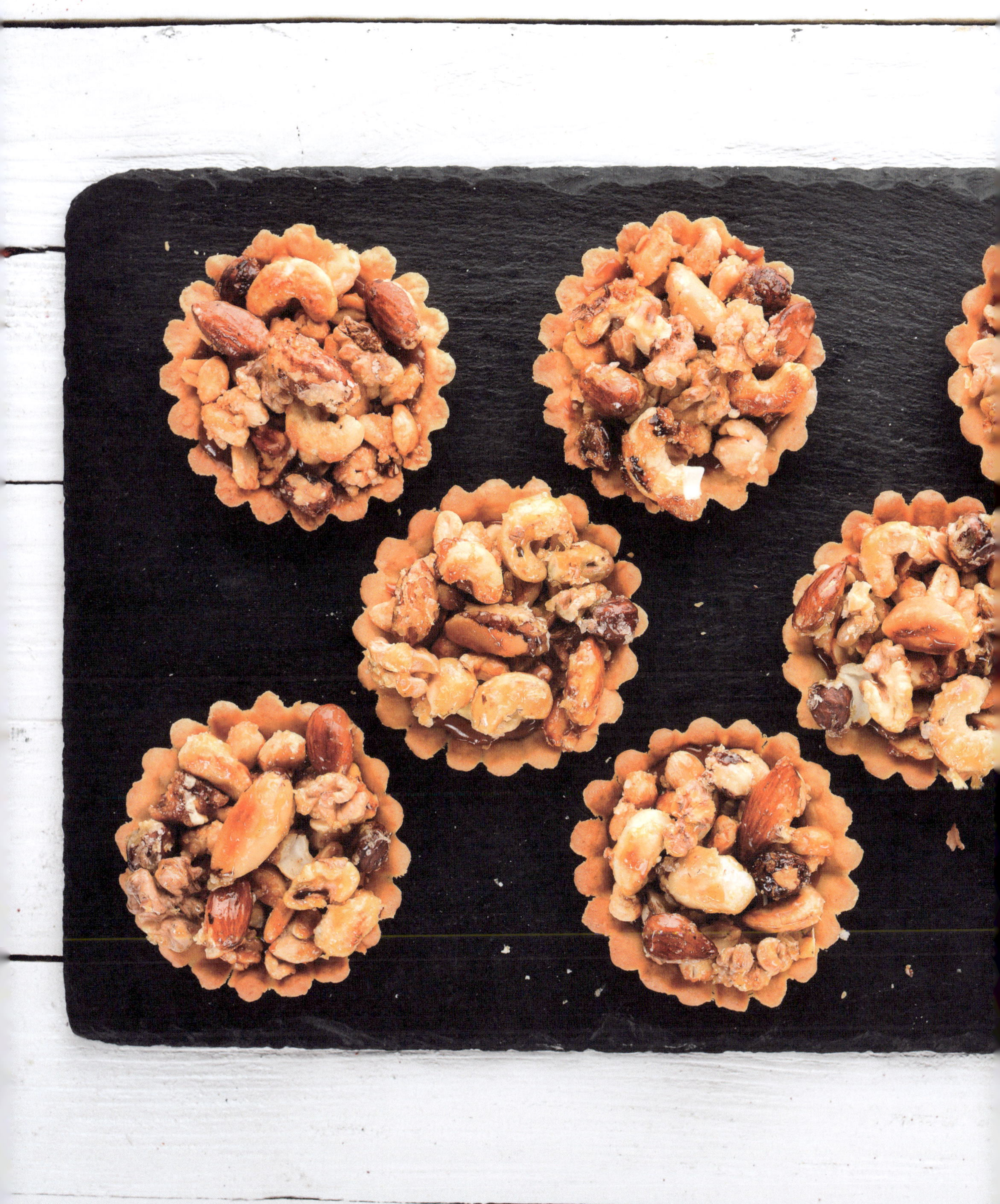

Index

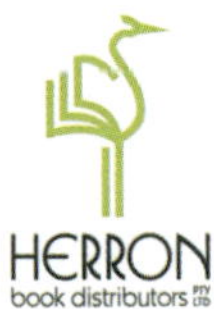

First Published in 2021 by Herron Book Distributors Pty Ltd
14 Manton St
Morningside
QLD 4170
www.herronbooks.com

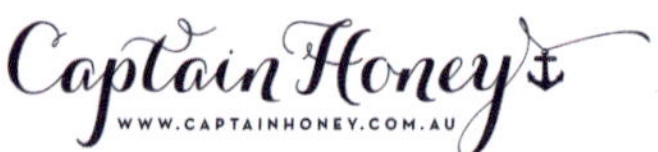

Custom book production by Captain Honey Pty Ltd
12 Station St
Bangalow
NSW 2479
www.captainhoney.com.au

Cataloguing-in-Publication. A catalogue record for this book is available from the National Library of Australia

ISBN 978-1-922432-14-8

All images used under license from Shutterstock.com
Printed and bound in China

5 4 3 2 1 20 21 22 23 24

NOTES FOR THE READER

All reasonable efforts have been made to ensure the accuracy of the content in this book. Information in this book is not intended as a substitute for medical advice. The author and publisher cannot and do not accept any legal duty of care or responsibility in relation to the content in this book, and disclaim any liabilities relating to its use.